Exercise Testing and Exercise Training
in Coronary Heart Disease

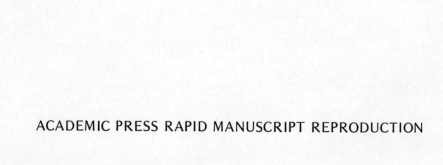

Exercise Testing and Exercise Training in Coronary Heart Disease

Edited by

John Naughton, M.D.
Herman K. Hellerstein, M.D.

Irvin C. Mohler
Coordinating Editor

1973

ACADEMIC PRESS   New York   San Francisco   London

A Subsidiary of Harcourt Brace Jovanovich, Publishers

ACADEMIC PRESS, INC.
111 Fifth Avenue, New York, New York 10003

United Kingdom Edition published by
ACADEMIC PRESS, INC. (LONDON) LTD.
24/28 Oval Road, London NW1

Library of Congress Cataloging in Publication Data
Main entry under title:

Exercise testing and exercise training in
    coronary heart disease.

    Based on a postgraduate course on the physiology
and psychology of exercise testing and training of
coronary disease patients and coronary-prone subjects,
held during the spring of 1972 at the Airlie
Conference Center, Warrenton, Va.
    1.   Coronary heart disease—Congresses.
2.   Cardiovascular patient—Rehabilitation—Congresses.
3.   Gymnastics, Medical—Congresses.   I.   Naughton,
John, ed.   II.   Hellerstein, Herman K., ed.
[DNLM: 1.   Exercise test—Congresses.   2.   Exercise
therapy—Congresses.   3.   Myocardial infarct—Rehabilitation—Congresses.   WG300 A298e   1972]
RC685.C6E9   616.1'23'0624   73–9440
ISBN 0–12–515050–4

CONTENTS

FOREWORD

The Rehabilitation Services Administration has a mission in coronary heart disease. More Americans are disabled by disorders of the heart than any other cause and, unfortunately, there is too little information available concerning the vocational rehabilitation needs of cardiac patients. Evaluation techniques are available in relatively few geographic areas for the assessment of patients with disorders of the heart to determine their ability to work, the characteristics of the work they may safely perform, or the prescription for physical training they need to work safely. Furthermore, the same problem prevails in our attempt to determine the appropriateness of the nonwork activities necessary to full community interaction.

Evaluation techniques must become more readily available to those who are disabled by heart disease and to those who think they are disabled by these disorders. I shall encourage the State-Federal Vocational Rehabilitation Program to participate more actively in the development of such resources, and to make full use of them by referring clients of the program for evaluation services. Such evaluations are the starting point for the entire constellation of vocational rehabilitation services; they must be made more readily available to the public for those in need of such services.

In addition, the research, demonstration, and training programs will give heart disease problems priorities appropriate to the seriousness of the social, situational, and vocational problems resulting from these disorders.

It was not until 1969 that the public rehabilitation program in the United States began to classify coronary heart disease (CHD). In July of 1969, a report was issued by the Department of Health, Education, and Welfare Secretary's Task Force on Physical Activity and Health. This report acknowledged the fiscal limitations upon the American Heart Association and the American College of Cardiology which made unlikely their support of the comprehensive studies needed to assess the practical value of heart rehabilitation programs, as well as the role rehabilitation centers could have in the development of such programs. Moreover, one of the options in the Task Force report was the creation of seminars to help define the problems of establishing a coronary heart disease prevention study, including the necessary rehabilitation of patients with cardiac impairments.

The Task Force on Barriers to the Rehabilitation of Persons Disabled by CHD, sponsored by the Rehabilitation Committee of the American Heart Association, met in New York City to consider the rehabilitation of persons disabled by acute myocardial infarction (MI). The participants of this Task Force agreed that too little information was available concerning rehabilitation achievement, as well as the barriers to full rehabilitation.

A strong beginning to fill this information gap was made, internationally, through the deliberations and proposals of the 1969 and 1971 Cardiac Rehabilitation Conferences in Yugoslavia.

The Airlie Conference on Physiology and Psychology of Exercise Testing and Training of Coronary Disease Patients and Coronary-Prone Subjects, sponsored by interested organizations, was another step in the right direction.

This volume is designed to meet the needs of the members of the health and rehabilitation programs involved in the organization, development, and application of rehabilitation and physical reconditioning programs. It is hoped that it will help to vitalize programs that can serve a vast public with needs that are not being met: the cardiac patients, persons with probable future cardiac impairments, and those persons who often believe they have heart disorders, but in reality do not.

We in the Rehabilitation Services Administration are pleased to have the opportunity to work on this important national health problem.

Edward Newman, Ph.D.

PREFACE

The concept of a postgraduate course in which the latest information could be assimilated and distributed about multiple aspects of the rehabilitation process for patients with myocardial infarction was realized in the spring of 1971, by means of grants from the Social and Rehabilitation Service of the Department of Health, Education, and Welfare, to its Regional Rehabilitation and Training Center Number 9, and from the American Heart Association. The title selected for the course was "Physiology and Psychology of Exercise Testing and Training of Coronary Disease Patients and Coronary-Prone Subjects: Principles, Techniques, Applications and Effects." It has since been identified as the "Airlie Conference in Exercise Testing and Training of Coronary Patients," because it was conducted in the beautiful Virginia countryside during the spring of 1972 at the Airlie Conference Center near Warrenton, Virginia. This monograph results, with the updated contributions of the faculty of that conference, and with an analysis of the teaching-learning experiment in the education of health professionals concerned with the expanding field of health care, now identified as Cardiac Rehabilitation.

The purposes of the postgraduate course were to develop a sound curriculum and teaching aids, and to offer an opportunity for personal exposure of the multidisciplinary participants to the physiology, psychology, and methodology of physical reconditioning and rehabilitation of coronary heart disease patients and of normal coronary-prone subjects. Participants included international authorities and members of the health professions actively involved in the organization, development, and application of rehabilitation and physical reconditioning community programs. Included were biochemists, physiologists (basic science, sports), cardiologists, internists, physical educators, and therapists; lawyers, economists, and rehabilitation counselors.

The core curriculum was so designed that participants would carry away not only sound ideas but practical personal experiences in exercise testing and training techniques, assessment of coronary risk factors, cardiopulmonary resuscitation, problem solving, medical literature, and knowledge to apply in their particular professional areas.

With full awareness of the magnitude of this educational challenge, we incorporated into the design of the course not only theory and practice but also several features to assess our efforts. This included pre- and postcourse testing of the participants' attitudes and knowledge of selected basic concepts, item analysis to identify the areas which merited further clarification and emphasis for the various health professionals, instruction and certification of participants in cardiopulmonary resuscitation, assessment by the participants of the content and design of the course and of the individual faculty members for their pedagogy: content, clarity of presentation, and ability to communicate, and for favorable interdisciplinary exposure in small and large tutorial groups, in informal and formal groupings, facilitated by the gemütlich environs of Airlie House.

Although the immediate impact of these novel features of this educational effort was striking (see Chapter 29), a better measure of the true value of this course and of this monograph will be found in the long-term and judicious utilization of their principles and techniques in practical application and in continuing education.

We are grateful to the faculty who enthusiastically participated and contributed to this effort; to the participants who made it an exciting educational experience; to the two universities who permitted and encouraged our collaboration; to those organizations who joined with the Social and Rehabilitation Service as sponsors to insure the realization and success of the program; and to Mr. Joseph LaRocca for his herculean efforts toward making sure that we met our commitments and realized our ambitions.

We hope that this monograph adequately reflects the effort and the input of the faculty, and that you, the reader, will also be rewarded.

John Naughton, M.D.
Herman K. Hellerstein, M.D.

Editors' Note

The use of "O$_2$ intake" was agreed upon for the sake of uniformity during the original styling of this monograph. This was prior to the publication of *Glossary on respiration and gas exchange*, in the Journal of Applied Physiology, vol. 34, no. 4, April 1973, which gave "oxygen uptake" as the preferred usage. Since the major part of the book was already in print, a changeover in the terminology in question was not feasible.

PLANNING COMMITTEE

John C. Bish, Ed. D.
  Bethesda, Maryland

Henry Blackburn, M.D.
  Minneapolis, Minnesota

Samuel M. Fox, III, M.D.
  Washington, D.C.

Walter Goo, M.D.
  Washington, D.C.

Patrick A. Gorman, M.D.
  Washington, D.C.

William L. Haskell, Ph.D.
  Palo Alto, California

Richard E. Hurley, M.D.
  New York, New York

Larry Hurwitz, M.D.
  Washington, D.C.

Joseph LaRocca
  Washington, D.C.

Irvin C. Mohler
  Washington, D.C.

Nanette K. Wenger, M.D.
  Atlanta, Georgia

CURRICULUM COMMITTEE

Elsworth Buskirk, Ph.D.
  University Park, Pennsylvania

Samuel M. Fox, III, M.D.
  Washington, D.C.

Ernest H. Friedman, M.D.
  Cleveland, Ohio

Menard Gertler, M.D.
  New York, New York

Fred Heinzelmann, Ph.D.
  Washington, D.C.

Herman K. Hellerstein, M.D.
  Cleveland, Ohio

Albert Kattus, M.D.
  Los Angeles, California

John Naughton, M.D.
  Washington, D.C.

Karl Stoedefalke, Ph.D.
  University Park, Pennsylvania

Merritt Stiles, M.D.
  Spokane, Washington

xi

FACULTY

Joseph E. Acker, M.D.
Knoxville Cardiovascular Group
Knoxville, Tennessee

Ezra A. Amsterdam, M.D.
University of California
School of Medicine,
Davis, California

Tage Astrup, Ph.D.
The Washington Clinic
Washington, D.C.

Henry Blackburn, M.D.
University of Minnesota
Minneapolis, Minnesota

James L. Breen, Ph.D.
George Washington University
Washington, D.C.

Sterling B. Brinkley, M.D.
Department of Health, Education,
and Welfare
Washington, D.C.

Loring Brock, M.D.
Spalding Rehabilitation Center
Denver, Colorado

Robert A. Bruce, M.D.
University of Washington
School of Medicine
Seattle, Washington

John Bruhn, Ph.D.
University of Oklahoma
Medical Center
Oklahoma City, Oklahoma

Daniel Brunner, M.D.
Government Hospital
Donolo, Jaffa, Israel

Elsworth Buskirk, Ph.D.
Pennsylvania State University
University Park, Pennsylvania

Mary Ellen Caplin
George Washington University
Medical Center
Washington, D.C.

K. K. Datey, M.D.
St. George's Hospital
Bombay, India

Henri Denolin, M.D.
University Libre de Bruxelles
Brussels, Belgium

Stephen E. Epstein, M.D.
National Institutes of Health
Bethesda, Maryland

Stanley H. Fisher, Ed.D.
University of Connecticut
Storrs, Connecticut

Samuel M. Fox, III, M.D.
George Washington University
Medical Center
Washington, D.C.

Ernest H. Friedman, M.D.
Case Western Reserve University
Cleveland, Ohio

Victor Froelicher, M.D.
University of Alabama
Birmingham, Alabama

Menard Gertler, M.D.
New York University Medical Center
Medical Center
New York, New York

Alberto Goldbarg, M.D.
University of Chicago
Pritzer School of Medicine
Chicago, Illinois

Walter Goo, M.D.
George Washington University
Medical Center
Washington, D.C.

Alden Gooch, M.D.
Deborah Hospital
Browns Mills, New Jersey

Patrick A. Gorman, M.D.
George Washington University
Medical Center
Washington, D.C.

Thomas P. Hackett, M.D.
Massachusetts General Hospital
Boston, Massachusetts

William L. Haskell, Ph.D.
Preventive Medical Center
Palo Alto, California

Fred Heinzelmann, Ph.D.
Department of Justice
Washington, D.C.

Herman K. Hellerstein, M.D.
Case Western Reserve University
Cleveland, Ohio

John O. Holloszy, M.D.
Washington University
School of Medicine
St. Louis, Missouri

Jan J. Kellermann, M.D.
Tel-Hashomer Government Hospital
Tel-Hashomer, Israel

Kris Lange-Andersen, M.D.
International Biological Programme
Oslo, Norway

John E. Merriman, M.D.
University of Saskatchewan,
Saskatoon, Canada

Lars Mogensen, M.D.
Council on Rehabilitation of
Cardiac Patients
Stockholm, Sweden

John Naughton, M.D.
George Washington University
Medical Center
Washington, D.C.

Edward Newman, Ph.D.
Department of Health, Education,
and Welfare
Washington, D.C.

Ivan Pinto, M.D.
University of Bombay
Bombay, India

Cedomil Plavsic, M.D.
Institute for Thalassotherapy
Opatija, Yugoslavia

Howard R. Pyfer, M.D.
Cardio-Pulmonary Research Institute
Seattle, Washington

Corbett Reedy
Department of Health, Education,
and Welfare
Washington, D.C.

W. A. Seldon, M.D.
Prince of Wales Hospital
Randwick, Australia

Thomas Semple, M.D.
The Victoria Infirmary
Glasgow, Scotland

Gerald H. Siegel, Esq.
American Heart Association
Brooklyn, New York

Stanley M. Silverberg, M.D.
Chevy Chase, Maryland

James Snyder, M.D.
Washington Cardiovascular
Evaluation Center
Washington, D.C.

Melvin Stern, M.D.
George Washington University
Medical Center
Washington, D.C.

Karl Stoedefalke, Ph.D.
Pennsylvania State University
University Park, Pennsylvania

Hugh G. Welch, Ph.D.
University of Tennessee
Knoxville, Tennessee

Nanette K. Wenger, M.D.
Emory University
School of Medicine
Atlanta, Georgia

Lenore R. Zohman, M.D.
Montefiore Hospital
Bronx, New York

SPONSORS

American Association for Health, Physical Education,
and Recreation

American College of Cardiology

American College of Sports Medicine

American Heart Association

Case Western Reserve University School of Medicine

The George Washington University School of Medicine

Scientific Council on The Rehabilitation of Cardiac
Patients of The International Society of
Cardiology

Social and Rehabilitation Service,
Department of Health, Education, and Welfare

Washington, D.C. Heart Association

SUPPORTERS

Metropolitan Washington Regional Medical Program

Stuart Pharmaceuticals of ICI America, Inc.

Vertek Corporation

Quinton Instrument Corporation

Marquette Instrument Corporation

Schwinn Bicycle Company

Physiometrics Corporation

INTRODUCTION

THE STATE-FEDERAL VOCATIONAL REHABILITATION
PROGRAM IN CARDIAC REHABILITATION

One of the most significant events in rehabilitation in this country in 1972 was the Airlie House Conference on Cardiac Rehabilitation. The Rehabilitation Services Administration of the Department of Health, Education, and Welfare was indeed honored to be a cosponsor. Dr. Brinkley and I will outline information about the rehabilitation program we represent.

My long interest and identification with cardiac rehabilitation include service for a number of years on the American Heart Association's Rehabilitation Committee, with Dr. Fred Whitehouse. It is both refreshing and challenging to return to this specific subject. Vocational rehabilitation, a goal-oriented program, has various aims of competencies: physical, social, vocational, and economic. At the core, of course, is orientation toward helping the disabled person select, prepare for, and enter a suitable occupation—an occupation that is suitable to his physical, mental, and health needs; to his vocational interests and abilities; and to his economic needs.

A great debate is going on in this country on how we should deal with the problem of dependency. In the United States, some 30 million persons are considered dependent. On the one hand, there are those who believe that a guaranteed income from public funds would be the solution. Others, in my opinion constituting the majority, believe that self-support through work is the solution of choice. There is no question that dependency is one of the greatest concerns at present in the United States.

Mary Switzer, former director of rehabilitation in this country, said, "Dependency is a creeping cancer in our society." Disability leading to unemployment is a major cause of dependency. A great majority of Americans share deep convictions about work, even for the disabled. These convictions are well-stated in a mission-and-goals statement of the State Federation Program of Rehabilitation:

Work is one of the basic ingredients of American culture. Everyone has the right and the need to work, and disabled people frequently present unique employment problems. Work directly or indirectly satisfies many basic needs. It enables man to acquire the means of subsistence. It is a symbol of status. Work satisfies the urge to create. It satisfies the urge to be one of the group. It erases the feeling of being a receiver only, which is the usual lot of one who is unable to secure and hold employment. This idea of work is basically humanitarian since it emphasizes the values to the individual.

I must confess no patience with the ideas often expressed today that the responsibility to work and the benefits from work are outmoded. A compassionate society willingly supports its dependent children, its aged, and the chronically ill. However, a society is not compassionate when it forces dependency on an individual, denying him an opportunity for a job.

Rehabilitation of the disabled, then, is a widely held national goal, an expression of new national policy in dealing with the problem of disability and dependency. This expression in the Congress is in terms of a 10-year goal, that will enable us to offer rehabilitation to those who need, and can profit by it. It is an expression endorsed by numerous professionals, such as those at the Airlie House Conference; by the rehabilitation, health, and social agencies of this country; and increasingly by the average citizen. It has been said that rehabilitation is a profound movement in our society. It is more than a process, more than a program or a profession.

The former director of the Institute for Crippled and Disabled in New York, Colonel John Smith, provided our most adequate definition of rehabilitation as it is practiced today ... "Rehabilitation is a composite science to which all related professional and social groups must contribute their knowledge and skills." These groups that combine to make rehabilitation a composite science include medicine in all its specialities (including physical medicine and its corollaries), physical and vocational rehabilitation, psychiatry, mental hygiene, clinical psychology, and prosthetics. The new science also includes family case work, psychiatric and medical social work, recreation, and social group work.

On the educational and vocational levels it includes vocational and academic guidance and training in industry, sheltered workshop employment, and job placement. This defines the scope of modern rehabilitation in very comprehensive terms.

The State Federal Program of Vocational Rehabilitation is a jointly supported program in all the States. The public program of rehabilitation has been called *new federalism* at its best, because it combines State and Federal support with a great deal of flexibility on the part of the States. This program has just entered its second half-century, having been authorized by legislation in 1920. In 1972, a total enrollment was expected of more than one million disabled persons in the public rehabilitation programs. It was expected that at the end of Fiscal Year 1972, our record for rehabilitating disabled persons for employment would exceed the national goal of 312,000 for the year. These are people who will complete their programs of rehabilitation and return to work. The cost of this program is slightly in excess of $800 million.

It required 42 years for this program to reach the level of rehabilitating 100,000 persons a year. That happened in 1962. From 1962 to 1972, there has really been a boom in rehabilitation in all its dimensions. The number of people rehabilitated has risen to 312,000, an increase of 212,000 in 10 years, compared with 100,000 in the first 42 years. The States' role in this partnership is to provide services to the individual.

Of the principal activities in the Federal rehabilitation program, the first is awarding grants for rehabilitation. There are five types of grants: (1) aid to the States (the largest bulk of the funds); (2) special service project grants for innovations and expansions; (3) research grants and innovative demonstrations; (4) grants for employment and developmental training; and (5) grants for facilities. The Federal role includes that of preparing and issuing regulations, guidelines, and policies about the public program; exercising national leadership in planning, legislation, and evaluation; technical assistance to the States and other constituents; and introducing the principles, methods, and philosophy of rehabilitation (as widely as possible) into the human services programs.

Thus, the vocational rehabilitation system, the public program of rehabilitation, has evolved into a vast network of services to which many agencies, professions, and different kinds of enterprises make contributions.

Growth has been witnessed in recent years of that which is termed cooperative programming. It includes mental health, special education, public welfare, correctional agencies, employment agencies, and numerous other entities. Thus, for disabled people, including the cardiac client, vocational rehabilitation potentially offers a vast array of services.

The day I began to plan this presentation, a letter in the *Washington Star* presented a familiar situation. The letter stated, "My husband has worked in a factory most of his life. He had a heart attack several weeks ago, and we are worried that he may not be able to go back to his old job. If his old job turns out to be too hard, where can he find a new job that he could hold with his condition?" This typical rehabilitation problem shows the concern of both patients and their families after the experience of cardiac attack.

The newspaper reply was, "First of all, you will get help from your physician, and likely under his service, you will know whether to go back to your job or not." The reply stated further, "If you are lucky enough to live in one of the 18 states that has a work evaluation unit, then you could get a very highly sophisticated, comprehensive evaluation as to your work suitability." Then, buried deep in the article was a very casual reference to the vocational rehabilitation program. I can assure you, we read that with some chagrin!

What about the vocational rehabilitation program and the cardiac patient? How is the vocational rehabilitation program assisting the cardiac patient? What are the future prospects?

After a myocardial infarction, work is of great concern to the cardiac patient, to his physician, and to his family. This has been well-established. Vocational rehabilitation does not treat acute illness. Rather, it deals with the residual impairment of illness, a congenital defect, or effects of other traumatic conditions. With respect to rehabilitation services for the cardiac patient, which can be sponsored through any of the rehabilitation programs in the 50 States, five broad types of services are very specific. Included are corrective surgery, reconditioning therapy (which is, of course, the focus of this conference), therapy for psychological trauma, job counseling, training and placement, and resocialization services to combat dependency and withdrawal, which is a very ordinary and common symptom associated with disability.

We estimate that today we are serving 20,000 cardiac patients and rehabilitating 7,400 per year. Services provided have held steady for the last 3 years, even though the total number of persons served and rehabilitated continues to rise sharply. In all truth, we are not very happy with this picture. The capacity of the program is much larger. The number of persons disabled by cardiac conditions is far greater. This relatively low number of cardiac clients on our case rolls exists in spite of our greatest source of referrals for disabilities in general being the physician. We can only conclude that a serious gap in communication and understanding exists between those in the vocational rehabilitation program and those concerned about the treatment of cardiac patients.

Apparently we have a situation where knowledge and technique of rehabilitation are far advanced, but the use of this knowledge is still too limited. How many cardiac patients get no rehabilitation at all? It could well be a majority.

Ten years ago, we were excited about work classification units, reconditioning programs, and special rehabilitation facilities to serve the cardiac patient in the public program of rehabilitation. This excitement has now subsided. It appears that the movement to expand the rehabilitation possibilities for the cardiac patient needs rehabilitation. We are deeply interested in moving forward in this area. Perhaps the Airlie House Conference, focusing as it has upon rehabilitation of the cardiac patient, will provide the stimulus for this rebirth.

Corbett Reedy

PART I

Epidemiology, Physiology, and Biochemistry

1

RELATIONSHIP OF ACTIVITY HABITS TO CORONARY HEART DISEASE

Samuel M. Fox, III, M.D.

Physical inactivity, permitted or encouraged by modern mechanization, is among the listed factors which contribute to the reported major increase in coronary heart disease (CHD) morbidity and mortality in many developed and developing countries. As is true of most all the presently identified coronary risk factors, the evidence suggests that *correction* of the risk factor abnormality will be helpful, even though acceptable proof is clearly lacking.

The objectives of a preventive program should include the extension of life, and provide an opportunity for preserving and enhancing the quality of life. Nearly all individuals find that an increase in habitual physical activity will produce an increase in physical (and perhaps mental) vigor, stamina, and enthusiasm and that it may enhance creativity and optimism as well. Research in these important but difficult study areas is urgently needed.

The idea that man prospers best with a life of movement has been with us since the time of Plato. In the *Dialogues*, Timaeus tells Socrates, ". . . Concerning the mode of treatment by which the body and mind are to be preserved . . . moderate exercise reduces to order, according to their affinities, the particles and affections which are wandering about the body . . . "

More than 2,000 years later, still lacking is a definitive demonstration of just how much physical activity is worth an investment in time, effort, and other resources. Recently, Laurence J. Peter, Ed.D., who had previously enunciated *The Peter Principle*,[1] published a book, *The Peter Prescription*. Prescription I is: "Revitalize Your Body" and in the explanation he states, "Daily vigorous exercise is an important ingredient in the revitalization of your body and the maintenance of your health" [1].

More information is needed so that the most desirable *intensities, durations* and *frequencies* of various *types* of activities productive of an optimal response can be defined specifically. It is not known how to determine whether a particular individual should, for example, walk, jog, or run. Nor is it known what influence such activity might have on his longevity and the lessening of

---

[1] *The Peter Principle*: In a Hierarchy Every Employee Tends to Rise to His Level of Incompetence.

probabilities that he would fall victim to various diseases, or whether a particular level of exercise, pursued according to a specified schedule, is indeed optimal for enhancing health in a broader context.

The opportunity for examining the potential for health enhancement in the larger sense commands our attention, since great benefit might accrue to individuals and their leadership groups (labor, management, government), if convincing evidence were developed indicating that an increase in habitual physical activity enhances total human performance and productivity, as well as conserving health values.

Data Relative to Physical Activity and CHD Prevention

The first persuasive evidence demonstrating a statistically significant relationship between physical activity and CHD was that reported by J.N. Morris and colleagues in 1953 [2]. It is indicated in Fig. 1 that conductors in the London Transport System, presumably more active than the drivers, since they collected tickets, had 70 percent of the age-corrected incidence of all CHD manifestations. The relative psychic stresses and strains of driving and ticket collection were not assessed. The same authors compared London postmen and less active postal clerks and reported a similar reduced incidence of coronary manifestations in the more physically active postmen. It is encouraging that the postmen did not climb many flights of stairs, nor indeed be strenuously active in making their rounds.

In reviewing this data, it is important to recognize, as Morris and colleagues did, that this is an *association* of less CHD with more occupational physical activity and is not necessarily a cause-and-effect relationship. Morris, in a subsequent article [3], indicated that there were some factors of personal and system selection, such as height limitation for conductor applicants, which might have had an influence on the eligibility of individuals for the respective jobs. It was noted that drivers on entering employment were of greater average girth for a given height than conductors. The same group [4] published data in 1966 indicating that serum lipid and blood pressure levels appeared to make the greatest contribution to the differences in manifestations. It was not considered possible to determine if an increase in physical activity had contributed to the lesser levels of blood pressure and cholesterol.

In observational studies it is difficult to rule out personal and other selection factors that might be operative in respect to the differences in CHD noted. This comment in no way diminishes the honor we should accord the epidemiologists, who have recognized these limitations. They are, in fact, among the strongest proponents of the *controlled intervention studies* which are now needed to convince an appropriately skeptical scientific community of the power of specific preventive proposals.

Among the many studies which followed Morris's pioneer work, the majority of investigators report a statistically significant difference, or a definite trend toward an association, between groups of males with more physical activity of occupation or total life pattern and decreased CHD in terms of incidence, prevalence, severity and mortality (Figs. 1, 2).

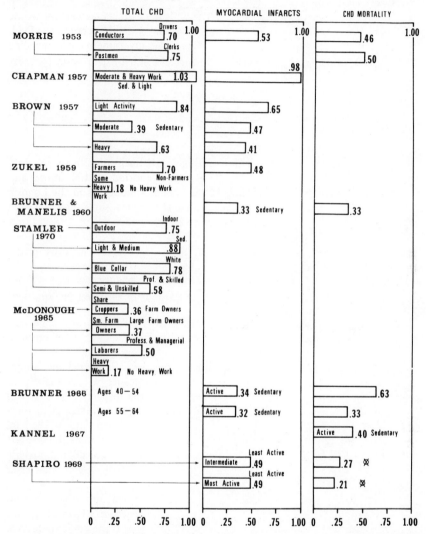

Data from many observational studies comparing groups of differing habitual physical activity. The horizontal bars, and the numbers near their end, represent the relative occurrence of a coronary heart disease manifestation in those of presumed or measured greater physical activity as compared to their more sedentary colleagues. A bar representing the experience of the more sedentary group would, in each case, extend exactly to the line labeled 1.00. Except for Chapman's data there is a lesser occurrence of coronary manifestations in those of greater habitual physical activity.

Fig. 1   Physical activity and coronary heart disease

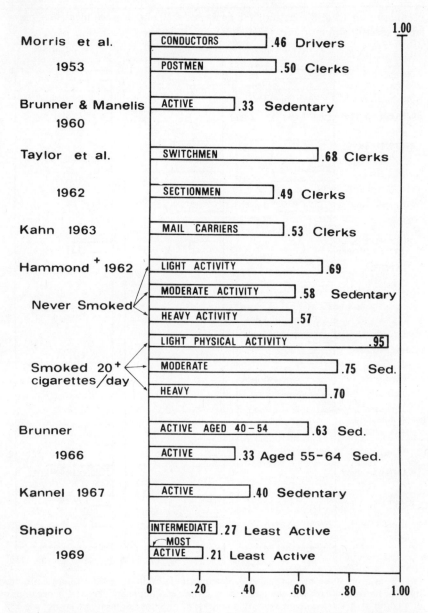

Data concerning coronary mortality relative to previous levels of physical activity from many, but not all relevant observational studies. This graph includes some of the data from Fig. 1 and has the same design.

Fig. 2. Physical activity and coronary mortality

Zukel and colleagues [6] reported a striking difference in the incidence between persons performing heavy work and those doing almost no physical work. Later analysis [7] of Zukel's data revealed that persons doing from 1 to 2 hours of heavy physical activity a day had only 13 percent the incidence of coronary events as those whose usual life pattern included no heavy work. These data are insufficient to derive any difference that might be associated with periods of heavy physical activity less than 1 hour in duration every day. This would be particularly relevant to the question of what type of recreational activity, either in games, individual jogging, bicycling, or swimming is required to stimulate meaningful changes.

Chapman [8] reported no difference in total CHD manifestations or myocardial infarctions (MI) in a population of Los Angeles civil servants. It is possible that true differences may be masked by grouping some individuals who were habitually physically active with many others having job classifications suggesting that they were more active than was truly the case. Chapman indicated [9] that this is unlikely. The ouside-of-work physical activities of those workers in sedentary jobs that might tend to overwhelm occupational differences were not documented.

Dr. Oglesby Paul's data [10] from the Western Electric study in Chicago shows no overall differences but ". . . after eight years the more active men in Code 4 indeed showed fewer coronary deaths than those in the less active Code 2, but, unfortunately, also relatively more infactions with survival." This tendency to have an associated reduction in severity of disease manifestations is encouraging, but a preventive approach should influence sublethal manifestations as well as total mortality.

Stamler [11] reports a consistent trend to less CHD manifestation in those Chicago utility workers who were presumably physically more active, but the small population studied did not make the difference statistically significant. That occupational differences can provide an associated difference in the prevalence of disease manifestations even in later years was emphasized by Brown and colleagues [12] who studied a group of men in Birmingham, England, over age 65.

Brunner and Manelis [13] evaluated CHD differences in workers in the Kibbutzim of Israel where most individuals received meals in a common dining facility. The meat ration was usually the same but the more active persons made up their greater caloric needs with grains and other foods which might have had a contributory effect to help produce the reported lower rate of CHD. In this respect, therefore, the Brunner studies do not represent a situation in which dietary factors were completely controlled.

The study of death certificates by Breslow and Buell in California [14] indicated there was little difference when a simple comparison was made between previous occupational physical activity related to mortality. After "correction" for the strong association of increased general mortality with increased physical activity of work (which may be social class-dependent), the usual inverse relationship (less physical activity-more CHD) became significant except for some cases of Medium General Mortality Risk.

Taylor and associates [15] reported greater CHD rates among railroad workers of sedentary categories compared to switchmen and particularly to section repairmen. Although differential job transfers (the more active changing to less active jobs) could explain some of the differences, this does not seem to be sufficient to eliminate the significance of the differences. As the study participants aged it was apparent that differences in atherosclerotic manifestation were reduced [16]. It was not documented that the more physically active men became less active with seniority but such is a reasonable assumption.

Kahn [17] documented the association of less CHD in the postal deliverymen in Washington, D.C. compared to the presumably more sedentary clerical personnel (similar to findings in the London postal workers). His major contribution may be the statement: "There is a suggestion here that physical activity of 5, 10, or 15 years ago may not be associated with change in current mortality risk." Thus, past physical activities may not last long as "credit in the bank for continued health."

In a study primarily directed toward elucidating factors contributing to cancer mortality, Hammond [18] analyzed all other causes of death and found that 47 percent of all deaths were due to CHD. It was his conviction that no other variable contributing to death appeared as amenable to significant alteration as physical inactivity except for abstention from smoking cigarettes.

In a community of blacks and whites, McDonough et al [19] reported some striking differences, but only after correcting for social class. It is of interest that Skinner et al [20], working with a subsample of the same Evans County study population, confirmed that the prevalence of CHD was significantly less in the more active groups, but that they did not demonstrate any difference between the treadmill-elicited work capacity of members of the inactive compared to the physically active groups.

In Framingham, Massachusetts, Kannel and colleagues [21] reported that those subjects with higher indices of physical activity developed manifestations of CHD less frequently during this extensive prospective study. These indices included non-occupational physical activity as does the assessment of physical activity in the Health Insurance Program (HIP) in New York which Shapiro, Weinblatt, Frank, and Sager reported [22]. The same trends are reported from both these studies including the lack of any significant difference in the occurrence of angina pectoris (AP) relative to reported physical activity.

Angina Pectoris

The usual finding—the more active have fewer manifestations of CHD—is not found in relation to AP, at least in the earlier studies. The groups of both Morris and Zukel had almost twice the incidence of AP in the more active subjects. Only Brunner's report [23] indicates a significantly reduced occurrence of AP in the more active groups. A satisfactory explanation of this enigma is not available. It is not apparent that the greater exertion of the more active persons differentially elicited AP symptoms. Nor is there proof of the optimistic hypothesis that members of the active group are living with this less threatening manifestation (AP) of the total CHD spectrum which otherwise would have produced MI or a lethal outcome had they not stimulated some protective adaptation by their greater involvement in physical activity. In most studies, AP accounts for approximately 12-18 percent of all reported manifestations of CHD.

Athletic Participants

It is difficult to assess the importance of studies reporting lesser incidence, prevalence, and/or severity of CHD or its manifestations in lifelong athletes. This is due, in part, to the possibility that those who succeed athletically have a generalized or constitutional superiority that enhances their chances for survival without developing disease manifestations. Differences in *life-style*, aspirations, and relative values may be of great significance. The lifelong athlete may be more prudent concerning smoking, diet, body weight, and the psychic stress to which he exposes himself or the manner in which he handles it (all of which may operate through mechanisms not specifically connected to his increased habitual physical activity). The reports of Montoye [24], Paffenbarger et al [25], Pomeroy and White [26], and Pyörälä et al [27] reinforce the argument that habitual physical activity is probably beneficial. The review and data of Polednak and Damon [28] showing no difference after a long-term followup of athletes and non-athletes leaves the situation unclear.

Autopsy Studies

The few reported autopsy studies indicate that usual occupational physical activity may have only a modest influence on the degree of atherosclerosis occurring in the major coronary arteries. Morris and Crawford [29] reported that in the hearts of 3,800 men aged 45 to 70, dying from causes not including CHD, there were more healed infarcts, fibrous patches, scars, and coronary occlusions in individuals who had engaged in "light" as compared to "active" or "heavy" job-related work throughout the major part of their lives. Less difference was observed in the frequency of severe atherosclerosis in the large coronary vessels.

This study confirmed the previous report of Spain and Bradess [30]. Little difference was observed in the degree of atherosclerosis (determined by the degree of encroachment upon the lumen and the amount of surface area involved) present in the coronary arteries of those who died suddenly and unexpectedly from accident, homicide, or suicide, regardless of their previous level of occupational physical therapy.

It may be that the hearts of those conditioned by higher energy expenditures will adapt by developing larger coronary arteries less likely to be compromised by a given amount of atheromatous deposition. There is no convincing data as yet to support this hopeful hypothesis, but it is an intellectually attractive jusitification for vigorous athletics during the formative years of youth.

Limitations of Data

Results of population studies generally support the hypothesis that individuals who are selected for, or who themselves select, more active occupations and leisure time activities experience fewer and less severe CHD episodes. These data provide only indirect support for the main hypothesis in question: Will an increase in habitual physical activity by previously sedentary adults reduce the possibilities of the development of the clinical manifestations or premature death from CHD?

In all the published studies, individuals could have made a personal selection for, or have been selected for, different activity groups as a result of factors that may also influence the frequency or severity of CHD. Such factors may include the nature of their general health in early life, body type and weight, blood pressure, responses to environmental stress, motivation, and other psychological factors.

The types of physical activity which contribute most to classifying individuals as being more, instead of less, physically active in many population studies, include walking on the level and upstairs, lifting relatively light objects, operation of machinery or appliances, gardening or working around the house, and participating in a limited variety of games or sports. Participation in physical fitness programs contributes almost nothing to this classification in the studies reviewed. In most studies, only on-the-job physical activity was used for classification purposes, but common sense and the HIP Study data [22] indicate that both occupational and non-job physical activity must be considered if the relationship to CHD is to be determined accurately.

These studies, and their limitations, are discussed in greater detail in some reviews [5, 31-38]. The criticism of Keys [35] is partly justified, and should serve as a useful stimulus for necessary further work.

Amount of Increased Physical Activity

Most of the reported studies suggest, but do not prove, that the amount of exertion required to evoke whatever protective mechanism may exist need not be of the type, intensity, duration, or frequency which would prevent its reasonably widespread acceptance into the lives of even our time-pressured colleagues, as well as most other citizens. It must, however, create tangible rewards. Skinner and colleagues [20] calculated that the difference in daily caloric expenditure of groups of men classified as "inactive" as compared to "active" was in the range of 400 to 500 kilocalories (hereafter given as calories) per day. The railroad occupations studied by Taylor [39] showed a difference in energy expenditure associated with a considerably lessened occurrence of CHD of as little as 500 calories a day, 5 days a week. On the other hand, Paffenbarger et al [40] found only a 25 percent reduction in CHD death rates associated with a 925 calorie per day increase in energy expenditure.

An average 70 kg (154 lb) man burns 1.2 calories/min sitting at rest, uses approximately 3 times that amount (3 METS) walking 4 km (2.5 miles)/hr. A 70 kg man burns about 144 excess calories/hr walking at 4 km/hr, 324 excess calories/hr walking at 5.5 km/hr and 576 km/hr either by bicycling on the level at 21 km/hr (13 mph) or running or jobbing at 9 km/hr (a rate of 1 mile in 10 to 12 minutes calculated at 9 METS). It is important to establish what can be considered a useful minimum of physical activity that will offer long-term help at an acceptable commitment of time, effort, and resources rather than that which gives impressive changes in a brief period of time. Details concerning the energy costs of various physical activities are documented in other reports [5, 41].

Among relatively inactive workers the questionnaire-elicited data of Shapiro et al [22] and Rose [42] suggest an even lesser energy requirement, usually achieved in large part at a low intensity of effort such as walking. Rose reported a strong association between the prevalence of "ischemic type" ECG findings and the duration of the walk to work taken by 8,948 British male civil servants, aged 40-54 (excluding men with dyspnea and AP, and messengers). Fig. 3 indicates that those individuals who walked 20 or more minutes a day on their way to work had only approximately two-thirds the prevalence of ischemic type ECGs (4.18/6.33) as did those who did not walk at all on their way to work. The Ponderal index (a relationship of height to weight) was not significantly different between these groups.

In his commentary Rose further states:

> The association could not be accounted for in terms of differences in age, smoking habit, grade of employment, blood pressure, serum cholesterol, or glucose tolerance; those who walked less tended to be a little more overweight. It remains to be seen whether the duration of the walk to work is merely an indicator of some other etiological characteristic (*e.g.*, a generally greater level of physical activity). Alternatively it would be encouraging if further studies were to show that as little as 20 minutes walking each day might help protect a man from CHD. A controlled trial would be needed to test this hypothesis.

Most workers in the area of coronary risk prevention recognize that a controlled trial with random allocation of individuals at various levels of risk with disease, or with the prognostic markers of later disease, must be undertaken to develop the type information that will be truly persuasive. Lacking this information, it appears "prudent" that individuals attempt to reduce their risk of CHD manifestations with programs of increased physical activity. Although the exact mechanisms whereby this physical activity might modify CHD risk are not yet well defined, the following information seems relevant.

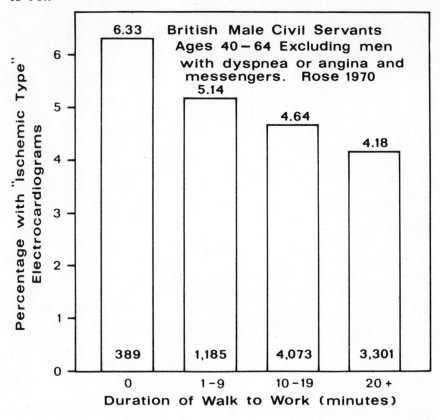

Fig. 3. Individuals walking 20 or more min/day to work had only an approximate two-thirds the prevalence of ischemic type ECGs as those who did not walk to work.

Possible Mechanisms of Preventive Benefit

Mechanisms by which an increase in habitual physical activity *may* reduce the occurrence or severity of CHD are listed in TABLE I. It is appropriate to emphasize that the available data are inadequate or inconclusive relative to most of the listed possibilities as they may relate to middle-aged persons in developed countries.

Development of significant collateral passages carrying oxygenated blood around coronary obstructions has been reported in experimental animal work. A few arteriographic studies before and after exercise programs have demonstrated that some middle-aged persons with coronary obstructions can develop interarterial collaterals. It is also well established that these collaterals do form occasionally with or without exercise in the presence of obstructive atherosclerotic disease. As-yet-unpublished angiographic studies of post-infarct patients under-

TABLE I

Mechanisms by which physical activity may reduce CHD risk

Physical activity may:

Increase	*Decrease*
Coronary collateral vascularization	Serum lipid levels
Vessel size	Triglycerides
Electron transport capacity	Cholesterol
Myocardial efficiency	Glucose intolerance
Efficiency of peripheral blood	Obesity-adiposity
distribution and return	Platelet stickiness
Blood oxygen content	Arterial blood pressure
Red blood cell mass and blood volume	Heart rate
Fibrinolytic capability	Vulnerability to dysrhythmias
Thyroid function	Neurohormonal overreaction
Growth hormone production	"Strain" associated with psychic
Tolerance to stress	"stress"
Prudent living habits	Chronic catecholamine
"Joie de vivre"	production

going physical reconditioning for periods of less than a year have not reported these desired changes to be very frequent. The duration of physical training and the time between coronary angiograms may have been too brief. Possibly, the beneficial effects may have been more significant in those blood vessels too small for adequate visualization. This last explanation is probably not valid for explaining why such collaterals have not been demonstrated. It is also important to recognize that in the presence of generalized ("three vessel") obstructive coronary disease, whatever the stimulus placed on the myocardium to establish a means of better blood supply, it is unlikely that an adequate flow adaptation will occur. It may be that where one vessel is severely involved, a potential exists for collaterals to expand from relatively uninvolved coronary arteries nearby.

Encouraging reports of peripheral vascular improvements on exercise programs suggest that benefits can occur even late in the course of atherosclerotic disease [43, 44].

Work with young animals suggests that physical training will increase the size of the coronary vessels, but there are no reports of similar studies undertaken in humans. The report by Currens and White [45], finding unusually large coronary vessels in the famous marathon runner, Clarence DeMar, after his death from cancer, may only mean that he succeeded with a superior endowment. That coronary vessels can become larger, and therefore less likely to be compromised by atheromatous deposits, will remain conjectural until further studies are reported.

Improved myocardial efficiency—greater work performed at lesser cost—is suggested by some data [46, 47, 48, 49], particularly in respect to an increased stroke volume and slower heart rate at a given workload after training. Animal studies indicate that physical activity may also improve myocardial efficiency by increasing available potassium and cytochrome oxidase supplies and the ability to utilize lactate [50, 51, 52]. An increase in electron transport capacity, as reported by Holloszy in rats after 12 weeks of treadmill training, may have an equivalent in man [53]. A small, but possibly significant increase in thyroid function has been mentioned in unpublished verbal reports [54, 55]. The possibility of a useful stimulation of growth hormone with favorable serum lipid reduction might also be of benefit.

The apparent reconditioning of the mechanisms controlling peripheral blood distribution and return and, perhaps, a slightly increased blood volume, might act principally by preventing secondary complications (hemorrhage or hypotension with inadequate venous return, etc.) after an accident or infarct than by preventing damage (thrombosis and/or electrical failure).

Changes in the constituency of blood associated with physical training indicate greater arterial oxygen content can be acquired [49].

Physical activity of a light or moderate intensity (Master's Step Test, 10-12 minute walk at 3 mph, or an 8-minute walk at 3.5 mph and 5 percent grade) significantly increases, at least temporarily, fibrinolytic activity [56, 57, 58]. Data on more strenuous activity [59], especially competitive games, is less consistent with some investigators observing increases in fibrinolytic activity or related parameters while others have observed an opposite effect [60, 61]. Some of this inconsistency in results may be due to the means by which the blood clotting mechanism is evaluated and the type of exercise performed. There is some suggestion that a moderate increase in habitual physical activity may have a favorable chronic effect on blood clotting or fibrinolytic mechanisms [62] while unaccustomed strenuous exercise tends to shorten blood clotting time temporarily [63]. A decreased tendency for platelet aggregation with acute moderate exertion has been observed [64].

Psychological Aspects

Depending on the importance attributed to the psychological aspects of CHD there is a varying potential for benefit resulting from improvement in personal self-image, *joie-de-vivre*, and tolerance to stress that is reported by many, but not all, who invest their energies in an endurance-enhancing activity program [65, 66]. Physical activity may be a highly desirable tranquilizer for many subjects. The late Howard Sprague of Harvard often said, "You see no charwomen troubled with insomnia."

Preserving and building self-esteem may be an important part of any preventive program. Weight lifting and isometrics may contribute to such efforts, although they have little apparent direct relationship to CHD risk reduction. In today's stressful world, reinforcing "self-image" may be important as a means of promoting health-related efforts. Great care must be taken, however, to avoid taxing blood pressure responses that often accompany straining against significant resistance [67, 68, 69].

The relationship between physical activity and serum lipid levels, especially serum cholesterol, is not established. In some earlier studies where exercise was reported to exert a lowering effect on cholesterol levels, little or no information was available on the subjects' dietary habits and many subjects had greater loss in body weight than could be accounted for by the increase in physical activity [70, 71]. Other reports include both a reduction and no change in cholesterol with an increase in physical activity when body weight was held constant [72, 73, 74, 75]. Some of the differences in these reports may be due to changes in dietary habits not accurately recorded by some subjects, differences in initial cholesterol levels, or a variation in the characteristics of the physical conditioning programs (type, amount, and intensity of activity). Studies are needed where diet is stringently controlled and sufficient subjects are available so that the effects of conditioning programs of varying intensities and durations on individuals with different initial cholesterol levels can be investigated.

Tooshi [76] reported that middle-age men who walked, jogged, and ran for 15 min/day showed an improvement in fitness; those exercising 30 min/day improved body composition as well (more muscle, less fat per given weight); but a significant lowering of cholesterol levels was found only in the group exercising at the same intensity for 45 min/day, 5 days a week. Except for the report by Mann et all [75], studies on the influence of increased serum triglyceride levels that generally accompany post-prandial hyperlipidemia [79, 80, 81]. The reduction in fasting triglyceride levels by exercise, even if the exercise must be performed every 2 to 3 days to maintain a lower serum level, is encouraging since hyperlipidemia has been associated with accelerated blood clotting, increased blood viscosity and adhesiveness and aggregation of platelets [82, 83, 84]. Also, impaired myocardial oxygen extraction, decreased coronary blood flow, decreased physical performance capacity, and AP attacks are reported to occur in humans during alimentary hyperlipidemia [85, 86]. Although there is still a question about the relative importance of cholesterol and triglycerides as markers of increased coronary risk there is a growing tendency to include triglycerides as important, if not of equal importance, as cholesterol determinations [87]. We do not know if the physically active person can tolerate eating more saturated fats than the less active or if he can indulge in other dietary indiscretions beyond enjoying the extra calories his activity consumes. Increased physical activity can be a useful adjunct to dietary efforts to reduce adiposity.

Elevated blood pressure as a CHD risk factor, and its reduction as a preventive approach, is one of the most accepted concepts in CHD control efforts at present. Some investigators report a reduction in systemic blood pressure following participation in a physical conditioning program [88]. This has not been a significant or major finding in most controlled studies. Boyer and Kasch report considerable improvement in a recent report but their patients were not randomly allocated into exercising and non-exercising groups. The "operational blood pressure" with which we live, work, and love may be more important than the casually recorded resting blood pressure.

Following endurance-stimulating physical reconditioning there is usually a reduction of heart rate at rest and more impressively so at various levels of submaximal exertion. The mechanisms producing this training bradycardia are not defined but this effect appears to be a reliable indicator of cardiovascular adaptation of a desirable type. Bradycardia and a reduced blood pressure level (and the heart rate-systolic blood pressure product calculated from their multiplication) may be the major contributors to the markedly increased tolerance to, and capacity for, exertion after physical training in patients with AP [48]. The available data are too meager to determine whether conditioning protects the myocardium against further damage or enhances chances for survival after a further insult.

Neurohormonal influences, including those which affect lipid-carbohydrate metabolism, tend to change in a direction that is considered salutary, but such changes are not proven to be associated with a reduction in CHD occurrence. If catecholamine responses to both physical and psychic stress can be appropriately modified, this might have significance in the "over-pressured" lives to which the coronary prone may expose themselves.

There is a suggestion [22, 90] that sudden death may be less frequent among the habitually more physically active, particularly among men under age ,65. A reduced incidence of cardiac dysrhythmia or decreased myocardial vulnerability to such disturbances is postulated, but too little data are available. Sudden death was not decreased in an otherwise encouraging diet intervention study among survivors of MI [91]; this represents a specific reason for accelerating the definitive evaluation of the contribution of physical activity among the factors that may affect CHD risk.

These possibilities command the attention of investigators, who need to improve techniques of measurement as well as conduct properly controlled studies.

Summary

The available scientific evidence suggests that an increase in habitual physical activity is beneficial. Likely benefits may be more in the area of an improved quality of life than in life extension. If acceptance levels of preventive regimens can be categorized as the Possible, the Prudent, and the Proved, there is sufficient reason to place habitual physical activity among the Prudent actions to be recommended at present. Habitual lifetime physical activity is apparently important; the past physical activity pattern may be of value, but it may be the actual activity, rather than the degree of "fitness" achieved, that is influential in favorably affecting cardiovascular health. The favorable effect appears to persist into later life and the amount of activity required appears to be acceptable for inclusion in the lives of most persons in present-day time-pressured circumstances. More studies are urgently needed to determine whether increased physical activity will contribute to cardiovascular and general health enhancement, increased total human performance, and a vigorous, creative society.

While studies develop better definition, it is now possible with exercise stress testing to "clear" individuals relative to the intensity of exertion that involves an acceptably low hazard of acute cardiac catastrophe yet will provide an almost predictable improvement in physiologic capability. It is possible to prescribe the intensity of activity from recently developed information concerning heart rate responses, and to make useful recommendations as to the type, frequency, and duration of various activities on an individual basis that will fit with the subject's interest and desired life-style.

REFERENCES

1. Peter, L.J. *The Peter Prescription: How to be Creative, Confident, and Competent*, p. 75. New York, Morrow, 1970.

2. Morris, J.N., Heady, J.A., Raffle, P.A.B., Roberts, C.G., and Parks, J.W. Coronary heart disease and physical activity of work. *Lancet* 2:1053, IIII, 1953.

3. Morris, J.N., Heady, J.A., and Raffle, P.A.B. Physique of London busmen: Epidemiology of uniforms. *Lancet* 2:553, 1966.

4. Morris, J.N., Kagan, A., Pattison, D.C., Gardner, M.J., and Raffle, P.A.B. Incidence and prediction of ischemic heart disease in London busmen. *Lancet* 2:553, 1966.

5. Fox, S.M., Naughton, J., and Haskell, W.L. Physical activity and the prevention of coronary heart disease. *Ann. Clin. Res.* 3:404-432, 1971.

6. Zukel, W.J., Lewis, R.H., Enterline, P.E., Painter, R.C., Ralston, L.S., Fawcett, R.M., Meredith, A.P., and Peterson, B. A short-term community study of the epidemiology of coronary heart disease. *Am. J. Public Health* 49:1630, 1959.

7. Fox, S.M., and Haskell, W.L. Physical activity and health maintenance. *J. Rehabil.* 32:89, 1966.

8. Chapman, J.M., Goerke, L.S., Dixon, W., Loveland, D.B., and Phillips, E. The clinical status of a population group in Los Angeles under observation for two to three years. *Am. J. Public Health* 47:33, 1957.

9. Chapman, J.M. Personal communication.

10. Paul, O., Lepper, M.H., Phelan, W.H., Dupertuis, G.W., McMillan, A., McKean, H., and Park, H. A longitudinal study of coronary heart disease. *Circulation* 28:20, 1963.

11. Stamler, J., Berkson, D.M., Lindberg, H.A., Whipple, I.T., Miller, W., Mojonnier, L., Hall, Y.F., Soyugenc, R., and Levinson, J.M. Long-term epidemiologic studies on the possible role of physical activity and physical fitness in the prevention of premature clinical coronary heart disease. *In,* Brunner, D., and Jokl, E., Eds., *Physical Activity and Aging*, pp. 274-300. Baltimore, University Park Press, 1970.

12. Brown, R.G., Davidson, L.A.G., McKeown, T., and Whitfield, A.G.W. Coronary artery disease influence affecting its incidence in males in the seventh decade. *Lancet* 2:1073, 1957.

13. Brunner, D., and Manelis, G. Myocardial infarction among members of communal settlements in Israel. *Lancet* 2:1049, 1960.

14. Breslow, L., and Buell, P. Mortality from coronary heart disease and physical activity of work in California. *J. Chronic Dis.* II:421, 1960.

15. Taylor, H.L., Klepetar, E., Keys, A., Parlin, W., Blackburn, H., and Puchner, T. Death rates among physically active and sedentary employees of the railroad industry. *Am. J. Public Health* 52:1967, 1962.

16. Keys, A. Physical activity and the epidemiology of coronary heart disease. *In,* Brunner, D., and Jokl, E., Eds., *Medicine and Sport.* Vol. 4, *Physical Activity and Aging*, p. 264. Baltimore, University Park Press, 1970.

17. Kahn, H.A. The relationship of reported coronary heart disease mortality to physical activity of work. *Am. J. Public Health* 53:1058, 1963.

18. Hammond, E.C. Smoking in relation to mortality and morbidity. Findings in first thirty-four months of follow-up in a prospective study started in 1959. *J. Nat. Cancer Inst.* 32:1161, 1964.

19. McDonough, J., Hames, C., Stulb, S., and Garrison, G. Coronary heart disease among negroes and whites in Evans County, Georgia. *J. Chronic Dis.* 18:443, 1965.

20. Skinner, J.S., Benson, H., McDonough, J.R., and Hames, C.G. Social status, physical activity and coronary proneness. *J.Chronic Dis.* 19:773, 1966.

21. Kannel, W.B. Habitual level of physical activity and risk of coronary heart disease. In, Proceedings of the International Symposium on Physical Activity and Cardiovascular Health. *Can. Med. Assoc. J.* 96:811, 1967.

22. Shapiro, S., Weinblatt, E., Frank, C.W., and Sager, R.V. Incidence of coronary heart disease in a population insured for medical care (HIP). *Am. J. Public Health* 59, Suppl. to June 1969.

23. Brunner, D. The influence of physical activity on incidence and prognosis of ischemic heart disease. *In,* Raab, W., Ed., *Prevention of Ischemic Heart Disease: Principles and Practice,* p. 236. Springfield, Ill., Thomas, 1966.

24. Montoye, H. Summary of research on the relationship of exercise to heart disease. *J. Sports Med. Phys. Fitness* 2:35, 1962.

25. Paffenbarger, R.S., Jr., Nothin, J., Krueger, D.E., Wolf, P.A., Thorne, M.C., Lebauer, E.J., and Williams, J.L. Chronic disease in former college students. II. Methods of study and observations on mortality from coronary heart disease. *Am. J. Public Health* 56:962, 1966.

26. Pomeroy, W., and White, P.D. Coronary heart disease in former football players. *J.A.M.A.* 167:711, 1958.

27. Pyörälä, K., Karvonen, M.J., Taskinen, P., Takkunen, J., and Kyronseppa, H. *Cardiovascular Studies on Former Endurance Runners.* Helsinki, Inst. of Occupat. Health, 1965. (Rpt. 19)

28. Polednak, A.P., and Damon, A. College athletics, longevity and cause of death. *Hum. Biol.* 42:28, 1970.

29. Morris, J.N., and Crawford, M.D. Coronary heart disease and physical activity of work. *Br. Med. J.* 2:1485, 1958.

30. Spain, D., and Bradess, V. Sudden death from coronary atherosclerosis: Age, race, sex, physical activity and alcohol. *Arch. Int. Med.* 100:228, 1957.

31. Holloszy, J.O. The epidemiology of coronary heart disease. National differences and the role of physical activity. *J. Am. Geriatr. Soc.* 11:718, 1963.

32. Davies, C., Drysdale, H., and Passmore, R. Does exercise promote health? *Lancet* 2:930, 1963.

33. Fox, S.M., and Paul, O. Physical activity and coronary heart disease. *Am. J. Cardiol.* 23:298, 1969.

34. Skinner, J.S. The cardiovascular system with aging and exercise. `In,` Brunner, D., and Jokl, E., Eds., *Medicine and Sport.* Vol. 4. *Physical Activity and Aging,* p. 100. Baltimore, University Park Press, 1970.

35. Keys, A. Physical activity and the epidemiology of coronary heart disease. *In,* Brunner, D., and Jokl, E., Eds. *Medicine and Sport.* Vol. 4. *Physical Activity and Aging,* p. 264. Baltimore, University Park Press, 1970.

36. Stamler, J., Berkson, D.M., Lindberg, H.A., Whipple, I.T., Miller, W., Mojonnier, L., Hall, Y.F., Soyugenc, R., and Levinson, M.J. Long-term epidemiologic studies on the possible role of physical activity and physical fitness in the prevention of premature clinical coronary heart disease. *In,* Brunner, D., and Jokl, E., Eds. *Medicine and Sport.* Vol. 4. *Physical Activity and Aging,* pp.274-300. Baltimore, University Park Press, 1970.

37. Leon, A.S. Comparative cardiovascular adaptation to exercise in animals and man and its relevance to coronary heart disease. In, Bloor, C.M., Ed., *Comparative Pathophysiology of Circulatory Disturbances,* pp.143-174. New York, Plenum, 1972.

38. Froelicher, V.F., and Oberman, A. Analysis of epidemiologic studies of physical inactivity as risk factor for coronary artery disease. *Prog. Cardiovasc. Dis.* 15:41-65, 1972.

39. Taylor, H.L., Blackburn, H., Puchner, T., Vasquez, C.L., Parlin, R.W., and Keys, A. Coronary heart disease in selected occupations of American railroads in relation to physical activity. *Circulation* 40, Suppl. 3:202, 1969.

40. Paffenbarger, R.S., Jr., Laughlin, M.E., Gima, A.S., and Black, R.A. Work activity of longshoremen as related to death from coronary heart disease and stroke. *N. Engl. J. Med.* 282:1109, 1970.

41. Fox, S.M., Naughton, J., and Gorman, P.A. Physical activity and cardiovascular health. *Mod. Concepts Cardiovasc. Dis.* 41:17-30, 1972.

42. Rose, G. Current developments in Europe. *In*, Jones, R.J., Ed., *Atherosclerosis: Proceedings Second International Symposium*, p. 310. New York, Springer-Verlag, 1970.

43. Ericsson, B., Haeger, K., and Lindell, S.E. Effect of physical training on intermittent claudication. *Angiology* 21:188, 1970.

44. Larson, O.A., and Malmborg, R.O., Eds., *Coronary Heart Disease and Physical Fitness*, 277 pp. Baltimore, University Park Press, 1971.

45. Currens, J.H., and White, P.D. Half a century of running. *N. Engl. J. Med.*, 265:988, 1961.

46. Katz, L.N. Physical fitness and coronary heart disease: Some basic views. *Circulation* 35:405, 1967.

47. Frick, M.H. Coronary implications of hemodynamic changes caused by physical training. *Am J. Cardiol.* 22:417, 1968.

48. Epstein, S.E., Redwood, D.R., Goldstein, R.E., Beiser, G.D., Rosing, D.R., Glancy, D.L., Reis, R.L., and Stinson, E.B. Angina pectoris: pathophysiology, evaluation and treatment. *Ann. Intern. Med.* 75:263, 1971.

49. Detry, J.R., Rousseau, M., Vandenbroucke, G., Kusumi, F., Brasseur, I.A., and Bruce, R.A. Increased arteriovenous oxygen difference after physical training in coronary heart disease. *Circulation* 44:109, 1971.

50. Gollnick, P.D., and Hearn, G.H. Lactic dehydrogenase activities of heart and skeletal muscle of exercised rats. *Am. J. Physiol.* 201:694, 1961.

51. Raab, W. The nonvascular metabolic myocardial vulnerability factor in coronary heart disease. *Am. Heart J.* 66:685, 1963.

52. Hearn, G.R. The effects of terminating and detraining on enzyme activities of heart and skeletal muscle of trained rats. *Int. Z. Angew. Physiol.* 21:190, 1965.

53. Holloszy, J.O. Biochemical adaptations in muscle: effects of exercise on mitochondrial oxygen uptake and respiratory enzyme activity in skeletal muscle. *J. Biol. Chem.* 242:2278, 1967.

54. Register, U.D. Personal communication.

55. Teraslinna, P. Personal communication.

56. Cash, J.D. Effect of moderate exercise on the fibrinolytic system in normal young men and women. *Br. Med. J.* 2:502, 1966.

57. Menon I.S., Burke, F., and Dewar, H.A. Effect of strenuous and graded exercise of fibrinolytic activity. *Lancet* 2:700, 1966.

58. Rosing, D.R., Brakman, P., Redwood, D.R., Goldstein, R.E., Beiser, G.D., Astrup, T., and Epstein, S.E. Blood fibrinolytic activity in man. Diurnal variation and the response to varying intensities of exercise. *Circ. Res.* 27:171, 1970.

59. Epstein, S.E., Rosing, D.R., Brakman, P., Redwood, D.R., and Astrup, T. Impaired fibrinolytic response to exercise in patients with type IV hyperlipoproteinemia. *Lancet* 2:631, 1970.

60. Fearnley, G.R., and Lacker, R. The fibrinolytic activity of normal blood. *Br. J. Haematol.* 1:189, 1955.

61. Ikkala, E., Myllylä, G., and Sarajas, H.S. Platelet adhesiveness and ADP induced platelet aggregation in exercise. *Ann. Med. Exp. Biol. Fenn.* 44:88, 1966.

62. Guest, M., and Celander, D. Fibrinolytic activity in exercise. *Physiologist* 3:69, 1960.

63. Egeberg, O. The effect of exercise on the blood clotting system. *Scand. J. Clin. Lab. Invest.* 13:8, 1963.

64. Hames, C.G. Personal communication relative to Evans County, Georgia, study. To be published.

65. Durbeck, D.C. et al. The NASA-USPHS health evaluation and enhancement program. *Am. J. Cardiol.* 30:784-790, 1972.

66. Heinzelmann, F., and Bagley, R.W. Response to physical activity programs and their effects on health behavior. *Public Health Rep.* 85:905, 1970.

67. Lind, A.R. Cardiovascular responses to static exercise. (Isometrics, Anyone?). *Circulation* 41:173, 1970.

68. Nutter, D.O., Schlant, R.C., and Hurst, J.W. Isometric exercise and the cardiovascular system. *Mod. Concepts Cardiovasc. Dis.* 41:11-15, 1972.

69. Muller, E.A. Physiologic methods of increasing human physical work capacity. *Ergonomics* 8:409, 1965.

70. Rochelle, R. Blood plasma cholesterol changes during a physical training program. *Res. Q. Am. Assoc. Health Phys. Educ.* 32:538, 1961.

71. Romanova, D., and Barin, P. The influence of physical exercise on the content of serum protein, lipoprotein and total cholesterol in persons of middle and elderly age with symptoms of atherosclerosis. *Kardiol. Pol.* 1:36, 1961.

72. Taylor, H.L. Relationship of physical activity to serum cholesterol concentration. *In,* Rosenbaum, F., and Balknap, E., Eds. *Work and the Heart,* p.111. New York, Hoeber, 1959.

73. Naughton, J., and McCoy, J.F. Observations on the relationship of physical activity to the serum cholesterol concentration of healthy men and cardiac patients. *J.Chronic Dis.* 19:727, 1966.

74. Goode, R., Firstbrook, J., and Shephard, R. Effects of exercise and a cholesterol-free diet on human lipids. *Can. J. Physiol. Pharmacol.* 44:575, 1966.

75. Mann, G.V., Garrett, H.L., Farhi, A., Murray, H., and Shutte, E. Exercise to prevent coronary heart disease. *Am. J. Med.* 46:12, 1969.

76. Tooshi, A. Effects of three different durations of endurance exercises upon serum cholesterol (abstract) *Med. Sci. Sports* 1:1971.

77. Holloszy, J.O., Skinner, J., Toro, G., and Cureton, T. Effects of a six-month program of endurance exercise on the serum lipids of middle-aged men. *Am. J. Cardiol.* 14:753, 1964.

78. Garrett, H.L., Prangle, R.V., and Mann, G.V. Physical conditioning and coronary risk factors. *J. Chronic Dis.* 19:899, 1966.

79. Cohen, H., and Goldberg, C. Effect of physical exercise on alimentary lipemia. *Br. Med. J.* 2:509, 1960.

80. Nikkilä, E., and Konttinen, A. Effects of physical activity in postprandial levels of fats in serum. *Lancet* 1:1151, 1962.

81. Cantone, A. Physical effort and its effects in reducing alimentary hyperlipemia. *J. Sports Med. Phys. Fitness* 4:32, 1964.

82. Buzina, R., and Keys, A. Blood coagulation after a fat meal. *Circulation* 14:854, 1956.

83. McDonald, L., and Edgill, M. Coagulability of blood in ischemic heart disease. *Lancet* 2:457, 1957.

84. Williams, A., Higginbotham, A., and Knisely, M. Increased cell agglutination following ingestion of fat, a factor contributing to cardiac ischemia, coronary insufficiency and anginal pain. *Angiology* 8:29, 1957.

85. Regan, T., Binale, K., Gordon, S., DeFazio, V., and Hellems, H. Myocardial blood flow and oxygen consumption during postprandial lipemia and heparin-induced lipolysis. *Circulation* 23:55, 1961.

86. Hellerstein, H.K., Hornsten, T.R., Baker, R.A., and Hoppes, W.L. Cardiac performance during postprandial lipemia and heparin-induced lipolysis. *Am. J. Cardiol.* 20:525, 1967.

87. Carlson, L., and Böttiger. Ischaemic heart disease in relation to fasting values of plasma triglycerides and cholesterol. *Lancet* 1:865-868, 1972.

88. Naughton, J., Shanbour, K., Armstrong, R., McCoy, J., and Lategola, M. Cardiovascular responses to exercise following myocardial infarction. *Arch. Intern. Med.* 117:541, 1966.

89. Boyer, J.L., and Kasch, F.W. Exercise therapy in hypertensive men. *J.A.M.A.* 211:1668, 1970.

90. Rosenman, R.H. The influence of different exercise patterns on the incidence of coronary heart disease in the Western Collaborative Group Study. *In,* Brunner, D., and Jokl, E., Eds., *Physical Activity and Aging,* p.272. Baltimore, University Park Press, 1970.

91. Leren, P. The Oslo diet-heart study: eleven-year report. *Circulation* 42:935, 1970.

2

CARDIOVASCULAR ADAPTATION TO PHYSICAL EFFORT IN HEALTHY MEN

E. R. Buskirk, Ph.D.

Introduction

The cardiovascular system has been the subject of investigation for many years, but only recently has the functioning of the cardiovascular system during exercise been examined intensively. This examination has included the oxygen transport function of the circulation, cardiac output, and regional distribution of blood flow including flow to the skeletal musculature.

Although cardiac output and heart rate are linearly related to metabolic demands at all but the highest workloads, the stroke volume of the heart appears to reach a maximal value at about one-third of aerobic capacity. The increase in cardiac output during exercise is achieved primarily by an increase in heart rate and to a lesser extent by an increase in stroke volume. Heart rate frequently provides a useful index of physiological strain as does the heart rate systolic blood pressure product. Both have been so used in a variety of investigations.

Distribution of blood flow during exercise among the body regions is controlled largely by changes in regional vascular resistance which insures that the brain, heart, and working muscles are adequately perfused. Flow through regions other than working muscle and the brain can be drastically reduced. Total peripheral vascular resistance decreases during exercise largely because of vasodilation in working muscle. Arterial systolic and mean blood pressure both increase with the intensity of exercise, but diastolic pressure is altered little. An exception is the performance of static or isometric exercise where the reflex pressor response insures some blood perfusion during sustained muscular contraction.

Variability in the cardiovascular response to exercise in men is associated with a variety of factors including: age, physical conditioning and training, obesity, diet, drugs, heat, and cold. The impact of these factors acting independently or in concert has been incompletely studied.

The circulation is a complicated transport system under intricate neural and humoral control involving feedback mechanisms responding to signals produced in the organs and tissues subjected to movement or alteration by exercise. The circulation handles numerous transport tasks. The blood carries metabolic substrates such as free fatty acids and glucose to the exercising muscles and removes metabolities such as carbon dioxide and lactic acid. In addition, the circulation carries hormones to end organs in muscle, and participates in the dissipation of heat produced during exertion. The heart muscle, during its contraction, develops force which builds up pressure facilitating perfusion of the several organs and acting as a driving force for diffusion of various substances through the capillary wall. The central arterial pressure increases during exercise, and is vital for augmented perfusion and metabolite exchange in working muscles.

Physical Conditioning as an Adaptation

A definition of physiological adaptation as used in the title is important; it is defined as: "any property or response of an organism which favors survival in a stressful environment." It includes all those changes in physiological responses and morphology of organs and tissues resulting from environmental exposure. The primary environmental factor of concern here, considered a stress by some, is physical work or exercise. Adaptation takes time, involves genetic components together with environmental components, and is responsive to the type, frequency, intensity, and duration of exercise. Adaptation is an expected and useful biological phenomenon and in this specific instance is associated with physical conditioning. Thus, physical conditioning involves the general physiological process of adaptation to exercise. The studies of Hettinger and colleagues [11] on strength development point out that optimal adaptation to stress implies that:

1. An intensity duration threshold must be exceeded to achieve an optimal rate of response,
2. Near continuous exposure facilitates adaptation, and
3. Intermission allows some deadaptation to occur which may be physiologically beneficial.

Although the term training has been used extensively by physiologists, training to coaches and those involved with athletes relates to improvement of performance including the acquisition and development of skill. Thus, the term physical conditioning is a more appropriate term to use here for it relates to the repeated participation in bouts of exercise to enhance one's physical capabilities including cardiovascular.

The comprehensive review by Grande and Taylor [9] covers the anatomical and physiological changes associated with conditioning in animals and man in more detail than this summary. The discussion which follows emphasizes the circulatory changes related to oxygen transport resulting from conditioning. A selected review of the literature is presented. Interpretation has been drawn from several key references [1, 4, 5, 7, 9, 13, 15].

Responses to Exercise

The distribution of blood flow to the various tissues during exercise has been summarized by several workers—perhaps most recently by Finch and Lenfont [7]. The tissue potential for an incremental increase in blood flow under maximal exercise conditions may approximate the following multiples over resting conditions: working skeletal muscle, +18X; heart, +4X; skin, +2X; brain, no change; liver, -4X; kidney, -4X; and other tissues combined, -6X.

Before onset of exercise there may be an anticipatory increase in heart rate and a small increase in cardiac output. With onset of exercise the heart rate and cardiac output generally increase in proportion to the workload. There is a widening of the arteriovenous oxygen difference as more oxygen is transferred from hemoglobin to myoglobin and the mitochondria in the working muscles to accommodate increased metabolism. In terms of the various contributions made by components of the oxygen transport system to working muscle, the incremental increase during the transition from rest to maximal exercise may approximate the following multiples: oxygen intake, +12X; cardiac output, +4X; heart rate +2.7X; stroke volume, +1.4X; and the arteriovenous oxygen difference, +3X.

A similar tabulation can be made for the change in hemodynamic values during the transition from rest to maximal exercise. The incremental increases in terms of multiples over rest may approximate the following: systolic blood pressure, +1.6X; diastolic blood pressure, +1.1X; mean blood pressure, +1.4X; systemic resistance, -2.7X; and pulmonary resistance, -2X. Thus, perfusing pressure is increased and vascular resistance decreased. Of the changes mentioned, many are proportional to the relative workload. A notable exception is stroke volume in many men, for stroke volume may increase with the first increments in workload and not increase thereafter—a curvilinear response.

At the onset of exercise an increase occurs in both the central and peripheral circulation which is modified somewhat as the adjustments approximate the controlled requirements for the particular workload [1]. The rate of change in function is somewhat different for each circulatory function, e.g., using heart rate as an illustration during the transition from rest to moderate exercise, the heart rate assumes a controlled level after 2-3 minutes, in strenuous exercise from 5-8 minutes, and in exhausting exercise the heart rate reaches a maximal level within 1.5 minutes and may not change as exercise continues or may increase slightly until exhaustion. Cardiac output increases as exercise begins and usually stabilizes within 1½-2 minutes over a wide range of workloads.

Blood flow in the pulmonary circulation is equal to that in the systemic circulation although the pressures and pressure gradients are much smaller. Pulmonary arterial pressure rarely exceeds 30 mm Hg but it may be somewhat higher in older men. It is vital that pulmonary capillary pressure remain low if effusion of fluid into the interstitium and alveoli, leading to pulmonary edema, is to be prevented.

As exercise begins, there is a marked vasodilation in the arterioles of working muscle and an increase in the number of open capillaries. Resistance to muscle blood flow decreases. A compensatory vasoconstriction in nonworking muscles and other tissues takes place which prevents a precipitous drop in total peripheral resistance. The overall reduction in total peripheral resistance is, however, proportional to the exercise intensity. If cardiac output remains constant, total peripheral resistance is directly related to the mean blood pressure. Aging involves higher mean pressures and hence, higher total peripheral resistances during exercise because of a loss of distensibility and elasticity of the resistance vessels. There is little evidence that exercise hyperemia in skeletal muscle is caused by a reduction in sympathetic constrictor activity or by an increase in dilator activity. Presumably humoral factors such as potassium ions override any increase in constrictor tone [12].

The word exercise implies to most people dynamic rhythmic exercise and not static exercise or sustained contractions. Yet many tasks involve static exercise. The cardiovascular system reflects the tension developed in the activated muscle groups by an increase in heart rate, cardiac output, and particularly blood pressure. Mechanical compression by the skeletal muscle fibers may completely or partially occlude the local blood vessels. There is a pronounced reflex to sustained contraction which causes a sharp increase in blood pressure to maintain some perfusion. The pressor response to static exercise involving two or more muscle groups is established by the muscle group operating at the highest proportional tension. Because the relative sustained workload determines the magnitude of the pressor response, the maximal strength of the muscle group is important [14].

Physical Conditioning

The circulatory responses to exercise of well-conditioned men or athletes are qualitatively similar to those of less well-conditioned men, but differ quantitatively (Fig. 1). The increase in cardiac output ($\dot{Q}$) with increasing metabolic requirements is similar in both groups, with the range described for the athletes covering somewhat lower $\dot{Q}$ values at each submaximal work level. Both maximal oxygen intake ($\dot{V}_{O_2}$ max) and maximal cardiac output ($\dot{Q}$ max) are higher in the endurance event athletes, reaching extreme values of from 5-6 l/min and more than 40 l/min (depicted by separate points in Fig. 1), respectively. The changes in the arteriovenous oxygen concentration difference (C [a–v] O_2) are correspondingly similar in both groups, with the conditioned men or athletes having somewhat higher O_2 extraction at each $\dot{V}_{O_2}$ level. A more distinct difference between the groups is in stroke volume (SV); the upright sedentary men reach their maximal or near-maximal SV at low workloads with little change at higher loads. In contrast, the SV of the athletes keeps rising with increasing workloads. It can be deduced from this difference that exercising sedentary men increase their $\dot{Q}$ primarily by an increase in HR, while athletes utilize an increase in SV to a greater extent as an increase in HR [1, 6].

Cardiovascular morphological characteristics such as heart weight/body weight, heart volume, blood volume, and total hemoglobin also tend to be

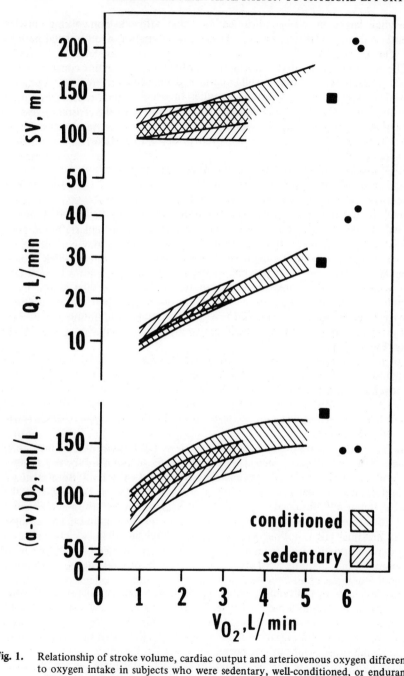

Fig. 1. Relationship of stroke volume, cardiac output and arteriovenous oxygen difference to oxygen intake in subjects who were sedentary, well-conditioned, or endurance athletes in training (individual points, 6). (Summary of results from literature [1])

somewhat larger in well-conditioned men and athletes than in age-matched sedentary men (TABLE I) [4, 9]. These characteristics are correlated to $\dot{V}_{O_2}$ max, $\dot{Q}$ max, and SV.

The demonstrated differences in the cardiovascular functions and morphological characteristics between well-conditioned and sedentary men presented are derived mostly from cross-sectional studies in which different groups of men were compared. Genetic endowment perchance skewed the distribution of values pertaining to the well-conditioned men and athletes. Their values may have been higher than those of sedentary men even prior to their engagement in conditioning and sports.

It is possible that preselection determines those people whose cardiovascular system responds to exercise in a certain way, or who possess large cardiovascular dimensions, and who respond to conditioning quantitatively more or become athletes in the first place. Recently, the need has been partially met for longitudinal studies in which the same men are tested before and after extensive conditioning or intensive training for athletic competition. Several longitudinal studies of physical conditioning have demonstrated increases in maximal aerobic capacity ranging from 4-37 percent of the preconditioning values [5, 10, 16]. This wide variation in improvement can be explained by differences in the frequency, intensity, and duration of the conditioning program, as well as by the activity level of the participants prior to conditioning. The more active individuals prior to conditioning show less improvement than their sedentary counterparts (Fig. 2) [3].

An increase in both maximal arteriovenous oxygen difference and in $\dot{Q}$ max contributes to the improvement in $\dot{V}_{O_2}$ max with physical conditioning. The improvement in $\dot{Q}$ max is primarily due to a higher SV, which in turn has been shown to be positively related to an increase in heart and blood volume after a 2-month conditioning program, at least in young men (i.e., those still growing and developing) [1].

It has been reported that maximal HR in superbly conditioned men is no higher than in sedentary men [2]. On the basis of pooled evidence there is probably little alteration of maximal HR with physical conditioning. It is important to realize that the methodology by which maximal HR is determined affects the result obtained. $\dot{V}_{O_2}$ max can be reached before maximal HR is established, and by measuring the HR at a workload corresponding to $\dot{V}_{O_2}$ max, a true maximal HR is not necessarily achieved. Such an effect has been observed in sedentary middle-aged men who have undergone an 18-month conditioning program in our laboratory. This decrease may be attributed to a decreased sympathetic input or an increased vagal output.

The explanations advanced so far regarding the mechanism involved in the development of conditioning bradycardia during submaximal exercise are not satisfactory. One school of thought attributes this phenomenon to the autonomic nervous system (vagal or cholinergic dominance, with or without sympathetic inhibition), while others correlate it with the modest amount of myocardial hypertrophy of the well-conditioned man or athlete, which is accompanied by larger SV, and therefore, lower HR for a given workload.

TABLE I

Average cardiovascular values for sedentary and well-conditioned men

	Heart wt. g. Body wt. kg	Heart volume[1] ML	Blood volume liters	Total hemoglobin G
Sedentary men	5.8	769	5.3	805
Well-conditioned men	6.5	986	7.5	1130
Δ	+0.7	+217	+2.2	+325

[1] Resting, presystolic

[as summarized by Grande & Taylor]

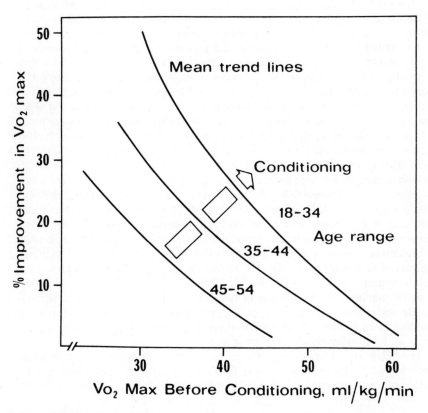

Fig. 2. Relationsnip of changes in maximal oxygen intake with physical condition and age [3].

As a result of physical conditioning, muscle blood flow through working muscle is apparently decreased during submaximal work and increased during maximal work [4, 12]. In the liver, kidney, and perhaps the skin, blood flow may be relatively greater after, than before, conditioning when submaximal work is performed. Apparently vascular control within skeletal muscle becomes more precise with conditioning.

Summary

To summarize the results of physical conditioning of sufficient intensity, duration, and frequency to induce physiological changes, perhaps the following could be listed for maximal work: an increase in heart size and volume brought about particularly during the maturational and developmental years; an increase in the maximal cardiac output brought about primarily by an increase in stroke volume; an increase in the maximal arteriovenous oxygen difference; an increase in myocardial pressure work capacity; and a possible improved synchroneity of the myocardial contractile pattern during heavy work.

During submaximal work the following changes have been observed to result from physical conditioning: a decreased heart rate at a fixed workload or alternatively an increased workload at a fixed heart rate, a reduced systolic and mean blood pressure at a fixed workload, a decreased heart rate blood pressure product, and a decreased cardiac output at a fixed workload. The decreased cardiac output is of lesser relative magnitude than the decrease in heart rate with the result that stroke volume is increased slightly.

With regard to the peripheral circulation, physical conditioning produces an increased maximal skeletal muscle blood flow but a relatively reduced blood flow during a fixed level of submaximal work. Blood flow to the kidneys and liver may be increased at a fixed workload following physical conditioning. There may well be a reduction in sympathetic arteriolar tone as well as in venous or capacitance vessel tone. The morphological changes with physical conditioning may well involve an increase in skeletal muscle capillary density, skeletal muscle hypertrophy, increased quantity of skeletal muscle involved under conditions of maximal work, increase in total circulating hemoglobin and skeletal muscle myoglobin, and increase in left ventricular wall thickness in diastole resulting in an increased heart muscle mass. The latter finding is of more prominence in the growing, developing young man.

The relatively favorable changes in the oxygen transport system resulting from physical conditioning increase man's work capacity; hence, the general statement "healthy man can be conditioned at any age" appears to have validity.

REFERENCES

1. Bar-Or, O., and Buskirk, E.R. The cardiovascular system and exercise. *In*, Johnson, W.H., and Buskirk, E.R., Eds. *Science and Medicine of Exercise and Sports*, 2nd edition. New York, Harper and Row, 1973.

2. Benestad, A.M. Trainability of old men. *Acta Med. Scand.* 178:321-327, 1965.

3. Buskirk, E.R. An introduction to exercise and performance evaluation. *J. S. C. Med. Assoc.* 65:Suppl., 4-7, 1967.

4. Clousen, J.P. Effects of physical conditioning. *Scand. J. Clin. Lab. Invest.* 24:305-313, 1969.

5. Ekblom, B. Effect of physical training on oxygen transport system in man. *Acta Physiol. Scand.* Suppl. 328:9-44, 1969.

6. Ekblom, B., and Hermansen, L. Cardiac output in athletes. *J. Appl. Physiol.* 25:619, 1968.

7. Finch, C.A., and Lenfont, C. Oxygen transport in man. *N. Engl. J. Med.* 286:407-415, 1972.

8. Frick, M.H. Coronary implications of hemodynamic changes caused by physical training. *Am. J. Cardiol.* 22:417-425, 1968.

9. Grande, F., and Taylor, H. Adaptive changes in the heart, vessels, and patterns of control under chronically high loads. *In, Handbook of Physiology—Circulation III*, Chap. 74. Washington, D.C., Am. Physiol. Soc., 1965.

10. Hartley, L.H., Grimby, G., Kilbom, A., Nelsson, N.J., Astrand, I., Bjure, J., Ekblom, B., and Saltin, B. Physical training in sedentary middle-aged and older men. III. Cardiac output and gas exchange at submaximal and maximal exercise. *Scand. J. Clin. Lab. Invest.* 24:335-344, 1969.

11. Hettinger, T. *Physiology of Strength*. Springfield, Ill., Thomas, 1961.

12. Kjellmer, I. Studies on exercise hyperemia. *Acta Physiol. Scand.* 64:Suppl. 244: 1, 1964.

13. Larsen, O.A., and Malmbarg, R.O., Eds. *Coronary Heart Disease and Physical Fitness*. Baltimore, University Park Press, 1971.

14. Lind, A.R., Taylor, S.H., Humphreys, P.W., Kennelly, B.M., and Donald, K.W. The circulatory effects of sustained voluntary muscle contractions. *Clin. Sci.* 27:229, 1964.

15. Rowell, L.B. Cardiovascular limitations to work capacity. *In*, Simonson, E., Ed. *Physiology of Work Capacity and Fatigue*, pp. 132-169. Springfield, Ill., Thomas, 1971.

16. Siegel, W., Blomquist, G., and Mitchell, J.H. Effects of a quantitated physical training program on middle-aged sedentary men. *Circulation* 41:19-29, 1970.

3

THE DETERMINANTS OF PHYSICAL PERFORMANCE
CAPACITY IN HEALTH AND DISEASE

Kris Lange-Andersen, M.D.

In order to describe the effects of variations in motor activity, the concept of physical performance capacity (PPC) must be considered. The PPC of an individual comprises different elements [1] :
1. Maximum aerobic power and endurance. Maximum aerobic endurance is usually defined as the maximum time a certain fraction of the maximum aerobic power can be sustained. It can also be measured in terms of the workload at which (a) normal metabolic homeostasis no longer can be maintained, and (b) signs and symptoms of impaired coronary circulation occur.
2. Maximum anaerobic power and capacity.
3. Maximum muscular strength and endurance.
4. Neuromuscular coordination.
5. Subjective exercise tolerance.
Methods for measurements of these elements have been developed, especially for maximum aerobic power and endurance [2], for maximum muscular strength and endurance [3], and for subjective exercise tolerance [4].

Maximum Aerobic Power

Principles of Measurement

Maximum aerobic power is assessed by measurement of the maximum oxygen intake attained in dynamic muscular exercise. It can be measured directly or indirectly. Direct measurement is based on performing muscular exercise with increasing intensity and establishing a work rate above which a further increase in work output does not bring about an increase in oxygen intake. This plateauing of oxygen intake is used as a criterion of the maximum value (Fig. 1).
Indirect measurement is based on establishing a linear relationship between the heart rate and the oxygen intake measured when the metabolic rate, circula-

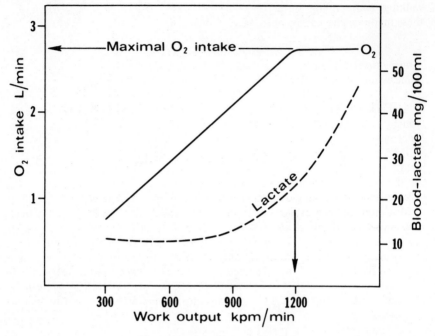

Fig. 1. Principle for the direct determination of maximal oxygen intake. *Steady state* values for oxygen intake are measured at increasing submaximal workloads, and the level established at which a further increase in work rate does not result in any increase in oxygen intake. Note the increase in blood lactate at progressively higher loadings.

tion, and respiration have reached the *steady state* at submaximal work, and with subsequent extrapolation to the maximum heart rate (Fig. 2).

Empirically established age-dependent mean maximum values for a given population are often used as an approximation for the maximum heart rate (TABLE I).

The indirect method can be simplified by establishing the linear relationship between the work rate (e.g. on a bicycle ergometer) and the heart rate, with a subsequent extrapolation to the maximum heart rate. In this way the work rate corresponding to the maximum oxygen intake can be estimated.

The accuracy in predicting the maximum oxygen intake by the indirect method varies among laboratories, but is no better than ±10 percent when individuals are tested, but as good as ±5 percent when groups of subjects are considered.

The maximal aerobic power is related to the amount of muscle mass being used in the particular exercise stress. Work with the arms yields considerably lower results than work with the legs (TABLE II).

The critical muscle mass that must be activated to measure the *true* maximum value cannot be stated at this time. Pedaling a bicycle ergometer, stepping, walking, and running are activities commonly employed. Within certain limits, these methods give comparable results (TABLE III).

*Interrelations of Structural and Functional Attributes
to Maximum Aerobic Power*

The maximum aerobic power in healthy subjects is correlated to body size (weight and height); body composition, particularly to lean body mass; and to functional dimensions of the oxygen transport system (TABLE IV).

It is possible with the aid of these variables to predict normal values for maximum aerobic power and to define limits of normal variation. Normal values for the relationship between aerobic power and body size, heart volume, lung volume, and total hemoglobin have been reported from different laboratories.

Maximum oxygen intake is related to heart rate, stroke volume, and arterio-venous oxygen difference through the equation:

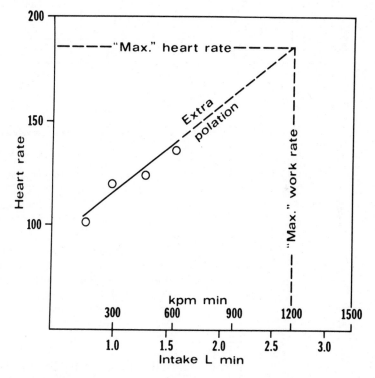

Fig. 2.   Principle for the indirect determination of maximal oxygen intake. Submaximal heart rates are determined, the linear relationship between heart rate and oxygen intake or work rate established with subsequent extrapolation to the maximal heart rate.

TABLE I
Norms for maximal heart rate

AGE IN YRS.	MAX. HEART RATE		
	LOWER LIMIT	MEAN	UPPER LIMIT
10	190	205	200
15	185	203	218
20 - 29	173	193	213
30 - 39	165	185	205
40 - 49	156	176	196
50 - 59	148	168	188
60 - 69	141	161	181
70 - 79	133	153	173
80 - 89	125	145	165

TABLE II
Maximal O_2 intake by crank and legwork (mean $\pm$ S.E. and S.D.)

V_{O_2} - MAX	LEGWORK		SIMPLE CRANK WORK		DOUBLE CRANK WORK	
	MEN	WOMEN	MEN	WOMEN	MEN	WOMEN
L/MIN	4.22 ± 0.17	2.63 ± 0.10	3.07 ± 0.11	1.89 ± 0.05	3.05 ± 0.10	2.12 0.09
	0.5	0.3	0.3	0.2	0.3	0.3
IN % OF V_{O_2} - MAX BY LEGWORK	100	100	73.1 ± 2.50	71.3 ± 3.01	73.2 ± 3.84	83.7 4.62
			7.5	9.0	11.5	13.9

TABLE III
Maximum oxygen intake in three types of exercise tests

TEST	(V_{O_2}) MAX (L/MIN STPD)	HEART RATE (BEATS/MIN)	LACTATE LEVEL (MG/100ML)
TREADMILL	3.84 ± 0.76 (2.54 – 5.84)	190 ± 5 (178 – 197)	122 ± 21 (78 – 166)
BICYCLE	3.56 ± 0.71 (2.57 – 5.23)	187 ± 9 (167 – 207)	112 ± 15 (89 – 143)
STEPS	3.68 ± 0.73 (2.66 – 5.59)	188 ± 6 (170 – 195)	105 ± 26 (45 – 165)

Shephard, et al. Bull. W.H.O., 1968

TABLE IV
Increase of maximal aerobic power 3 months after an acute cardiac episode

MAXIMAL O_2 INTAKE	PATIENT GROUP	INCREASE		SIGNFICANCE, P	
		6 MONTHS	9 MONTHS	6 MONTHS	9 MONTHS
V_{O_2} L/MIN	TRAINING	109 ± 3.9	115 ± 2.5	< 0.05	< 0.001
	SEDENTARY	108 ± 3.9	109 ± 2.2	n.s.	< 0.01
	TOTAL	109 ± 2.7	112 ± 1.8	< 0.01	< 0.001
V_{O_2} ML/MIN KG BODY WEIGHT	TRAINING	111 ± 3.8	119 ± 2.8	< 0.05	< 0.001
	SEDENTARY	109 ± 4.5	110 ± 1.5	n.s.	< 0.001
	TOTAL	111 ± 2.8	115 ± 2.1	< 0.01	< 0.001
V_{O_2} ML/MIN EMBODY HEIGHT	TRAINING	109 ± 3.9	115 ± 2.6	< 0.05	< 0.001
	SEDENTARY	108 ± 4.0	109 ± 2.3	n.s.	< 0.01
	TOTAL	109 ± 2.8	112 ± 1.9	< 0.01	< 0.001

A.M. Benestad, 1971

$$\dot{V}_{O_2} \max = f_h \times SV \times AVD$$
$$f_h = \text{heart rate}$$
$$SV = \text{stroke volume}$$
$$AVD = \text{arteriovenous oxygen difference}$$

$\dot{V}_{O_2}$ max is reached when the combination of these variables is optimal. In steady exercise of short duration (less than 10 minutes), the heart rate is linearly related to the oxygen intake almost up to the maximum heart rate, when the line may plateau. The stroke volume usually increases in the transition from rest to work. The magnitude of the increase is determined by the distribution of blood volume within the capacitance vessels. When work is continued, the stroke volume remains unchanged up to the maximum levels of work intensity. The magnitude of the stroke volume is determined by size of the heart (radiographical heart volume) and filling and emptying of the heart.

Factors Influencing the Level of Maximum Aerobic Power

The maximum aerobic power of an individual is determined by his inherited constitution, but a number of environmental factors are known to modify it.

Age. Age exerts a considerable influence upon the maximum aerobic power; this has been established in a number of populations. Absolute values increase during childhood and adolescence at approximately the same rate as the weight and height. The peak values are reached in early adulthood. In man, a steady decline in peak heart rate associated with age occurs after age 25-30, and at age 70, the maximum aerobic power approximates 50 percent of that at the age of

20. For women, the peak value is reached closely after maturity; the absolute value remains fairly constant during the fertile part of life, after which it declines at about the same rate as in men.

Sex. In early childhood there are no sex differences in aerobic power. At the onset of adolescence a divergence takes place, resulting in higher values for boys, and at the end of adolescence the maximum aerobic power per kg for girls is only about 70 percent of that for boys (Fig. 3).

Ethnic differences. Few studies have been reported in which the subjects were selected according to ethnic origin and the methods used were comparable. The available information indicates a similarity in aerobic power between the various ethnic groups. Not only do they average about the same, but also the variability measured by the standard deviation is quite similar, giving a variability

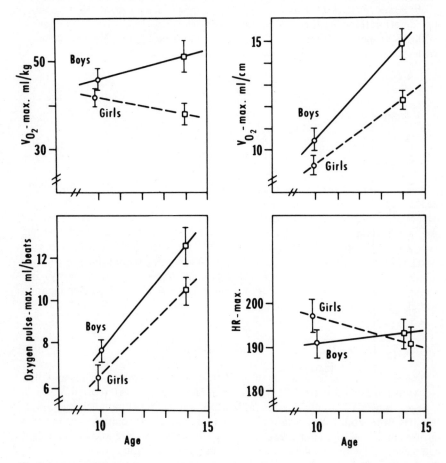

Fig. 3. Sex differences in the development of maximal values for oxygen intake, oxygen pulse, and heart rate during adolescence.

coefficient for the maximum aerobic power per kg body weight of about 10 percent.

Small but significant differences, however, have been established between populations with different genetic backgrounds. At present, it is not possible to state the extent to which such differences are genetically or environmentally determined.

Climate. Short-term exposure to heat or cold does not appear to create differences in the maximum aerobic power. Differences, however, are observed between arctic and tropical populations, the former having higher values at all ages for both sexes.

Nutrition. A number of experimental studies on man have shown that undernutrition and malnutrition reduce the maximum aerobic power; however, it is quickly restored to its normal value when the food supply becomes adequate.

Hypoxia (altitude). When sea-level dwellers are exposed to altitude, there is no deterioration in their maximum oxygen intake up to an altitude of 1200-1800 meters. After that, deterioration takes place at a rate that increases with the altitude. At 3000 meters the reduction is about 20 percent (Fig. 4).

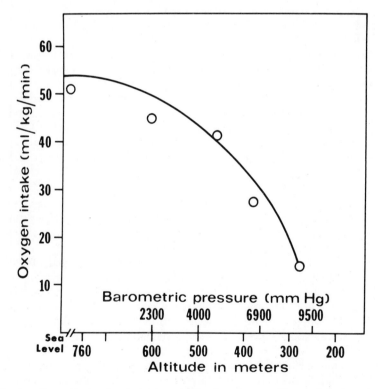

Fig. 4.   The reduction in maximal oxygen intake when ascending to altitude. Approximate figures.

Acclimatization to altitude can occur. The performance capacity is improved after a few weeks of dwelling at high altitudes. Acclimatization is known to proceed for at least a year, but it is doubtful if full compensation can be acquired within a man's lifetime, even at a moderate altitude (2000-2500 m).

Populations that have for generations adapted themselves to a life under hypoxic conditions have bodily characteristics making them particularly fit for work at high altitudes. A comparison between genetically similar lowland and high-altitude populations (3000 m) has revealed a similar maximum aerobic power in these two populations when tested in their own environments.

Habitual physical activity. In the clinically healthy, well-nourished man, the level of habitual physical activity is probably the most important behavioral factor influencing maximum aerobic power. The level of maximum oxygen intake in population groups that differ with regard to habitual physical activity deserves attention.

There are great differences in the energy requirements of different occupations. Studies of the relationship between the maximum oxygen intake of workers and their occupational energy expenditure reveals a great similarity between workers in occupations requiring different levels of energy expenditure. Lumberjacks, for example, have an aerobic capacity which is only 10-15 percent higher than that of office workers. This difference may, at least partly, be attributed to selection.

Considerable information is available about the maximum aerobic power of up to 80 percent above the average of sedentary people. Athletes are certainly a highly selected group, probably with distinct genetic characteristics.

Leisure-time activity may be very vigorous in some population groups of industrialized societies. Comparisons have been made between groups of middle-aged men in professions requiring a low level of energy expenditure. One group was extremely physically active during its leisure, the other more sedentary. The results revealed that maximum aerobic power was 30 percent greater in the group given to more physical activity, but again selection may have played a role.

Pathological conditions. Considerable evidence is available to demonstrate deterioration in the maximum oxygen intake in acute and chronic disease states. This deterioration may be a result of the pathological condition, but is also due to the physical activity that results from bed rest (Fig. 5).

The maximal oxygen intake in patients suffering from myocardial infarction has been measured 3, 6, and 12 months after the acute episode, and results indicate the deteriorative effect of the pathological condition. A 10-percent improvement was observed during convalescence, which could be increased up to 20 percent by the application of physical reconditioning (TABLE IV).

The maximal aerobic power has been systematically studied during convalescence in patients admitted to a small rehabilitation center in Norway with various acute and subacute disease states. On admission it was found that the maximal oxygen intake was less than 75 percent of a standard mean value in 25 percent of the cases. Participation in sports activities and the routine of exercise therapy normalized the physical performance capacity in most of these patients.

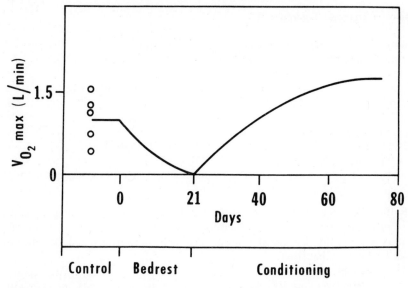

Fig. 5. Curvilinear response of maximal oxygen intake to bedrest and conditioning

Endurance for Prolonged Work

The physiology of prolonged work has not been well-investigated, and there are many unsolved problems with regard to the limiting factors.

When lactic acid concentration is measured in arterial blood, it is usually found that little or no elevation takes place before the workload exceeds 50-60 percent of the maximal aerobic power. Further increase above this level results in progressive elevation of the blood lactate, and consequently, the acid-base balance is altered and the blood pH decreased. This breaking point defines the level of work in relation to the maximum aerobic power where normal metabolic homeostasis can no longer be maintained. It has been reported that healthy subjects can work at the 50 percent relative load for about an hour without becoming exhausted and with maintenance of steady circulation and respiration. Work at a higher level usually exhausts the subjects within an hour, and circulation and respiration cannot maintain a steady state. There are some indications showing that the *exhaustion* point corresponds to the time when the glycogen content in the working muscles is depleted. However, fatigue during prolonged work is also related to numerous other physiological parameters, such as water balance, temperature balance, electrolyte balance, and the enzyme systems in the muscle cells and other tissues.

Experiments indicate that the well-trained individual can work at a higher relative load before lactate enters the circulating blood. This mechanism, therefore, may also contribute to the trained individual's better fitness for prolonged work.

Subjective Exercise Tolerance

Borg [5] describes a simple rating scale concerning the degree of perceived exertion during physical work. The latest version of this scale is [6]:

6		13	Somewhat hard
7	Very, very light	14	
8		15	Hard
9	Very light	16	
10		17	Very Hard
11	Fairly light	18	
12		19	Very, very hard
		20	

Rating of perceived exertion (RPE) is related in a fairly linear manner to heart rate and to workload. Furthermore, the use of the scale gives complementary information about exhaustion, since RPE between 18 and 20 indicates a high degree of exhaustion.

The maximal oxygen intake, but not the heart rate, declines with *age* at a given load. However, the RPE values, contrary to the heart rates, increase with age for the same workload, which is explained by the fact that the maximal heart rate decreases with age.

Use of RPE-Scale in Ergometric Testing of Patients

In the progressive submaximal exercise test, the recording of perceived exertion provides additional information to the usually measured physiological criteria, making it possible to define the subjective exercise tolerance limit. For many purposes this limit may be established at a value of 15. This value corresponds approximately to the work level at which a measurable amount of anaerobiosis occurs.

In a study by Borg and Linderholm [7], the relationship between heart rates and RPE-values were calculated for various patients, with coronary heart disease, or with arterial hypertension, or with vasoregulatory asthenia. These three groups were then compared with healthy control groups of comparable age. The results of the study indicated that patients with vasoregulatory asthenia rated the exertion to be less severe in relation to the heart rate than did the control group. This was especially true for low-intensity levels. The same result, although less distinct, was reported for patients with arterial hypertension. However, the group of patients with coronary heart disease rated the exertion to be higher in relation to heart frequency, particularly at high-rating levels. In comparison with the healthy controls, there was a smaller increase in heart rate in relation to a given increase in rating of perceived exertion for all patient group studies. The differences reported between various patient groups, especially between patients with coronary heart disease and those with the vasoregulatory asthenia syndrome is, therefore, of differential discriminatory value.

Nordeik et al (unpublished data) made an intensive study of perceived exertion during graded exercise on patients in a mental hospital. These patients have, in general, a low physical performance capacity, but it turned out that the RPE-value in relation to heart rate was not different from that in healthy persons.

REFERENCES

1. Andersen, K.L., Shephard, R.J., Denolin, H., Varnauskas, E., and Masironi, R. *Fundamentals of Exercise Testing.* Geneva, W.H.O., 1971.
2. Andersen, K.L., and Magel, J. Physiological adaptation to a high level of habitual physical activity during adolescence. *Int. Z. Angew. Physiol.* 28:209-227, 1970.
3. Andersen, K.L. The effect of altitude variation on the physical performance capacity of Ethiopian men. In Press.
4. Andersen, K.L. Work capacity of selected populations. *In*, Baker, P.T., and Weiner, J.S., Eds. *The Biology of Human Adaptability.* Oxford, Clarendon Press, 1966.
5. Borg, G. *Physical Performance and Perceived Exertion.* Lund, Gleerup, 1962.
6. Borg, G. Perceived exertion as an indicator of somatic stress. *Scand. J. Rehabil. Med.* 2:92-98, 1970.
7. Borg, G., and Linderholm, H. Exercise performance and perceived exertion in patients with coronary insufficiency, arterial hypertension and vasoregulatory asthenia. *Acta Med. Scand.* 187:17, 1970.

SELECTED RELATED REFERENCES

Andersen, K.L., Benestad, A.M., and Segrem, N. Maximal oxygen uptake. *In*, Andersen, K.L., and Wilson, O., Eds. *A Field Study of Physiological Adjustment to Increased Muscular Activity With and Without Cold Exposure.* Lund, Gleerup, 1966.

Andersen, K.L., and Ghesquiere, J. Sex differences in the development of physical performance capacity during the puberty growth spurt period in a population unit at the west coast of Norway. *Hum. Biol.* In Press.

Cotes, J.E., Davies, C.T.M., Edholm, O.G., Healy, M.J.R., and Tanner, J.M. Factors relating to the aerobic capacity of 46 healthy British males and females, ages 18 to 28 years. *Proc. Roy. Soc. Lond. B* 174:91-114, 1969.

Myhre, K., Vik, T., Hellstrøm, B., and Andersen, K.L. Adaptation to heavy muscular work. *Arct. Anthropol.* 7:44-49, 1970.

Shephard, R.J., Allen, C., Benade, A.J.S., Davies, C.T.M., di Prampero, P.E., Hedman, R., Merriman, J.E., Myhre, K., and Simmons, R. Standardization of submaximal exercise tests. *Bull. W.H.O.* 38:765-775, 1968.

W.H.O. Optimum performance capacity in adults. *W.H.O. Tech. Rep. Ser.* No. 436, 1969.

Andersen, K.L., and Smith-Sivertsen, J. Evaluation of work power and exercise tolerance. *In*, Yoshimura, H., and Weiner, J.S., Eds. *Human Adaptability and Its Methodology*, pp. 183-203, Tokyo, Japanese Society for the Promotion of Science, 1966.

Andersen, K.L. Fitness for work of convalescents improved by various types of constitutioning exercise. *In*, Evang, K., and Andersen, K.L. *Physical Activity in Health and Disease*, pp. 165-174. Oslo, Universitetsforlaget, 1966.

Asmussen, E., Heebøll-Nielsen, and Mollbech, S. Methods for evaluation of muscle strength. *Communication, Testing and Observation Institute of Danish National Association for Infantile Paralysis.* No. 5. 1959.

Benestad, A.M. The deteriorative effect of myocardial infarction upon physiological indices of work capacity. *Acta Med. Scand.* 191:67-75, 1972.

Benestad, A.M. Variation in hemoglobin and physical performance capacity within a healthy adult population. In Press.

Benestad, A.M. Treningsterapi ved koronare hjertesykdommer. Oslo, Universitetsforlaget (0.95), 1971.

Benestad, A.M. Sportshjertet. Moen fysiologiske og kliniske betraktninger. *T. Norsk. Laegeforen.* 84:969-972, 1964.

4

PRINCIPLES OF EXERCISE TESTING

Robert A. Bruce, M.D. FACC, FACP, FRSM

Objectives, Assumptions, and Classification of Methods

In cardiac rehabilitation by exercise conditioning or physical training, the primary purpose of exercise testing is not the diagnosis of cardiovascular disease, which is already established by the clinical methods of history, physical, and radiological examinations, as well as by interpretation of the resting electrocardiogram (ECG). Instead, the purpose of exercise testing is to evaluate the severity of disease, reveal unexpected responses to exertion, and provide an appropriate baseline by which the effects of rehabilitation may be assessed physiologically. Accordingly, the *objectives* of an exercise test include:

a) The definition of IMPAIRMENT of functional aerobic power or maximal oxygen intake ($\dot{V}_{0_2\,max}$);

b) The determination of the MECHANISM of impairment;

c) The provision of a baseline to assess future CHANGES with the natural history of disease and its modification by clinical management.

Exercise testing can involve isometric or dynamic exercise. Because of the excessive pressor response which makes the former dangerous, only the latter is conventionally employed. Exercise testing involves these basic assumptions:

1. Only ambulatory patients without clinical contraindications are selected for testing.

2. The patient is provided with adequate information of the purpose, methods, risks, benefits, rights, and welfare to permit a truly informed consent[1]. A suitable statement of these principles should be read and signed by the patient, and witnessed by the supervising physician. This reinforces the doctor-patient relationship by identifying areas of concern, permitting the patient to ask questions, and the physician to provide appropriate information and reassurance.

---

[1] An example is found in the Appendix

3. Professional supervision should be provided, either clinically by a knowledgeable physician or indirectly by delegation to trained and supervised paramedical personnel. This involves monitoring the patient, his ECG, and blood pressure during and after exercise testing.

Risks, Precautions, and Benefits

For ambulatory persons without obvious contraindications, there may be occasional risks.

Arrhythmias. Either supraventricular or ventricular premature beats occur in 5-10 percent of both healthy persons or cardiac patients. More frequent premature beats are observed in cardiac patients, especially if treated with digitalis and/or diuretics which alter myocardial efflux of potassium during exercise. Serious tachyarrhythmias are less frequent; in over 10,000 tests at the University of Washington Hospital, ventricular fibrillation has occurred only twice, once in a normal subject after a hot shower [1], and once in a patient with angina pectoris (AP) immediately after exertion. Electrical defibrillation was performed successfully in each instance and both patients recovered.

Myocardial ischemia may be manifested by segmental ST depression in a precordial ECG, by tightness or pain (AP) in the chest, or by both. Despite ST depression in as many as 30 percent of individuals, varying directly with age and other risk factors, AP is observed in less than 1 percent of apparently normal persons.

Exertional hypotension may be mild, with inadequate rise in systolic blood pressure (less than 10 mm Hg), moderate or extreme, with a significant decrease in pressure. This decrease in blood pressure is an important sign in cardiac patients who develop symptoms. Occasionally, an apprehensive normal subject, when tested in a demonstration, may develop emotional hypertension at rest before exercise, and the pressure may fall with exertion as anxiety is allayed and no discomfort or limitation at low levels of exercise is encountered.

Injury should never occur; when it does, it is usually the result of an uninformed person stepping onto a treadmill without instruction, and without beginning his walk at a slow pace.

Myocardial infarction (MI) has been reported in less than 1 in 2500 properly selected patients; more commonly, it has occurred with the thermal stress of a hot shower after completion of an uneventful test. Indeed, the first example reported was in a presumably normal subject [1].

Cardiac arrest is equally rare associated with an exercise test, and is usually confined to patients with extensive coronary artery disease [2]. Actually, it is more frequently encountered after several weeks of physical training, than with testing.

Because of these risks, obvious safety precautions with which physicians should be acquainted include: (1) preliminary clinical examination just before testing; (2) professional monitoring during testing; and (3) criteria for stopping exercise.

Even in the absence of symptoms, exercise testing should be stopped immediately if a patient exhibits either 3 consecutive ventricular premature beats or develops an ataxic or staggering gait. The same precautions apply equally to the use of a step test or bicycle ergometer when neuromuscular coordination or pacing is disturbed.

Overall safety is ensured when morbidity, severe enough to require hospitalization, is less than 0.1 percent and mortality less than 0.01 percent. (In over 10,000 multistage-treadmill tests the mortality rate is zero.)

The benefits of exercise testing are at least twofold: it provides a more informative examination of the patient, not just at rest, but also under the stress and recovery from exercise; and provides more effective clinical management. This is particularly true when the effects of drug therapy need to be assessed. On some occasions, individually unpredictable, untoward effects are revealed and more judicious selection or dosage results. Another real benefit is the exclusion of possible cardiovascular disease in an anxious patient who otherwise exhibits normal responses and no functional impairment.

Types of Dynamic Exercise Tests

Basically there are two types of dynamic exercise-testing procedures (TABLE I). One is submaximal, with one or more workloads, whether performed continuously without rest periods or intermittently with intervening periods of rest. These tests always have some *predetermined* and *arbitrary* end

TABLE I

Dynamic exercise testing procedures

	Submaximal	*Maximal*
End-points	Arbitrarily determined (number of steps, heart rate, duration, etc.)	Individually determined after progressive increments in workloads
Observations	Usually ST segment, supine posture after exertion, various ECG leads	Symptoms, signs, changes in heart rate, rhythm, systolic pressure and ST segments in precordial ECG in upright posture
Examples	Double Master Two-Step Bicycle ergometry Heart rate–limited Graded treadmill test	Multistage Treadmill

points. The end points may be defined in terms of the workload, duration of exercise, heart rate and/or oxygen intake. Although such end points are sometimes adjusted for the type of individual, on the basis of sex, age, or body weight, they are not adjusted for the actual functional characteristics of the specific individual.

Oxygen requirements for five different types of submaximal exercise tests were recently defined for the same group of normal subjects [3]. Means, standard deviations, and coefficients of variation are tabulated in TABLE II. The least demanding, and most reproducible procedure of these five tests is the treadmill test at 3 mph and 5 percent grade of incline. The most demanding and most variable, despite adjustments for age and weight, is the double Master two-step test. In terms of multiples of the resting oxygen consumption they approximate 4 and 6 METS, respectively.

The other major type of exercise-testing protocol is the maximal exercise test. There is no arbitrary fixed end point, other than the individually determined limits of maximal possible or tolerated exertion. Alternatively this may be called *symptom-limited capacity*. When this limit is attained, intensity and duration of effort, heart rate, oxygen intake, and blood pressure are obsered to define the limits for the individual. In a direct comparison in 24 normal men, higher levels of oxygen intake, heart rate, and lactate were achieved with a treadmill than with either the bicycle ergometer or step-test methods (Fig. 1).

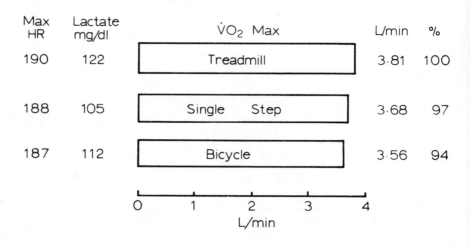

Adapted from Shephard et al, Bull WHO, 38, 757, 1968

Fig. 1. Comparative maximal exercise performance with discontinuous tests in 24 men 20-40 (26.4) years of age.

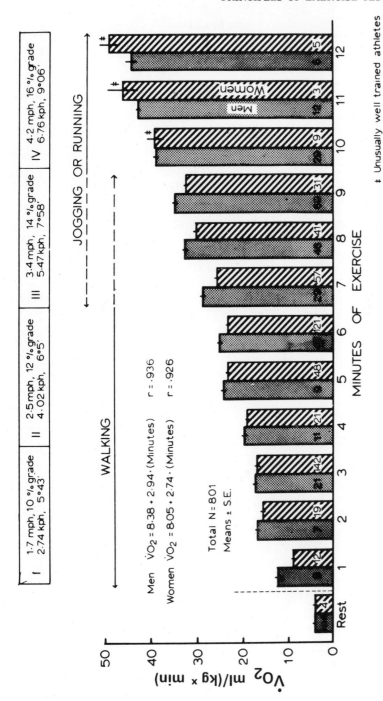

Fig. 2. Aerobic requirements of multistage-treadmill test (for submaximal only) [4]. (Reproduced with permission)

TABLE II

Comparison of 5 submaximal tests in 10 subjects [3]

3-Minute Tests	$\dot{V}_{O_2}$ ml/(kg · min)	Heart Rate	Comments
Double Master Two-Step			
9″ step	23.0 ± 3.1	122 ± 14	Highest cost
12″ step, 20 times	21.3 ± 2.4	117 ± 12	
9″ two-step, 40 times	20.4 ± 2.1	114 ± 14	
50 RPM bicycle, 600 KPM	18.9 ± 2.5	117 ± 14	
3 MPH treadmill, 5% grade	16.9 ± 1.6	105 ± 12	Least variable

The preferred testing procedure, in this author's experience, is a multistage treadmill test of both submaximal and maximal exercise [4]. Aerobic requirements, weight-adjusted, for healthy men and women are shown in Fig. 2 for the first four stages. Although the speed and grade are changed every 3 minutes, the oxygen intake increase is approximately linear with time. From the 5th to 9th minutes, for those who can continue beyond this time, oxygen intake in ml/(kg·min) averages 15 percent more in men than in women. This is consistent

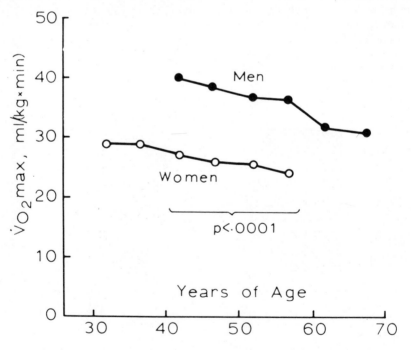

Fig. 3. Variations of $\dot{V}_{O_2}$ max with body weight and age.

with 12-13 percent greater values reported in three other studies of younger adults. The differences between men and women are attributed to differences in body dimensions, composition and metabolism [5, 6, 7].

Definition, Significance, and Reproducibility of $\dot{V}_{O_2}$max

$\dot{V}_{O_2}$max equals exactly the product of maximal cardiac output and maximal arterial-mixed venous oxygen difference [8]. Since $AV_{O_2}D_{max}$ varies little in heart disease, $\dot{V}_{O_2}$max virtually defines the pumping capacity of the heart. Therefore, it is of major importance in the evaluation of severity of heart disease. In health, $\dot{V}_{O_2}$max varies directly with body weight, especially lean body mass [9], and inversely with age [10]; it is higher in men than in women (Fig. 3), and higher in athletes than in sedentary persons [11, 12].

Average values of $\dot{V}_{O_2}$max in health and disease are shown in Fig. 4. In addition, major variations in relative aerobic requirement, weight-adjusted, are shown for the same external physical workloads, which reflects marked differences in capacity. Thus, three individuals may perform at the same workload; that which is only 45 percent of capacity for average normal men is 59 percent for women and 73 percent for cardiac men. This relationship defines the threshold for cardiorespiratory symptoms and the regulation of the distribution of cardiac output to the several regional circulations of the body [13]. Unless the capacity of each individual is actually measured, this relationship cannot be defined; when it is measured, the intensity of any submaximal exertion can be expressed quantitatively for any ambulatory person, whether or not heart disease is present.

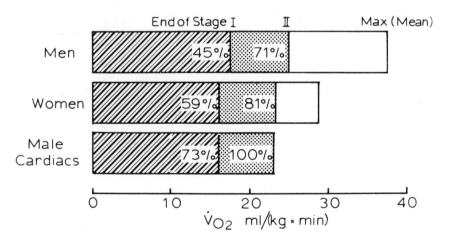

Fig. 4.   Relative aerobic requirements of multistage exercise [4].
(Reproduced with permission)

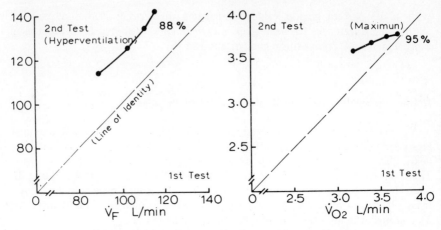

Fig. 5. Reproducibility of ventilation and oxygen intake.

(Classroom Demonstrations on Successive Days, 31 Year Old Healthy Male)

On successive days, $\dot{V}_{O_2}$ max of the same healthy person is more reproducible than $\dot{V}_{E max}$ or than $\dot{V}_{O_2}$ at any level of submaximal exertion or even at rest (Fig. 5). When tested days to weeks later, the correlation of $\dot{V}_{O_2}$ max is extremely high ($r = +.99$, N = 67, P $<$ .0001). When compared with the discontinuous method of Taylor and others [9], insignificantly higher values are obtained with the multistage-treadmill test within 10-15 minutes ($r = +.96$, N = 16, P $<$ .001) [14].

If the highest value of oxygen intake for the last 3-4 minutes of a multistage maximal test is taken as 100 percent, the percent relationship of values for the preceding 2 minutes is identical for men and women, even though the absolute values of $\dot{V}_{O_2}$ max, weight-adjusted, are quite different (Fig. 6) [14]. The same

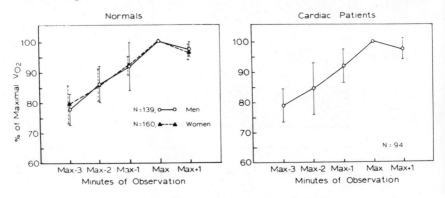

Fig. 6. Approach to maximal oxygen intake [14].
(By permission of the Amer. Heart Ass'n., Inc.)

applies to ambulatory patients with cardiovascular disease. Furthermore, for about 15 percent who can continue exertion for less than 1 minute after this peak value, the observed $\dot{V}_{O_2}$ is lower. This is because stroke volume is reduced.

Average values of $\dot{V}_{O_2}$max expected in healthy men and women can be predicted from these regression equations:

Active men = 69.7 − .612 (years of age) $(r = -.704)$ (Equation 1)
Sedentary men = 57.8 − .445 (years of age) $(r = -.659)$ (Equation 2)
Active women = 42.9 − .312 (years of age) $(r = -.634)$ (Equation 3)
Sedentary women = 42.3 − .356 (years of age) $(r = -.734)$ (Equation 4)

It should be noted that habitual physical-activity status is also included. If individuals do not engage in jogging or running games or enough exertion to develop sweating at least once a week regularly, they are considered sedentary.

Finally, because of the high correlation between duration of this multistage treadmill test of maximal exercise $[r = +.93,\ \text{SEE} = 4.9\ \text{ml}/(\text{kg} \cdot \text{min})]$, it is reasonable for clinical purposes to measure just the elapsed time and estimate $\dot{V}_{O_2}$max:

For men: 3.88 + .056[1] (duration in seconds) $(r = .920)$ (Equation 5)
For women: 1.06 + .056[1] (duration in seconds) $(r = .920)$ (Equation 6)

It should be noted that there are different intercepts for normal men and normal women.

Functional Aerobic Impairment

It is not enough to determine the $\dot{V}_{O_2}$max or functional aerobic power of any ambulatory person. It is also important to evaluate its relationship to expected values of appropriate peers. Thus, *a new concept of functional aerobic impairment* is introduced. This represents the percent difference of observed or estimated $\dot{V}_{O_2}$max and that predicted in health for a person of the same sex, age, and habitual activity status [4]:

$$\text{FAI} = \frac{\text{Predicted } \dot{V}_{O_2}\text{max} - \text{Observed } \dot{V}_{O_2}\text{max}}{\text{Predicted } \dot{V}_{O_2}\text{max}} \times 100 \qquad \text{(Equation 7)}$$

In order to simplify calculation of FAI, nomograms have been constructed (Figures 7A and B). The normal value of FAI is zero; this indicates that V_{O_2}max is 100 percent of average normal expected value. The 95 percent confidence interval is from −26 to +27. It should be emphasized that these nomograms apply to the multistage-treadmill test (Bruce) only; they should not be utilized for any other testing procedure. By addition of successive standard deviations, severity of FAI is defined as:

mild	27-40 percent
moderate	41-54 percent
marked	55-68 percent
extreme	more than 69 percent

[1] If duration is expressed in minutes, the slope coefficient should be multiplied by 60.

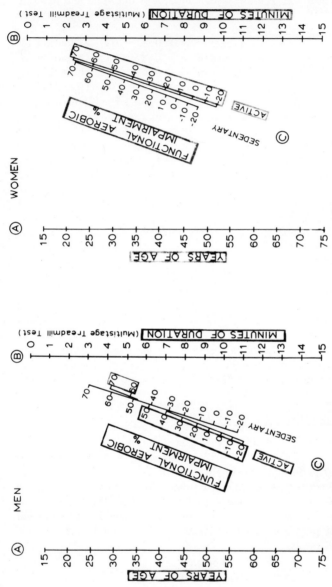

Fig. 7.   Nomograms for estimating functional aerobic impairment (FAI) [4].   (Reproduced with permission)

Nomograms for finding percent deviation of individual's estimated from average predicted values of $\dot{V}_{O_2}$max, in healthy middleaged men (A) and women (B).

$\dot{V}_{O_2}$max is estimated from equations 5 and 6. FAI is obtained by projecting a line from "age" to "duration of exercise" and reading the value at which this line intersects the diagonal which is appropriate for "habitual-activity status." Note that for *any given age* FAI varies markedly with duration of exertion, but less with habitual-activity status. Conversely, for any given *duration of exercise*, to the *same limit* of maximal exertion, FAI rises markedly with age, but less with habitual-activity status. These nomograms apply only for the multistage-treadmill exercise test.

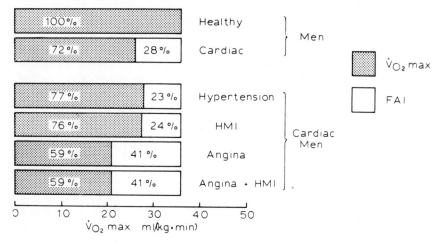

Fig. 8.   Comparative examples for middle-aged men [14].

To illustrate, patients with clinically uncomplicated hypertension have a mean FAI of 34 percent and the $\dot{V}_{O_2}$ max is only 66 percent of average normal expected value (Fig. 8).

Effects of Nitroglycerin

Unlike normal subjects, $\dot{V}_{O_2}$ max in patients with ischemic heart disease, whether manifested by AP or prior MI, can be increased acutely with 0.4 mg nitroglycerin sublingually (Fig. 9) [16]. Work capacity is also increased because

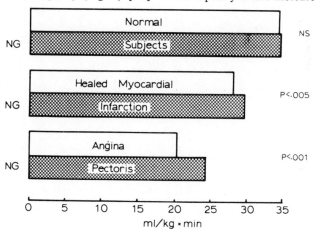

Fig. 9.   Acute effects of nitroglycerin (NG) on maximal oxygen intake [16]. (By permission of the Amer. Heart Ass'n., Inc.)

of the peripheral vasodilation of arterial resistance and venous compliance which reduce the afterload and preload, respectively, of the ischemic myocardium. It is also of interest to note the similarity in approach to percent $\dot{V}_{O_2}$ max in such patients when treated with nitroglycerin (Fig. 10).

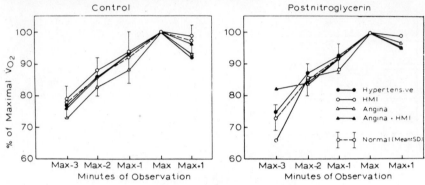

Fig. 10. Approaches to maximal oxygen intake [14].
(By permission of the Amer. Heart Ass'n., Inc.)

Circulatory Responses to Exercise

Cardiovascular responses to exercise may be quite variable at submaximal, but remarkably reproducible at maximal exercise (Fig. 11). This was clearly demonstrated where the same subject was exercised for classroom demonstration pur-

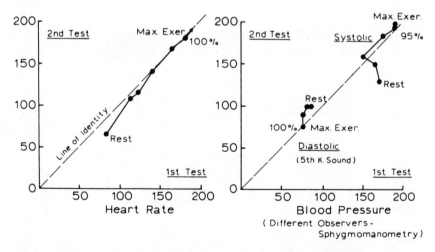

Fig. 11. Reproducibility of circulatory responses to exercise. (Classroom demonstration with a 31-year-old normal male)

TABLE III

Maximal exercise responses of men in relation to age and disease [4]

Variables	Healthy persons		Coronary patients		Additive effects of age and MI or AP
	Young adults n = 32	Middle-aged adults n = 117	With only healed myocardial infarction n = 28	With only angina pectoris n = 89	
Age, years	22.8 ± 3.4	51 ± 8	52 ± 9	52 ± 10	−21%
Duration, sec	755 ± 113	572 ± 108	400 ± 171	293 ± 156***	−45% −60%
FAI, %	−2 ± 11	2.9 ± 11	25 ± 19	45 ± 16	+25% −45%
Estimated $\dot{V}_{O_2}$max	44.6 ± 5.6	35.6 ± 5.3	26.1 ± 9.4	20.2 ± 8.6	−21% −45% −60%
Change in heart rate	125 ± 14	104 ± 16	75 ± 22	62 ± 20*	−14% −46% −49%
Maximal heart rate	197 ± 8	174 ± 14	155 ± 20	138 ± 22***	−11% −20% −29%
Change in systolic pressure	55 ± 22	55 ± 31	43 ± 24	30 ± 22**	+28% 0% −30%
Maximal systolic pressure	172 ± 23	183 ± 18	166 ± 27***	183 ± 28	+9% −1% −9%
Maximal pressure rate product /100	336 ± 40	316 ± 72	257 ± 75	252 ± 81	−3% −21% −22%
Maximal diastolic pressure	70 ± 7	69 ± 14	84 ± 14 (122%)	88 ± 15 (127%)	+22% +28%
Prevalence of ST segment depression, %	0	19	28	68	+19% +28% +68%

In comparison with middle-aged adults, $p < 0.05$ (*), $p < 0.01$ (**), and $p < 0.001$ (***)

poses on successive days. It was more remarkable when different observers recorded blood pressure, utilizing a clinical sphygmomanometer and stethoscope, and with no instructions about using the 4th versus 5th Korotkoff sound for the diastolic blood pressure values.

Heart rates at rest vary over an appreciable range, but there is no signficant difference between average values in relation to age or disease. In contrast, however, despite greater range of maximal heart rates, there are highly significant reductions with increasing age and particularly with coronary heart disease

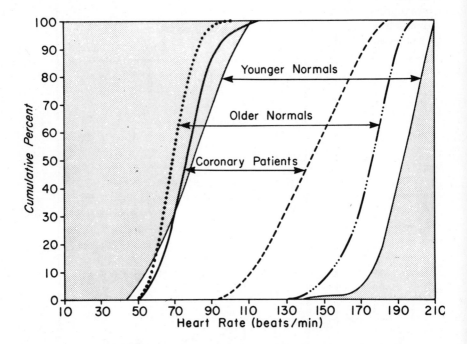

Fig. 12. Cumulative percent distribution curves for three classes of persons [17]. (By permission of the Amer. Heart Ass'n., Inc.)

(TABLE III). When cumulative percent distribution curves are used, the observed value for a given person may be expressed as percentile for his peer group (Fig. 12). The change in heart rate from rest to maximal exercise defines the chronotropic reserve of the heart [17]. Because there is little change in stroke volume, normally, this represents a crude index of changes in cardiac output.

Similarly, systolic blood pressure at rest and during exercise provides useful information. The change is normally about 60 mm Hg in men and only 30-35 mm Hg in women. This change is a crude index of the inotropic reserve of the heart [11]; because of the concomitant decrease in peripheral resistance, it underestimates the magnitude of increase in the contractile force of the heart.

Conclusions

Exercise testing represents an extension of the clinical examination of the ambulatory cardiac patient. Although arbitrary limits of submaximal dynamic exercise are commonly employed to assess function, much more information can be obtained simply, reliably, and safely with maximal testing to individually determined symptomatic limits of capacity. Maximal oxygen intake may be measured, or if a particular standardized multistage-treadmill procedure (Bruce test) is used, $\dot{V}_{O_2}$ max may be estimated. It can be evaluated in relation to appropriate peer groups of healthy persons by means of nomograms from elapsed duration of such exercise in terms of functional aerobic impairment. Cardiovascular mechanism of impairment can be assessed from changes in heart rate and blood pressure.

APPENDIX

INFORMED CONSENT [14]

Information Statement for Participants

In order to evaluate the *functional performance and capacity* of the heart, lungs, and blood vessels, each individual consents, voluntarily, to perform an exercise test. Before being tested, he is questioned and examined by a physician, and has an electrocardiogram recorded (to show whether or not testing should proceed), after which he walks on a treadmill, with speed and gradient increasing every 3 minutes, until the limits of fatigue, breathlessness, chest pain and/or other symptoms are of such severity that he should stop the effort. Blood pressure and electrocardiogram are monitored while he is exercising. In some instances expired air will be collected and oxygen intake determined.

Risks of testing include occasional changes in the rhythm of the heart beats and the possibility of excessive changes in blood pressure. There is a remote chance of fainting and an even more remote chance of a heart attack, particularly if the participant takes a hot shower shortly after strenuous exercise testing. Professional supervision protects against injury, by providing appropriate precautionary measures, and in the unlikely event that these precautions are insufficient, emergency hospital treatment is available.

Benefits of testing include quantitative assessment of working capacity and critical appraisal of the disorders or diseases that impair capacity, the knowledge of which facilitates better treatment, and more accurate prognosis for future cardiac events.

Both the *right* to withdraw from the tests at anytime with impunity and the right to withhold confidential information from nonmedical persons (such as employers and insurance agents) without consent are assured. The welfare of each person will be protected.

In addition to participating in this exercise test, each person permits his name to be registered for future followup studies.

Consent

Having read the information statement and had the opportunity to ask questions, I hereby willingly consent to be tested and enrolled in the Seattle Heart Watch Exercise Study.

Date _____   Signed _____

Time _____ a.m.   Witness _____
p.m.

REFERENCES

1. Bruce, R.A., Hornsten, T.R., and Blackmon, J.R. Myocardial infarction after normal responses to maximal exercise. *Circulation* 38:552, 1968.

2. Bruce, R.A., and Kluge, W. Defibrillatory treatment of exertional cardiac arrest in coronary disease. *J.A.M.A.* 216:653, 1971.

3. Blackburn, H., Winkler, G., Vilandré, J., Hodgson, J., and Taylor, H.L. Physical activity and aging. *In, Medicine and Sport*: vol. 4, p. 28. Basel, Kasser, 1970.

4. Bruce, R.A. Exercise testing of patients with coronary heart disease. *Ann. Clin. Res.* 3:323, 1971.

5. Booyens, J., and Keatinge, W.R. The expenditure of energy by men and women walking. *J. Physiol.* 138:165, 1957.

6. Cotes, J.E., et al. Factors relating to the aerobic capacity of 46 healthy British males and females, ages 18 to 28 years. *Proc. Roy. Soc. Lond. B.* 174:91, 1969.

7. Quenoville, M.D., et al. Statistical studies of recorded energy expenditure in men. I. Basal metabolism related to sex, stature, age, climate and race. *Commonw. Bur. Anim. Nutr.*, Tec. Comm. No. 17, 1969.

8. Mitchell, J.H., Sproule, B.J., and Chapman, C.B. The physiological meaning of the maximal oxygen intake test. *J. Clin. Invest.* 37:538, 1958.

9. Taylor, H.L., Buskirk, E., and Henschel, A. Maximal oxygen intake as an objective measure of cardiorespiratory performance. *J. Appl. Physiol.* 8:72, 1955.

10. Robinson, S. Experimental Studies of physical fitness in relation to age. *Arbeitsphysiologie* 10:251, 1938.

11. Åstrand, P.O. *Experimental Studies of Physical Working Capacity in Relation to Sex and Age*. Copenhagan, Munksgaard, 1952.

12. Hollman, Van W., and Grunewald, B. Der altere Mensch and der Sport. *Z. Allgemeinmed.* 43:1, 1967.

13. Rowell, L.B., Blackmon, J.R., and Bruce, R.A. Indocyanine green clearance and estimated hepatic blood flow during mild to maximal exercise in upright man. *J. Clin. Invest.* 43:1677, 1964.

14. Bruce, R.A., Kusumi, F., and Hosmer, D. Maximum oxygen intake and nomographic assessment of functional aerobic impairment in cardiovascular disease. *Am. Heart J.* 85:546, 1973.

15. Bruce, R.A. University of Washington Seattle. Unpublished data.

16. Detry, J-M.R., and Bruce, R.A. Effects of nitroglycerin on "maximal" oxygen intake and exercise electrocardiograms in coronary heart disease. *Circulation* 43:155, 1971.

17. Kasser, I.S., and Bruce, R.A. Comparative effects of aging and coronary heart disease on submaximal and maximal exercise. *Circulation* 39:759, 1969.

5

THE HEMODYNAMIC EFFECTS OF PHYSICAL CONDITIONING IN HEALTHY YOUNG, AND MIDDLE-AGED INDIVIDUALS, AND IN CORONARY HEART DISEASE PATIENTS

Victor F. Froelicher, Jr., M.D., Major, USAFMC

Introduction

Several reviews have been presented on the hemodynamics effects of physical conditioning [1, 2, 3]. New techniques now are available and new concepts recognized that make another review of this subject timely. This information is important for a number of reasons, including demonstration of the manner in which the cardiovascular system participates in the increased work capacity accompanying physical conditioning. This increased work capacity is important to patients with coronary heart disease (CHD) whose quality of life is reduced by the physical limitations imposed upon them by the disease process. However, if physical conditioning accelerates cardiac deterioration or abbreviates the quantity of life, then it is not a desirable mode of therapy. The hemodynamic studies give information regarding changes in cardiac function. Also, myocardial oxygen consumption can be indirectly estimated by changes in blood pressure, heart rate, stroke volume, ejection time, and myocardial contractility. Efficiency and changes in the peripheral circulation have been evaluated by oxygen and blood flow measurements. The results of these studies help to explain the cardiovascular response to physical conditioning and should support its clinical utilization.

The effects of physical conditioning can be studied by the cross-sectional approach, comparing athletes to normal people, and by the longitudinal approach comparing individuals before and after a training program. Both of these approaches have limitations and difficulties. The cross-sectional approach is easier since the trouble and expense of organizing a training program is avoided. However, athletes represent a population group endowed with biological attributes and motivation that make them capable of superior performance [4]. Also, they undergo long periods of physical training usually beginning at a young age when dimensional and morphological changes are more apt to occur

---

The views expressed are those of the author and do not necessarily reflect the views of the USAF.

[5]. This makes comparison with normal people rather tenuous since most trained normal individuals cannot reach the athletes' level of cardiovascular function or performance. For these reasons, only longitudinal studies are reviewed in this report.

Besides the expense and difficulty in organizing and maintaining a training program, there are other problems encountered in longitudinal studies. Volunteers often are athletic and differ from randomly selected normal people. The exercise program can affect other variables such as body weight and smoking habits, and the results can be biased by dropouts. In persons with CHD a placebo effect on hemodynamics has been documented [6] and the training program may select a healthier group.

In any training program, the end result depends upon a number of factors. These include the level of fitness, physical endowments, previous physical training, age, and health of the individual entering the program (TABLE I). The changes are greater in unconditioned individuals as compared to those somewhat physically fit, and greater in younger individuals than in older individuals [7]. It has been hypothesized that diseased hearts are not modified by chronic exercise and that peripheral circulatory changes associated with physical conditioning are more important in persons with CHD. The most important of these variables will be evaluated in this review by including normal trainees of different ages and individuals with CHD.

TABLE I

Effects of physical conditioning depend upon:

1. Level of fitness at onset of training
2. Genetic endowments
3. Previous training (especially regarding length of time and age it occurred)
4. Age
5. Health
6. Training program structure and length

The structure of an exercise program is important [7, 8, 9]. Intensity and duration of the work periods must be considered, as well as the overall time of training. Individuals with CHD must be carefully selected for an exercise program. During training they must be closely monitored and should follow a less demanding exercise protocol because of the danger of exercise-induced sudden death [10, 11, 12, 13, 14]. Physical training can be aimed at improving or increasing muscle strength and anaerobic or aerobic performance [4]. Only the latter effect is dependent upon the improvement of the oxygen transporting system (i.e., blood, lungs, heart, blood vessels) and is largely due to an improvement in the overall capacity of the cardiovascular system.

Muscle strength can be improved by repetitious isotonic or isometric muscle contractions of a few seconds duration against resistance. This type of exercise does not improve cardiovascular function as shown by the relatively normal-sized hearts, normal resting and exercise heart rates, and unexceptional maximal oxygen intakes of athletes who only train in this manner [4, 15].

Anaerobic capacity is necessary for short activities of high intensity or for activities that require more energy than is available from the oxygen transporting system. This energy is derived from high-energy phosphate compounds resulting from the breakdown of glycogen to lactic acid without oxygen utilization. Athletes, such as sprinters, who require relatively infrequent short bursts of high-intensity activity acquire this capacity and often do not improve their overall cardiovascular function. Training aimed at developing anaerobic capacity should consist of maximal work periods of short duration (10-60 sec). This type of training requires much motivation since it is difficult and painful. As mentioned, cardiovascular performance is not significantly improved.

Aerobic performance depends upon an increase in the oxygen transporting system and this is developed principally through adaptations in the cardiovascular system and the skeletal muscles. Large muscle masses should be called into play so the greatest demand for oxygen is made. Physical activity ranging from work periods of a few seconds repeated quickly and frequently up to hours of continuous work may induce an improvement in aerobic performance. The following patterns have been reported to be effective in this regard [5].

1. Dash training—maximal effort (i.e., running full speed preferably uphill) for 30-60 sec and repeated 5 to 10 times with several minutes of low-level activity between each dash. This pattern also improves anaerobic performance.

2. Interval training—slightly less effort than maximal (80% of dash effort) lasting 3-7 min repeated 3 to 7 times with low-level activity periods of 6-8 min between each interval.

3. Continuous training—submaximal effort for 45-75 min. Heart rates should range from 130 to 170 beats/min with maximal rates achieved at times.

These training patterns are applicable to walking, running, bicycling, swimming, or isotonic arm exercises. Isometric exercises such as weight lifting are not aerobic and they can be dangerous for CHD patients because of the excessive level of myocardial pressure work associated wth them. Monitored submaximal interval or continuous exercise with heart rates of 150 beats/min or less is recommended for most persons with CHD.

Surprisingly, there are only a few reported studies that have evaluated adequately the hemodynamic consequences of physical conditioning. These include arterial and venous catheterization during exercise testing, the Douglas bag technique for collection of expired air, accurate oxygen measurement, and the Fick or dye dilution technique for estimation of cardiac output. Cardiac catheterization is necessary for accurate pressure measurement and determination of cardiac output. Central aortic pressure is necessary for obtaining hemodynamic measurements to estimate myocardial oxygen consumption but most studies have been performed with brachial artery catheters. The Fick technique is the standard of reference for determining cardiac output but it requires right heart catheterization for sampling of mixed venous blood. The dye dilution technique is not as accurate as the Fick method but it does not require blood gas analysis or right heart catheterization. Currently, paramagnetic oxygen measurement techniques are very accurate, though the older chemical methods (Haldane, Scholander) are still the standards of reference. Direct gas flowmeter measurement of air flow during exercise is not sufficiently accurate to replace the Douglas bag technique. The validity of hemodynamic measurements during exercise with catheters has been established [16]. Even if the cardiac output, maximal oxygen intake, and heart rate are reduced in the catheterized exercising subject, the effect is consistent, influencing results similarly after as well as before physical conditioning. Most of the studies reviewed have utilized the above methodology and any unusual techniques will be mentioned. TABLE II lists the studies included for review along with the methods used. TABLE III summarizes the hemodynamic changes demonstrated by each study.

Review of the Studies

The Dallas Study included five male subjects aged 19 to 21 [16]. Three were classified by their activity habits as sedentary and two as active. The former had maximal oxygen intakes of 33 to 45 ml/kg/min prior to training and the latter 61 and 47 ml/kg/min. The training program lasted for 55 days with workouts held twice each weekday and once on Saturday. The workouts consisted principally of running and were either interval-patterned with periods of maximal effort for 2-5 min repeated 4 to 10 times with 2-min periods of rest, or continuous training with running at a constant pace until exhaustion for longer than 10 min. Before and after training, hemodynamic measurements were determined at rest and during exercise with catheters in a peripheral arm vein and in the brachial artery. Both treadmill and supine bicycle ergometer testing were performed at maximal effort and at workloads calculated to be 40, 60, and 80 percent of the maximal oxygen intake measured prior to training. The previously sedentary trainees had the greatest measured changes.

The Stockholm study included eight sedentary male subjects aged 19 to 27 [5, 17]. Maximal oxygen intakes prior to training ranged from 36 to 50 ml/kg/min. The training program lasted for 120 days and consisted of cross-country running three times a week in dash, interval, and continuous patterning. Before and after training, hemodynamics were measured. Testing was done with the subject sitting on a bicycle ergometer exerting maximal effort and at workloads calculated to be 25, 50, and 75 percent of the maximal oxygen intake measured prior to training.

Tabakin and colleagues, University of Vermont, studied nine members of the University cross-country team before and after 3 months of daily training in preparation for competition [18]. Training consisted of daily warmup exercises, sprints, and 5 miles of running. The radial artery and a peripheral vein were catheterized. Measurements were made at rest and while walking on a treadmill at 3 miles/hr on the level and at 4, 8, 12, and 14 degrees elevation. No changes

TABLE II

Studies of the hemodynamic effects of physical conditioning

Study	No. of Male Trainees	Age of Trainees	Interval Between Hemodynamic Studies	Type of Physical Conditioning	Methods
Dallas: Saltin et al, 1968	3 sedentary men and 2 athletes	18-21	55 days	interval and continuous; 6 days a week for 1½ hours a day	CO by dye dilution technique using indocyanine green (ICG). O_2 consumed using the Douglas bag (DB) and Scholander technique
Stockholm: Ekblom, 1969	8 sedentary men	19-27	120 days	continuous; 3 days a week for 1 hour a day	CO with ICG. O_2C with DB and Haldane technique
Vermont: Tabakin et al, 1965	9 athletes	18-24	90 days	dash and continuous; daily for 1-2 hours	CO with ICG. O_2C with DB and paramagnetic analyzer (PM)
Helsinki: Frick et al, 1963	14 sedentary men	19-26	60 days	hard basic military training	CO by dye injection and ear-lobe density measurement; no O_2C measurement
Stockholm-Gothenburg: Kilbom et al, 1969	15 sedentary men	38-55	63 days	interval and continuous; 2-3 days a week for 1 hour a day	CO with ICG; O_2C with DB and Haldane technique
Vermont. Hanson et al, 1968	7 sedentary men	40-49	200 days	competitive paddle ball for 1 hour 3 times a week	CO with ICG. O_2C with DB and PM analyzer
Gothenburg: Vernaukas et al, 1970	5 sedentary men with CHD	44-55	180 days	bicycle ergometer (BE) with progressive workloads for 1/2 hour, 3 times a week	CO by dye dilution technique using O_2C with DB and Scholander technique. AVO_2D calculated from CO and O_2 consumption.
Helsinki: Frick et al, 1968	6 sedentary men with AMI 2-4 mo. prior to PC	37-55	50 days	BE with progressive workloads 3 times a week; 15 min with HR 100, 10 min with HR 150	Right heart cath, CO by Frick method O_2C by DB and PM analyzer
Seattle-Louvain: Detry et al, 1971	6 men with documented AMI 6 men angina	34-68	90 days	submaximal endurance exercise for 45 min a day 3 times a week	Right heart cath, CO by Fick method; O_2C by DB and PM analyzer
Copenhagen: Clausen et al, 1970	7 sedentary men with CHD	46-60	30-70 days	intermittent progressive BE for 30 min a day 5 days a week	CO by dye dilution technique using iodohippurate (I^{131}); hepatic BM: hepatic vein cath and SVC cath, ICG; O_2C with DB and Haldane tech. BF in vastus lateralis with Xenon[133]

TABLE III

Hemodynamics post physical conditioning

STUDY	REST								SUBMAXIMAL EXERCISE										MAXIMAL EXERCISE							
	HR	SBP	DBP	CO	SV	O₂C	AVO₂D	TYPE OF EXERCISE	HR	SBP	DBP	CO	SV	O₂C	ME	LA	AVO₂D	INTENSITY OF EXERCISE	HR	SBP	DBP	CO	SV	MO₂	LA	AVO₂D	TYPE OF EXERCISE
Dallas (young normals)	↓	—	—	→	↑	→	↑	Supine & treadmill	↓	—	—	—	→	↓	—	—	—	Multiple levels	—	—	—	↑	↑	↑	—	↑	Supine & treadmill
Stockholm (young normals)	↓	—	—	→	↑	↑	↑	Sitting (bicycle ergometer) (BE)	↓	—	—	—	↑	↓	↑	→	↑	Multiple levels	↑	↑	↑	↑	↑	↑	↑	↑	Sitting (BE)
Vermont (young athletes)	→	—	→	↑	↑	↓	×	Treadmill	↓	—	→	→	↑	↑	↑		×	Low									
									↓	—	→	→	—	↑	↑		×	High									
Helsinki (young normals)	→	—	↑	↑	↑	↑	×	Supine	→	—	→	→	—	—	—	→	×	Moderate									
Stockholm-Gothenburg (older normals)	→	(mean) →		—	—	—	—	Sitting (BE)	→	(mean) →		↑	—	—	—	→	—	Multiple levels	→	(mean) —	—	↑	↑	↑	↑	—	Sitting (BE)
Vermont (older normal)	→	—	→	—	↑	→	×	Treadmill	→	↑	→	→	↑	↓	↑	→	×	Low	→	×	×	×	↑	↑	×	×	Sitting (BE) without catheters
									→	↑	→	→	—	↑	→		×	High									
Gothenburg (coronary artery disease) (CAD)	→	(mean) →		—	→	—	—	Sitting (BE)	→	(mean) →		→	↑	—	↑	→	↑	5 & 25 min during exercise									
Helsinki (CAD)	—	—	→	—	→	—	—	Supine	→	—	↑	↑	→	↑	→	→	—	Low									
									→	—	↓	↑	—	—	→	→	—	High									
Seattle-Louvain (CAD)	→	(mean) →		—	→	—	↑	Sitting (BE)	→	(mean) →		→	→	—	→	—	↑	Multiple levels	↓	×	×	× (	↑	↑	×	×	Bicycle or treadmill without catheters
Copenhagen (CAD)	→	—	→	↑	↓	—	×	Sitting (BE)	→	→	→	→	↑	—	—	—	×	Low									
									→	→	→	↓	—	—	—	—	×	High									

Legend: — no change   ↑ increase   → decrease   × not performed   ↗ slight increase   ↘ slight decrease

ME mechanical efficiency   O₂C oxygen consumption   O₂M maximal oxygen consumption   CO cardiac output   LA lactic acid concentration were noted other than a lowering of the cardiac output at the two lowest levels of exercise. The fact that the subjects were athletes explained this lack of significant change.

Frick and colleagues studied 14 men aged 19 to 26 before and after "hard basic military training" [19]. The exact nature of this training was not described. Oxygen consumption was not measured and cardiac output was estimated with Evans blue by a dye dilution technique using earlobe density changes. Physical work capacity was significantly increased posttraining. Hemodynamic measurements were made via a brachial artery catheter during supine bicycle exercise at 400 kgm/min for 6 min.

The Stockholm-Gothenburg study was designed to evaluate the effects of physical conditioning on middle-aged men [20, 21, 22]. Sixty-eight employees of an insurance company who considered themselves to be healthy but who were judged to be inactive by their response to a questionnaire, were asked to participate in a 10-week physical training program. The program consisted of 2 miles of intermittent or continuous running 2-3 times a week for a total time of about 18 hours and 55 miles of running. Twenty percent of the subjects dropped out for medical or other reasons. Of those who completed the program, half had significant orthopedic problems. Forty-two of the group had noninvasive studies performed [21] while 15 had venous and arterial catheterization [22]. Maximal effort and multiple predetermined levels of submaximal exercise were performed sitting on a bicycle ergometer.

Hanson and colleagues studied the hemodynamic response of 25 normal men aged 40-49 [23]. Ten of these men could not perform a 3-min walk at 3 mph and 14° elevation, and had a similar response to the treadmill test. They exhibited high resting oxygen consumption and stroke volume, then raised cardiac output excessively with level walking and maintained it throughout higher workloads. They demonstrated an initial overshoot and subsequent poor adaptation to exercise. These investigators assumed this response was due to prolonged physical inactivity. Seven of the 10 men completed a physical training program consisting of 3 hourly sessions a week of competitive paddle ball for 29 weeks [24]. Catheterization was repeated and hemodynamic measurements made while walking on a treadmill at 3-mph level and at elevations of 4, 8, 12, and 14 degrees. Maximal work capacity and maximal oxygen consumption were increased following training.

Varnauskas and colleagues, University of Gothenburg, studied the hemodynamics of five patients with CHD before and after 1 month [25] and then 6 months [26] of physical conditioning. CHD was diagnosed by clinical evaluation and coronary angiograms. The patients were exercised on a bicycle ergometer for 1/2 hour 3 times/week with the workload gradually increased according to individual tolerance and heart rate response. Measurements were made via catheters in the brachial artery and subclavian vein with the trainees sitting on a bicycle ergometer while at rest and at 5 and 25 min while pedaling against an individualized workload. The dye dilution technique using bromsulfopthalein was used to estimate cardiac output and the AV_{O_2} difference was calculated from the oxygen consumption and cardiac output. Plasma volume measured with I^{131}-tagged albumin, total blood volume, and red cell mass calculated from the hematocrit incrased with training. The hemodynamic changes were more significant after 6 months of training than after 1 month. Cardiac output decreased at the submaximal level and the AV_{O_2} difference increased. The investigators suggested that this favored a peripheral circulatory mechanism rather than a direct cardiac mechanism as the explanation for the increased work capacity in persons with CHD after training. However, Hanson and others have demonstrated this overshoot phenomenon in deconditioned persons. The exaggerated cardiac output and narrowed AV_{O_2} difference are returned to normal by physical conditioning just as they are in persons with vasoregulatory asthenia [27].

Frick and Katilla studied six men aged 37 to 55 before and after an exercise program which began 2-4 months after a documented myocardial infarction (MI) [28]. The exercise program consisted of pedaling a bicycle ergometer 3 times/ week at progressive workloads. Each session consisted of 15 min of exercise at a heart rate of 100 beats/min and then for 15 min at a heart rate of 150 beats/min or until chest pain. Hemodynamic measurements were made while pedaling a bicycle ergometer in the supine position for 6 min at one or two individualized submaximal workloads. The resting mean heart volume did not change for the group but two trainees with enlarged hearts had significant decreases in heart volume. Most of the subjects had abnormal hemodynamic measurements in response to acute exercise before and after the training program. This is in accord with the criteria of Donald and Reeves for cardiac output and pulmonary wedge pressure response to supine exercise [29]. However, all subjects developed an increased exercise tolerance and those with angina increased their angina-free work capacity.

Clausen and Trap-Jensen reported the effects of physical conditioning on hemodynamic measurements including hepatic and muscle blood flow during exercise in nine men with CHD [30]. The men were aged 36 to 57 and either had classically diagnosed MI or exertional chest pain. They accepted the work of other investigators as demonstrating hemodynamic alterations secondary to physical conditioning which reduced myocardial pressure work. Their aim was to determine the role of peripheral circulatory changes. They and others had demonstrated that in normal subjects abdominal viscera perfusion was less reduced during exercise in trained as compared to untrained subjects and that muscle blood flow was reduced during exercise after training [31]. The training program consisted of pedaling a bicycle ergometer in an intermittent pattern for periods of 30 min each, 5 days/week for 4-10 weeks. The workload was individualized, but progressively increased. For testing, catheters were placed in the brachial artery, superior vena cava, and right hepatic vein. Testing was performed sitting on a bicycle ergometer pedaling at workloads at first 60 percent of and then equal to the pretraining maximal workload. Hepatic blood flow was estimated using indocyanine green and blood gas analysis; cardiac output was estimated using I^{131}-tagged iodohippuric acid; and the blood flow in the vastus lateralis muscle was measured using the Xenon^{133} local clearance technique [32]. The cardiac output at the lowest exercise level clearly demonstrated the overshoot phenomenon and this hyperkinetic response was normalized after training. At the higher submaximal exercise level, there was no change in cardiac output. Muscle blood flow was reduced at submaximal loads and hepatic blood flow was less reduced during submaximal exercise after the training program. These changes were interpreted as supporting the concept that changes in peripheral circulation are important for reduction in myocardial pressure work secondary to physical conditioning.

Detry and colleagues collaborated for a joint study using patients from the University of Washington, Seattle, and the University of Louvain, Belgium [33]. Six men with angina pectoris (AP) and six men with documented healed MI underwent right heart catheterization and brachial artery cannulation before and after 3 months of physical training. Their ages ranged from 34 to 68 with a mean of 48 years. The exercise program consisted of 45 min sessions 3 times/week utilizing varius submaximal exercises including walking and running. Maximal exercise was done on a bicycle ergometer or treadmill prior to the hemodynamic studies. Hemodynamic measurements were made while sitting on a bicycle ergometer at rest and during 7 min exercise periods with workloads equal to 45 and then 75 percent of the pretraining maximal oxygen consumption. Surprisingly, arterial oxygen content was higher posttraining, indicating the possibility that improved oxygenation made possible the increased AV_{O_2} difference rather than improvements in the peripheral circulation. All of the trainees subjectively improved and two previously limited by symptoms of AP were no longer symptomatic at any exercise level. These investigators reported that their results favored a peripheral mechanism for the improved work tolerance of persons with CHD.

Discussion of Results

There were limited consistent changes posttraining in the hemodynamic measurements at rest. The resting heart rate was reduced in all trainees. Resting blood pressure was unchanged in normal individuals but was reduced in trainees with CHD. Studies have demonstrated physical conditioning to be helpful in the management of patients with hypertension [34,35] and a similar physiological mechanism may be in effect.

Hemodynamic measurements with catheterization were performed during maximal effort in two studies of young trainees and in one of older trainees, but in none of the CHD trainees. In the studies in which they were measured, cardiac output, stroke volume, and maximal oxygen consumption increased after training. Blood pressure was increased or unchanged. The increased maximal oxygen consumption in the young subjects was related to both an increase in cardiac output and in AV_{O_2} difference; in the older subjects it was related only to an increased cardiac output since the AV_{O_2} difference was unchanged. Maximal oxygen consumption was reported to be increased in the Seattle-Louvain trainees with CHD; however, invasive studies were not performed during maximal exercise. Measurement of maximal cardiac output and maximal AV_{O_2} difference in these trainees might have shown whether changes in cardiac function or in the peripheral circulation were more or equally important.

The submaximal testing demonstrated the most significant changes after training. All three classes of trainees exhibited a decreased heart rate for the same workload after training. The blood pressure response remained unchanged in the young trainees, was lowered in one of the two older trainee groups, and was lowered in most of the trainees with CHD. Stroke volume consistently increased in normal people and was increased in some of the trainees with CHD. Oxygen consumption remained the same for similar workloads posttraining and so total body mechanical efficiency remained unchanged (Fig. 1).

$$\frac{\text{Mechanical}}{\text{Efficiency}} = \frac{\text{Work Produced}}{\text{Energy expended}} \quad X \quad 100$$

$$(1 \text{ Liter } O_2 \cong 5 \text{ calories})$$

$$\text{M.E. of man} \cong 20\%$$

Fig. 1. Oxygen consumption and body mechanical efficiency.

From the submaximal testing results, it is apparent that peripheral adaptations to acute exercise secondary to physical conditioning are important. Lactic acid concentration during submaximal exercise was decreased in trainees of all three classes in spite of an unchanged or decreased cardiac output. Adaptations in the peripheral circulation were demonstrated by a decrease in active skeletal muscle blood flow and by less of a decrease in liver blood flow in conditioned normal people and in CHD trainees [30]. These changes in perfusion and aerobic metabolism are partially explained by morphological and enzymatic adaptations in skeletal muscle [31, 36].

The peripheral response to training is important for another reason. Clausen and Trap-Jensen have demonstrated that the training bradycardia is operative only when using trained skeletal muscles [37]. They trained two groups of men using similar bicycle ergometer protocols except that one group used their arms while the other used their legs. When tested with alternate arm and leg exercises after training, the trainees demonstrated a lower heart rate during exercise only when using the trained limbs. These investigators also trained individuals with fixed rate ventricular pacemakers. They responded to training with an increased work capacity in spite of a fixed ventricular rate. Interestingly, the atrial rate decreased after training in response to a similar submaximal workload. Frick has demonstrated that individuals with congenital bradycardia respond to training by increasing stroke volume [1]. These findings suggest that training induces a neural signal or a vascular response in the periphery that modifies the chronotropic and ionotropic control of the heart during acute exercise.

The AV_{O_2} difference was either increased or unchanged in normal people during submaximal exercise after training. In those patients with CHD, Detry

[33] and Varnauskas [25, 26] demonstrated an increase in the AV_{0_2} difference while Frick [28] found no change. Clausen [30] did not measure $A\overset{\circ}{V}_{0_2}$ but his data suggests that there was no change. Some investigators have suggested that the increase in AV_{0_2} difference supports the concept that peripheral changes rather than changes in cardiac function are of primary importance for the increased work capacity of trained CHD patients. It is conceivable that some hearts are so badly damaged that they cannot be modified by training. Certainly then, peripheral circulatory changes and enzymatic and morphological changes in skeletal muscle would be of primary importance. However, Frick demonstrated improvement in cardiac function in trained CHD patients. His data include changes in left ventricular stroke work versus pulmonary capillary wedge pressure during submaximal exercise or Sarnoff function curves, as well as increases in cardiac output for a given oxygen consumption in response to supine exercise [28, 38]. He also demonstrated an increase in diastolic left ventricular wall thickness using ultrasound [38] and an increase in the mean systolic ejection rate after training [28]. Thus, there appears to be evidence that physical conditioning can improve ventricular function in selected patients with CHD.

In normal people, Braunwald demonstrated that cardiovascular response to acute exercise involves the integrated effects on the myocardium of simple tachycardia, sympathetic stimulation, and the Frank-Starling mechanism [39]. The effects of physical conditioning on these responses, as well as on the morphology of the heart need delineation in man. Animal studies demonstrated exercise-induced ventricular hypertrophy and Aldinger and Scheuer showed that the exercise-hypertrophied rat heart has increased contractility [40, 41, 42]. An increase in sympathetic tone could also explain an increase in contractility with training. Evidence for an increase in contractility secondary to physical conditioning in man is limited; however, the mean rate of systolic ejection increases as does the dP/dt in the brachial artery [24]. Another point to be considered is that venous return could be facilitated by physical conditioning and the end diastolic volume for a given workload increased, and thus ventricular function increased.

Cardiac output was unchanged at identical submaximal workloads by physical conditioning in normal subjects except in the study by Hanson [23, 24]. However, this group of older normal trainees demonstrated a cardiac output overshoot phenomenon that was hypothesized to be secondary to prolonged physical inactivity. Approximately half the CHD trainees had a similar overshoot phenomenon and lowered their cardiac output response to submaximal exercise while the others did not. The correction of the exaggerated cardiac output and narrowed AV_{0_2} difference by physical conditioning was similar to its effects on the abnormal hemodynamics of vasoregulatory asthenia [27]. The lowering of cardiac output and widening of the AV_{0_2} difference in response to submaximal exercise are not the major effects of physical conditioning since this does not occur in all individuals who experience an increase in work capacity.

Measurement of myocardial oxygen consumption is technically difficult at rest and the problems of measuring it during exercise are insurmountable. However, it can be estimated by calculations using hemodynamic measurement [43,

44] (TABLE IV). Basically, these methods depend upon changes in blood pressure, heart rate, and ejection time. Blood pressure and ejection time can be

TABLE IV

Hemodynamic measurement calculations that approximate changes in
myocardial oxygen consumption

Cardiac effort = Mean Aortic Pressure X HR (mm Hg/min)

Time Tension Index = Area Under the Ventricular Pressure Pulse X HR
(mm Hg sec/min)

Triple Product = Aortic Systolic Pressure X HR X LVET (mm Hg sec/min)

Myocardial Work = Stroke Volume X Mean Aortic Pressure

lessened to some extent by physical conditioning but the major change is a
lowering of heart rate. Because of the lowering of heart rate, hemodynamic
calculations approximating changes in myocardial oxygen consumption will decrease after training. However, there is evidence that cardiac function improves
with training even in CHD patients. An increase in the contractile state of the
myocardium or an increase in end-diastolic volume (Frank-Starling mechanism)
would increase myocardial oxygen consumption and invalidate the approximations using hemodynamic calculations. Myocardial work is a determinant of
myocardial oxygen consumption; however, it is not sufficient to estimate this
alone. For instance, though calculated work might increase or not change if
stroke volume increased and blood pressure decreased, myocardial oxygen consumption would decrease. This is because myocardial flow work requires less
oxygen than pressure work.

The major determinants of myocardial oxygen consumption are depicted in
TABLE V [43, 44]. At this time, except for heart rate, not enough data are

TABLE V

Determinants of myocardial O_2 consumption (MVO_2)

1. Intramyocardial stress or tension
   $T = Pd/h$ ($\cong$ pressure X ventricular volume)
2. Contractile state
3. Heart rate
4. External work
   $MW = SV$ X P
   (but MVO_2 greater for pressure work than flow or volume work)

T	=	tension	d =	ventricular diameter
P	=	pressure (ventricular or aortic)	MW $\doteq$	myocardial work
h	=	ventricular wall thickness	SV =	stroke volume

available with respect to how these determinants are modified by physical conditioning. Ultrasound techniques can be used to measure left ventricular wall thickness [38], volume [45], and indices of contractility [46] at rest and could be adapted for use during exercise. Simultaneously, central aortic pressure and cardiac output could be measured via arterial catheterization. From these determinations, changes in myocardial oxygen could be estimated. However, even if myocardial oxygen consumption is not decreased by physical conditioning, the training bradycardia is an important physiological benefit. The concomitant increase in diastolic time increases the time available for myocardial perfusion.

Conclusion

The hemodynamic studies of the effects of physical conditioning support its clinical use in selected patients with CHD. However, the need for careful supervision and monitoring is apparent because of the possible orthopedic [20] and cardiac complications [10, 11, 12, 13, 14]. Changes in both cardiac function and the peripheral circulation are responsible for the increase in work capacity. However, in some CHD patients, the peripheral changes are most important. Myocardial oxygen consumption may not be changed by physical conditioning but the training bradycardia is an important consistent result which allows a longer time for myocardial perfusion.

REFERENCES

1. Frick, M.H. Coronary implications of hemodynamic changes caused by physical training. *Am. J. Cardiol.* 22:417-425, 1968.
2. Katz, L.N. Physical fitness and coronary heart disease. *Circulation* 35:405-414, 1967.
3. Saltin, B. Physiological effects of physical conditioning. *Med. Sci. Sports* 1:50-56, 1969.
4. Astrand, P. and Rodahl, K. *Textbook of Work Physiology*, pp. 375-430. New York, McGraw-Hill, 1970.
5. Ekblom, B. Effect of physical training on oxygen transport system in man. *Acta Physiol. Scand. Suppl.* 328, 1969.
6. Bergman, H., and Varnauskas, E. Placebo effect in physical training of coronary heart disease patients. *In*, Larson, O.A., and Halmborg, R.O., Eds. *Coronary Heart Disease and Physical Fitness*, pp.48-51. Baltimore, University Park Press, 1971.
7. Roskamm, H. Optimal patterns of exercise for healthy adults. *Can. Med. Assoc. J.* 96:895-898, 1967.
8. Siegel, W., Blomqvist, G., and Mitchell, J.H. Effects of a quantitated physical training program on middle-aged sedentary men. *Circulation* 41:19-29, 1970.
9. Shepard, Roy J. Intensity, duration and frequency of exercise as determinants of the response to a training regime. *Int. Z. Angew. Physiol.* 26:272-278, 1968.
10. Pyfer, H.R. and Doane, B.L. Cardiac arrest during exercise testing. *J.A.M.A.* 210:101-102, 1969.

11. Cantwell, J.D., and Fletcher, G.F. Cardiac complications while jogging. *J.A.M.A.* 210:130-132, 1969

12. Resnekov, L. Jogging and coronary artery disease. *J.A.M.A.* 210:126, 1969.

13. Bruce, R.A., and Kluge, W. Defibrillatory treatment of exertional cardiac arrest in coronary disease. *J.A.M.A.* 216:653-658, 1971.

14. Exercise and cardiac death. *In*, Jokl, E., and McClellan, J.T., Eds. *Medicine and Sport*, Vol. 5. White Plains, N.Y., Phiebig, 1971.

15. Reindell, H. *In*, Jokl, E., Ed. *Heart and Sport*, p. 25. Springfield, Ill., Thomas, 1964.

16. Saltin, B., Blomquist, G., Mitchell, J.H., Johnson, R.L., Jr., Wildenthal, K., and Chapman, C.B. Response to exercise after bed rest and after training. *Circulation* 38, Suppl. No. 7, 1968.

17. Ekblom, B., Astrand, P., Saltin, B., Stenberg, J., and Wallstrom, B. Effect of training on circulatory response to exercise. *J. Appl. Physiol.* 24:518-528, 1968.

18. Tabakin, B.S., Hanson, J.S., and Levy, A.M. Effects of physical training on the cardiovascular and respiratory response to graded upright exercise in distance runners. *Br. Heart J.* 27:205-210, 1965.

19. Frick, M.H., Konttinen, A., and Sarajas, H.S. Effects of physical training on circulation at rest and during exercise. *Am. J. Cardiol.* 12:142-147, 1963.

20. Kilbom, A., Hartley, L.H., Saltin, B., Bjure, J., Grimby, G., and Astrand, I. Physical training in sedentary middle-aged and older men. I. *Scand. J. Clin. Lab. Invest.* 24:315-322, 1969.

21. Saltin, B., Hartley, L.H., Kilbom, A., and Astrand, I. Physical training in sedentary middle-aged and older men. II. *Scand. J. Clin. Lab. Invest.* 24:323-334, 1969.

22. Hartley, L.H., Grimby, G., Kilbom, A., Nilsson, N.J., Astrand, I., Bjure, J., Ekblom, B., and Saltin, B. Physical training in sedentary middle-aged and older men. III. *Scand. J. Clin. Lab. Invest.* 24:335-344, 1969.

23. Hanson, J.S., Tabakin, B.S., and Levy, A.M. Comparative exercise-cardiorespiratory performance of normal men in the third, fourth, and fifth decades of life. *Circulation* 37:345-350, 1968.

24. Hanson, J.S., Tabakin, B.S., Levy, A.M., and Nedde, W. Long-term physical training and cardiovascular dynamics in middle-aged men. *Circulation* 38:783-799, 1968.

25. Varnauskas, E., Bergman, H., Houk, P., and Bjorntorp, P. Haemodynamic effect of physical training in coronary patients. *Lancet* 2:8-12 1966.

26. Bergman, H., and Varnauskas, E. The hemodynamic effects of physical training in coronary patients. *In*, Jokl, E., and Brunner, D., Eds. *Medicine and Sport*, Vol. 4., pp. 138-147. Baltimore, University Park Press, 1970.

27. Holmgren, A. Vasoregulatory asthenia. *In*, Larson, O.A., and Malmborg, R.O., Eds. *Coronary Heart Disease and Physical Fitness*, pp. 34-37. Baltimore, University Park Press, 1971.

28. Frick, M.H., and Katila, M. Hemodynamic consequences of physical training after myocardial infarction. *Circulation* 37:192-202, 1968.

29. Foster, G.L., and Reeves, T.J. Hemodynamic responses to exercise in clinically normal middle-aged men and in those with angina pectoris. *J. Clin. Invest.* 43:1758-1768, 1964.

30. Clausen, J.P., and Trap-Jensen, J. Effects of training on the distribution of cardiac output in patients with coronary artery disease. *Circulation* 42:611-624, 1970.

31. Clausen, J.P. Effects of physical conditioning, a hypothesis concerning circulatory adjustment to exercise (A review). *Scand. J. Clin. Lab. Invest.* 24:305-313, 1969.

32. Clausen, J.P., and Lassen, N.A. Muscle blood flow during exercise in normal man studied by the Xenon [133] clearance method. *Cardiovasc. Res.* 5:245-254, 1971.

33. Detry, J.R., Rousseau, M., Vandenbroucke, G., Kusumi, F., Brasseur, L.A., and Bruce, R.A. Increased arteriovenous oxygen difference after physical training in coronary heart disease. *Circulation* 44:109-118, 1971.

34. Boyer, J.L., and Kasch, F.W. Exercise therapy in hypertensive men. *J.A.M.A.* 211:1668-1671, 1970.

35. Kireloff, B., and Huber, O. Brief maximal isometric exercise in hypertension. *J. Am. Geriatr. Soc.* 19:1006-1012, 1971.

36. Holloszy, J.O. Morphological and enzymatic adaptations of training—a review. *In*, Larsen, O.A., and Malmborg, R.O., Eds. *Coronary Heart Disease and Physical Fitness*, pp. 147-151. Baltimore, University Park Press, 1971.

37. Clausen, J.P., Trap-Jensen, J., and Lassen, N.A. Evidence that the relative exercise bradycardia induced by training can be caused by extra cardiac factors. *In*, Larsen, O.A., and Malmborg, R.O., Eds. *Coronary Heart Disease and Physical Fitness*, pp. 27-28. Baltimore, University Park Press, 1971.

38. Frick, M.H., and Katila, M., and Sjogren, A.L. Cardiac function and physical training after myocardial infarction. *In*, Larsen, O.A., and Malmborg, R.O., Eds. *Coronary Heart Disease and Physical Fitness*, pp. 43-47. Baltimore, University Park Press, 1971.

39. Braunwald, E., Ross, J., and Sonneblick, E.H. Mechanisms of contraction of the normal and failing heart. *N. Engl. J. Med.* 277:964-966, 1967.

40. Froelicher, V.F. Animal studies of the effect of chronic exercise on the heart and atherosclerosis: a review. *Am. Heart J.* 84:496-506, 1972.

41. Aldinger, E.E. Effects of digitoxin on the development of cardiac hypertrophy in the rat subjected to chronic exercise. *Am. J. Cardiol.* 25:339-343, 1970.

42. Penpargkul, S., and Scheuer, J. The effect of physical training upon the mechanical and metabolic performance of the rat heart. *J.Clin. Invest.* 49:1859-1868, 1970.

43. Sonnenblick, E.H., and Skelton, C.L. Oxygen consumption of the heart: physiological principles and clinical implications. *Mod. Concepts Cardiovasc. Dis.* 40:9-16, 1971.

44. Braunwald, E. Control of myocardial oxygen consumption. *Am. J. Cardiol.* 27:416-432, 1971.

45. Pombo, J.F., Troy, B.L., and Russell, R.O. Left ventricular volumes and ejection fraction by echocardiography. *Circulation* 43:480-490, 1971.

46. Cooper, R., Karliner, J.S., O'Rourke, R.A., Peterson, K.L., and Leopold, G. Ultrasound determination of mean fiber-shortening rate in man. (Abstract) *Am. J. Cardiol.* 29:257, 1972.

6

METHODS OF EXERCISE TESTING*

John Naughton, M.D., and *Riaz Haider*, M.D.

Standardized exercise tests are administered using a wide variety of devices. The most commonly employed are steps, bicycle ergometers, and motor-driven treadmills. Since there are many indications for the performance of an exercise test, the methodology applied must be flexible and adaptable to the population receiving the service. In this chapter, some methods of exercise testing and ways in which various instruments are used will be reviewed.

Indications for Exercise Testing

Prior to World War II, exercise tests were usually employed by physiologists to determine performance capacity in athletes and by physicians as a diagnostic test for ischemic heart disease (IHD). In recent years, the indications for exercise testing have been broadened, and the application to clinical medicine increased as test designs were refined and improved equipment became available. At present, the usual indications for an exercise stress test include:

a. diagnosis of the etiology of previously undefined chest pain;

b. evaluation of an individual's capacity for work and/or sport; and

c. evaluation of a patient's response either to a therapeutic or a rehabilitation regimen [1].

Principles of Exercise Tests

Regardless of the instruments employed, a number of principles apply to all testing procedures:

---

*Supported in part by Grant RT 9 (C-5) from the Social and Rehabilitation Service, Department of Health, Education, and Welfare

An exercise test for a patient population should, insofar as possible, be of aerobic design. The design should be adequate to define the point at which a patient either attains his peak or maximal aerobic working capacity, or at which he develops some manifestations indicative of impairment, i.e., symptoms, signs, or ECG abnormality. Thus, an ideal exercise test initially requires a very low level of O_2 cost in terms of the resting metabolic state; the workload is increased gradually over time to insure maintenance of an aerobic state and to define more accurately a subject's end point for aerobic work.

An exercise test has specific end points. These include subjective end points such as exhaustion; symptoms such as chest pain, dyspnea, or palpitations; signs such as pallor, ataxia, or cold sweat; abnormal ECG changes such as arrhythmias or ischemic ST-T changes; or the attainment of a predetermined heart rate level. Some patients may experience more than one end point simultaneously while others may only attain one.

Every subject should have an appropriate cardiovascular history and examination prior to the exercise test. The subject should be tested either after an overnight fast or no earlier than 2 hours after a light meal. The patient should be instructed in the indications for the test, its methodology, potential hazards, and end points. **He should sign a written statement of informed consent.**

An exercise test is preceded by a warmup and recovery period to insure that the patient understands and can perform the proscribed test. The patient is allowed a sufficient period of recovery after the test, and is not permitted to take a hot shower for at least 1 hour after the testing procedure is completed.

Intermittent and Continuous Tests

Exercise tests can be either of intermittent (discontinuous) or continuous design. In an intermittent test a subject is evaluated at a specific workload and allowed a period of recovery before engaging in the next workload. This approach has the advantage that responses measured reflect adjustment to the defined workload. The disadvantage is that testing time and the time to attain either a near-steady or steady state adjustment are prolonged, especially as the intensity of external work is increased and nears or approximates a patient's aerobic working capacity.

In a continuous test the external workload is increased gradually at regular periodic intervals while the patient continues the procedure. The advantages of this approach are reduction in the testing time and the time required to develop near-steady state adaptation to each new workload [2]. The disadvantages include a *carry-over* O_2 debt from the previous workload, and the potential for fatigue of the utilized muscles preceding the attainment of cardiorespiratory limitations.

In a maximal exercise test, a subject works until he attains his threshold for O_2 intake; any additional increase in workload will not result in further increase in O_2 intake. This is an important physiologic concept underlying the development and application of all graded exercise tests. A submaximal exercise test is terminated before a subject attains his O_2 intake threshold, and the subject's peak aerobic working capacity is estimated by extrapolating the submaximally measured data to a predicted maximal response level.

Although many arguments have accrued among proponents of maximal and submaximal exercise tests, it should be remembered that in the clinical application of an exercise test, the end point is determined either by the development of a specific marker of impairment or the attainment of an age-predicted level of near-maximum or maximum heart rate. In these situations the point of termination, occasioned by the development of symptoms, may or may not correlate with the patient's maximal aerobic working capacity. In all likelihood, however, if the patient is tested to a defined end point, such as age-predicted heart rate, the correlation with maximal O_2 intake probably will be good.

Physiologic Measures

A number of physiologic events can be measured during the performance of an exercise stress test. It is generally recommended that the systemic blood pressure, heart rate, and at least a single-lead ECG be measured during each physiological condition or state. While it is ideal to measure respiratory gas exchange, particularly the O_2 intake, these measurements are much more difficult. It is well-documented that, as soon as a test is standardized by appropriate measurements of O_2 intake, the O_2 cost in ml/kg/min from subject to subject is relatively constant. Therefore, measurement of O_2 is not routine in most clinical facilities.

Since the mean O_2 intake in ml/kg/min at supine rest and at comparable levels of standardized exercise is relatively constant in various population groups, the MET is used to describe the resting O_2 intake. By definition, a MET approximates the resting O_2 intake in ml/kg/min. At supine rest a MET is assumed to represent 3.5 ml O_2/kg/min. Workload or work capacity can also be translated into METS. For instance, an individual who walks at 2 mph on a 3.5 percent slope will have an O_2 requirement of approximately 10.5 ml/kg/min or 3 METS (Fig. 1), and a subject whose work capacity is 31.5 ml/kg/min has an aerobic work capacity of 9 METS.

Blood pressure. The systemic blood pressure is usually measured by auscultation. The blood pressure cuff is attached to the upper arm in the normal fashion. Extrinsic noise is reduced if the tubing parallels the triceps muscle and hangs straight-down. An anesthetic diaphragm is used on the stethoscope and is secured with a strap over the impulse of the brachial artery. The examiner must be trained to filter any extraneous noise while listening for the Korotkoff sounds. The first sound detects systolic blood pressure. The first Korotkoff sound adequately and accurately reflects the systolic blood pressure recorded directly via catheter, but the diastolic blood pressure measurements are not accurate.

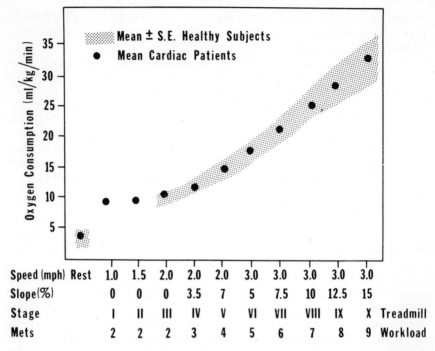

Fig. 1. The mean O_2 requirement for healthy subjects and cardiac patients at different workloads on a motor-driven treadmill.

The systolic blood pressure increases in proportion to work intensity. Only a few investigators have measured blood pressure response routinely as part of an exercise test; therefore, a minimum of normative data are available. In our laboratory the slope of systolic blood pressure increase with exercise approximates 7.5 mm Hg/MET with a peak of 12 mm Hg/MET. The mean peak systolic blood pressure attained by presumably healthy men in our laboratory is 240±20 mm Hg. We characterize the systolic blood pressure response as normal (physiologic), hypertensive, or hypotensive. An increase in excess of 12 mm Hg/MET is interpreted as a hypertensive response and one below 5 mm Hg/MET as a hypotensive response. A significant decrease in the level of systolic blood pressure with increasing work intensity is considered abnormal and an indication to terminate the test.

The normal diastolic blood pressure response to physical effort is characterized either by little significant change from that recorded during the control rest period, or with physically active subjects by a decrease in its level. A significant increase (>15 mm Hg) over that recorded during control rest is considered abnormal, and indicative of a hypertensive response.

Heart rate. The heart rate increases in proportion to the level of physical exertion (Fig. 2). The character of the heart rate response is related to a number of factors including the state of physical fitness and the degree of physiologic

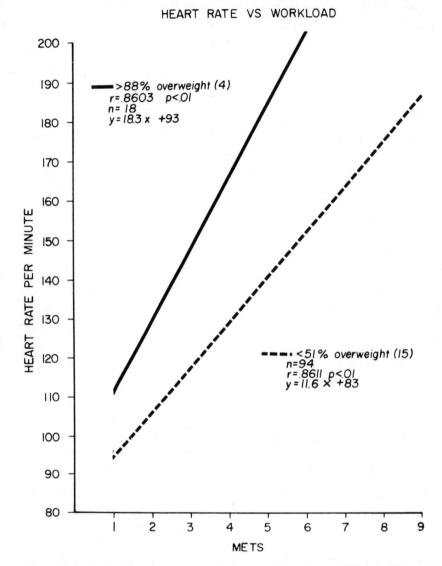

Fig. 2.   Heart rate slopes per MET in 15 girls whose ideal body weights are less than 51%
above ideal and in 4 girls who were more than 88% above ideal body weight.

impairment. In athletes the heart rate increases from 4-8 beats/MET while in
sedentary subjects the slope increases from 8-12 beats/MET. The slope for girls
with body weight 51 percent or less over ideal body weight approximates that of
sedentary healthy subjects; i.e., 11.6 beats/MET; the slope is 18.3 beats/MET for
girls with body weight in excess of 88 percent of ideal body weight.

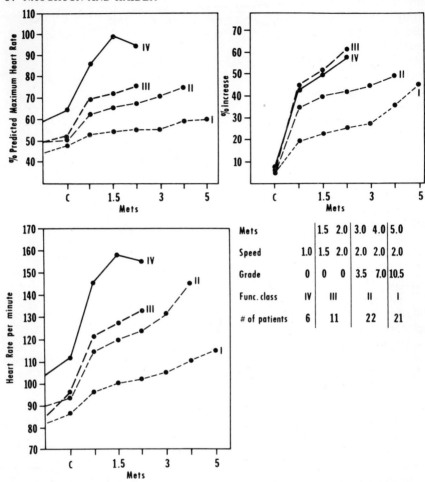

Fig. 3.   Absolute heart rate per min., percent of age-predicted maximum heart rate levels, and percent increase in heart rate over that measured at rest in cardiac patients of differing functional classification (NYHA).

Patients with cardiovascular disease have variable heart rate slopes depending upon their functional classification (New York Heart Association (NYHA)) [3]. Fig. 3 depicts the heart rate responses of 60 cardiac patients rated as Functional Class (F.C.)-I through -IV by their physicians. The slopes are characterized in terms of the absolute heart rates per minute, the percent of age-predicted maximum heart rate achieved, and the percent increase in heart rate level over that measured at rest. The F.C.-I patients had an absolute heart rate level significantly lower at rest and at comparable levels of external work than patients classified as F.C.-II, -III or -IV. This slope approximates that usually measured in healthy sedentary subjects. The slope for F.C.-II and -III patients did not differ significantly, but the F.C.-IV patients had higher heart rates at rest and at each comparable level of work. The F.C.-I patients achieved a 5 MET threshold with a mean rate that approximated 50 percent of their age-predicted maximum heart rate, and the F.C.-IV patients attained their maximum age-predicted heart rate levels at an estimated O_2 requirement of only 1.5 METS. When the heart rate response is characterized in terms of the percent increase over that measured at rest, the F.C.-II differ significantly from the F.C.-I patients, as do the F.C.-III and F.C.-IV patients. However, F.C.-III and -IV did not differ significantly in their responses.

The maximum heart rate decreases gradually with age (Fig. 4). The ability to achieve the age-predicted maximum heart rate is modified by cardiac or pulmonary disease, and most cardiac patients will have a reduced peak heart rate threshold. Fig. 4 depicts the peak heart rate levels attained by patients rated 1 through 4 as a result of their response to a treadmill test. Treadmill Group (T.G.)-1 were patients whose aerobic work capacity exceeded 22 ml O_2/kg/min; T.G.-2 from 16-22 ml O_2/kg/min; T.G.-3 10-16 ml O_2/kg/min; and T.G.-4 less than 10 ml O_2/kg/min [4]. T.G.-1 patients attained peak heart rates approximating those of young, healthy subjects whereas T.G-3 and -4 patients had significantly reduced peak heart rate responses. Those with regular sinus rhythm had peak heart rate levels nearer 50 percent of the age-predicted maximum while those with atrial fibrillation attained levels that approximated 80 percent of the age-predicted maximum. It is of interest that in these patients there was a correlation between age and work capacity. It appears that the reduction in age-related peak heart rate response is affected adversely by the presence of cardiac disease.

Electrocardiogram (ECG). The ECG responses to exercise will be reviewed elsewhere in this volume. The most commonly employed lead is the CM_5[1] (indifferent electrode (negative) attached to the manubrium of the sternum and exploring electrode at C_5 position). Its advantages are that it is reproducible; the electrodes can be placed on the chest with ease; and it usually senses the greatest amount of QRS voltage. Other single-lead systems have also been used. In terms of methodology, there is ample evidence that failure to record stable ECG is usually related to improper skin preparation and electrode placement, rather than the fidelity of the electronic equipment. The laboratory technician must clean the skin well with acetone. The electrode must be placed firmly over the cleansed area, and any tension on the electrode should be reduced. The skin resistance can be measured with an ohmmeter prior to applying an electrode. If the resistance is not sufficiently low to insure a quality ECG recording, the skin should be recleansed with acetone.

---

[1] This lead will not detect changes in the Z axis, i.e., from front to back, and will miss important changes in 5 to 15 percent of abnormal responses.

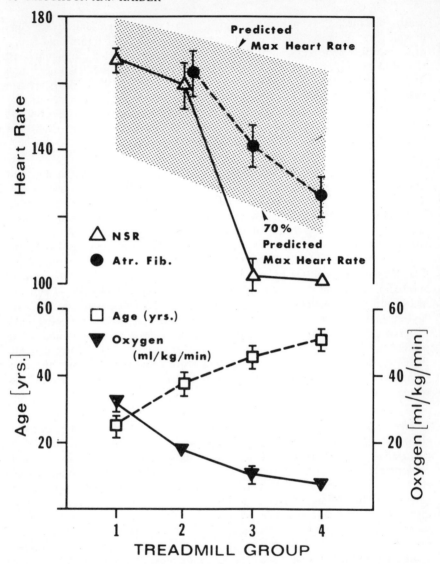

Fig. 4. Relationship of peak heart rate attained during treadmill exercise in cardiac patients of differing functional classification (NYHA) to that usually observed in a healthy population.

Step Tests

Steps are among the least expensive devices available for the administration of an exercise stress test. They usually require little space, are noiseless, and do not threaten or inhibit the patient.

The most commonly employed step test in clinical medicine is the Master's Step Test [5], which requires a platform of 2 steps: the first 9 inches high and the second 18 inches. Each stepping height is 9 inches. A patient walks up and down the steps at a given rate determined by age and sex. It is a diagnostic test and its duration is short (3 minutes).

The test is not adequate for measurement of aerobic work capacity. It is a single-stage test and external O_2 intake ranges from a low of 5 METS to a high of 7 METS [6, 7]. Therefore, it is not a standardized work test. Although it contributed vastly to the advance of exercise testing in clinical medicine, it is inadequately refined for meeting the multitude of indications for exercise testing previously listed. The test is also too strenuous for some cardiac patients and induces too little stress for many of the population. A literature review indicates that the mean peak heart rates induced with a Master's Double Step Test range from 115-130 heart beats/minute. Aronow [8] and others [9] have demonstrated that the diagnostic yield of IHD can be increased if a multistage testing procedure is employed in preference to the Master's test.

Nagle et al [7] developed a single platform which can be raised vertically to increase the external workload. This design paralleled the principles used in the design of treadmill tests. They developed two testing methodologies which maintained the initial stepping rate while the platform was raised vertically at periodic intervals (TABLE I). The first test required a stepping rate of 24/minute and the second, 30/minute. The cadence was maintained with a metronome. This methodology had the advantage that multiple physiologic responses could be measured simultaneously while the patient stepped up and down in the same

TABLE I

Graduated multilevel step test

Step Rate	24/min	30/min	Work Rates (METS)
	5	4	3
	12	8	4
	18	12	5
Step Height (cm)	25	16	6
	32	20	7
	35	24	8
	–	28	9
	–	32	10
	–	36	11
	–	40	12

Two-step test procedures. One procedure is performed at 24 steps/min., the other at 30 steps/min. A step is defined as one total ascent onto a platform and descent back to ground. The stepping rate is maintained while the step platform is elevated from one level to the next at periodic intervals.

place. One author (J.N.) witnessed a unique modification of the reported technique in a colleague's office. The physician simply replaced the examining table drawers with solid pieces of wood, each 3 inches in height. He applied the same principles by increasing the step height 3 inches at periodic intervals while maintaining a stepping rate of 24 steps/minute. When the test was completed the steps were simply placed back inside the examining table.

Steps have an advantage over the bicycle ergometer and treadmill in terms of test-retest reproducibility. This is supposedly related to the lack of noise and other fanfare; patients are, therefore, less anxious when tested with steps.

Bicycle Ergometers

The bicycle ergometer is more popular on the European continent than in the United States. Ostensibly, this is related to the fact that many Europeans cycle regularly and most Americans do not. Ergometers can be mechanical or electrical, and can be relatively inexpensive or inordinately expensive. They have the advantage of being stationary so that subjects can be evaluated and studied in the upright sitting position. Since subjects are required to pedal against a fixed external load or resistance, individuals with smaller muscle masses in the legs are at a disadvantage compared to healthy subjects, and most women are at a disadvantage compared to men. Many subjects suffer peripheral muscular fatigue before they actually achieve their cardiorespiratory limitation on a bicycle ergometer. The seat height must be adjusted for each subject to insure that the down leg is fully extended. Bicycle ergometers must be recalibrated at periodic intervals.

Mechanical bicycle ergometers are calibrated in kilopond meters (kpm) or kilogram meters (kgm) per minute. Electrical ergometers are calibrated in watt units. One watt approximates 6 kpm [10]. Each kpm requires approximately 2-2.4 ml O_2/kg/min. Therefore, a subject who exerts an energy expenditure of 25 watts is working at 150 kpm/min and requires from 300-360 ml O_2/min. The basal energy requirement approximates 300 ml; thus, total O_2 expenditure will range from 600-660 ml/min. Since the load is fixed, adjustments for estimating the external O_2 requirement must be made according to a subject's body weight. For instance, a 50-kg subject expending energy at a rate of 150 kpm/min will have an O_2 requirement of 12 ml/kg/min, while a 70-kg subject will require 8.5 ml O_2/kg/min, and a 100-kg subject 6.0 ml O_2/kg/min.

Some ergometers are constructed so that cycling rate is independent of the resistance load. Most investigators have determined that a pedaling rate of 50-70 rpm is preferable. Most bicycle tests are constructed so that the external workload is increased in increments of 50-150 kg at regular periodic intervals.

Treadmills

The motor-driven treadmill is assuming greatest popularity in the United States. It provides flexibility because the speed of the belt and the slope of the treadmill bed can be varied either independently or simultaneously. Subjects and patients perform a function which is near-physiologic, namely walking. The instrument can be used to simulate running or jogging if indicated. They are usually large and more expensive than steps or bicycle ergometers, and have a significant noise factor. Despite several physical disadvantages, they offer more flexibility than steps and bicycle ergometers.

A number of treadmill testing procedures have been developed and reported. Fig. 5 depicts a schema we developed from testing differing population groups. Three basic testing procedures are tabulated. Each is similar in that the speed is maintained while the slope of the treadmill bed is elevated in specified increments at periodic intervals. In the 2 mph test, the slope is increased 3.5 percent; in the 3 mph test, 2.5 percent; and in the 3.4 mph test, 2 percent. Each test design is set so that each new increment of work approximates an additional MET. The three tests overlap in MET equivalency from 4 through 7 METS, while the 3 and 3.4 mph tests overlap in MET equivalency from 4 through12 METS. The utilization of these three approaches provides a mechanism for applying identical principles to the evaluation of the extremely impaired and the extremely physically fit.

METS	1.6	2	3	4	5	6	7	8	9	10	11	12	13	14	15	16
TREADMILL TESTS — Speed				3.4 Miles Per Hour												
TREADMILL TESTS — %Grade *				2	4	6	8	10	12	14	16	18	20	22	24	26
TREADMILL TESTS — Speed			3.0 Miles Per Hour													
TREADMILL TESTS — %Grade *			0	2.5	5	7.5	10	12.5	15	17.5	20	22.5				
TREADMILL TESTS — Speed	1.0	2.0 Miles Per Hour														
TREADMILL TESTS — %Grade **	0	0	3.5	7	10.5	14	17.5									
METS	1.6	2	3	4	5	6	7	8	9	10	11	12	13	14	15	16
Ml. O_2/Kg/min	5.6	7		14		21		28		35		42		49		56
CLINICAL STATUS		Symptomatic Patients														
CLINICAL STATUS			Diseased, Recovered													
CLINICAL STATUS				Sedentary Healthy												
CLINICAL STATUS					Physically Active Subjects											
FUNCTIONAL CLASS	IV	III		II			I and Normal									

*Balke
**Naughton

Fig. 5. The relationship of work capacity attained on various treadmill procedures to METS, clinical status and functional classification.

In our experience most cardiac patients, symptomatic or asymptomatic, will achieve their limitations at 7 METS or less; most healthy, sedentary subjects at 10 METS or less, while physically active middle-aged subjects can attain thresholds between 10 and 16 METS. Obviously, some athletes will exceed 16 METS, and appropriate adjustments in either speed or grade of the treadmill slope can be made. The test results can be used to rate a subject's physiologic functional class (Fig. 5). Patients limited to 2 METS or less are rated F.C.-IV; to 3 or 4 METS, F.C.-III; 5 or 6 METS, F.C.-II; and 7 METS or greater as F.C.-I. Fig. 6 depicts the relationship between functional class as defined by the NYHA criteria and by treadmill criteria. The treadmill evaluation was of particular value in patients rated either F.C.-II or F.C.-III.

The data in Fig. 1 were obtained using another modification to treadmill testing. In these experiments the speed was maintained at 2 mph for three stages (0, 3.5, and 7 percent grades), then increased to 3 mph where it was maintained for the remainder of the procedure, while the slope of the treadmill bed was elevated periodically in 2.5 percent increments. This modification offers the advantage of interchanging speed for grade so that a patient does not become

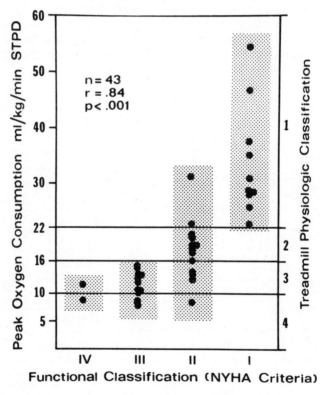

Fig. 6. The relationship of treadmill physiologic classification to clinical functional classification.

fatigued by either too fast a pace or too steep a grade. Again, the principle of gradually increasing the workload to MET increments was employed. The dashed area represents the mean O_2 intake ± standard error for healthy subjects who performed the test and the solid dots mean O_2 intake for cardiac patients. The data obtained for both groups of patients are similar.

In our laboratory the workload is increased in increments of 1 MET every 2 minutes. This methodology allows each patients ample time to assume a near-steady state and permits the investigator an opportunity to evaluate the subject's response critically.

Summary

The principles of developing an exercise test, the desired physiologic measurements, and the different available testing instruments are reviewed.

REFERENCES

1. Lange-Andersen, K., et al. *Fundamentals of Exercise Testing.* Geneva, W.H.O., 1971.

2. Nagle, F., Balke, B., Baptista, G., Alleyia, J., and Howley, E. Compatibility of progressive treadmill, bicycle and step tests based on oxygen uptake responses. *Med. Sci. Sports* 3(4):149-154, 1971.

3. Criteria Committee of the New York Heart Association. *Diseases of the Heart and Blood Vessels: Nomenclature and Criteria for Diagnosis*, 6th ed., pp. 112-113. Boston, Little Brown, 1953.

4. Patterson, J.A., Naughton, J., Pietras, R.J., and Gunnar, R.M. Treadmill exercise in assessment of the functional capacity of patients with cardiac disease. *Am. J. Cardiol.* 30:757, 1972.

5. Master, A.M., and Rosenfeld, I. Two step exercise test brought up-to-date. *N.Y. J. Med.* 61:1850, 1961.

6. Ford, A.B., and Hellerstein, H.K. Energy cost of the Master two step test. *J.A.M.A.* 164:1868, 1957.

7. Nagle, F.S., Balke, B., and Naughton, J.P. Gradational step tests for assessing work capacity. *J. Appl. Physiol.* 20:745, 1965.

8. Aronow, W.S. Thirty-month follow-up of maximal treadmill stress test in normal subjects. *Circulation* 47:287, 1973.

9. Bruce, R.A., and McDonough, J.R. Stress testing in screening for cardiovascular disease. *Bull. N.Y. Acad. Med.* 45:1288, 1969.

10. Fox, S.M., III, and Naughton, J.P. Physical activity and the prevention of coronary heart disease. *Prev. Med.* 1:92, 1972.

7

EXERCISE ELECTROCARDIOGRAPHY*

Patrick A. Gorman, M.D., *William S. Byers*, M.D.,
and *Riaz Haider*, M.D.

Introduction

The first widely used exercise test employing the ECG was developed by Master [1]. He found that by utilizing the ECG postexercise instead of heart rate and blood pressure changes, it was possible to detect evidence of subendocardial ischemia which was not present at rest. Since then, clinical experience has repeatedly confirmed the value of exercise-induced ST segment displacement in the diagnosis of myocardial ischemia. Today, study of the ECG response has been extended to include continuous ECG monitoring before, during, and after multistage exercise for heart rate, ST segment changes, arrhythmias, and conduction disturbances. These observations have increased the diagnostic value of exercise testing. Abnormal responses may be detected with minimal delay, thus reducing the risks of the procedure. Because of the diagnostic reliance placed on the exercise ECG, it is important that methods of recording and analysis be chosen with understanding of the physiologic, clinical, engineering, and economic aspects. Blackburn [2] has reviewed the subject in detail.

Lead Systems

The ECG lead systems commonly used in exercise are the standard 12 leads, bipolar leads, and orthogonal XYZ leads.

---

*This study was made possible by a grant to The George Washington University Rehabilitation Research and Training Center from the Social and Rehabilitation Services, Department of Health, Education, and Welfare, and by support from the Divisions of Cardiology and Rehabilitation Medicine, Department of Medicine, The George Washington University Medical Center.

In a review of the two-step exercise test, Master and Rosenfeld [3] recommended that leads V4, V5, V6 and lead II be recorded immediately, 2 min and 6 min after exercise. Robb and Marks [4] recorded leads I, AVL, and AVF in addition. The value of recording additional leads during postexercise recovery was demonstrated in patients with angina by Mason et al [5]. They used modified leads I, II, III, and V3-V6. In two-thirds of patients who developed ischemic ST depression, the abnormality appeared in more than one lead, and in only one lead in the remaining one-third. The results of a double two-step test and a graded ergometer test in the same patients were compared. Ischemic responses were found in 85 percent of ergometer tests, 61 percent of Master's test with in-exercise recording, and 56 percent where only postexercise ECGs were recorded.

A bipolar lead provides the simplest system. Blackburn [2] has stressed that the practical advantages include: minimal time required to prepare the subject; reduced amount of ECG data; reduced chance of motion artifact; and optimal ST segment display. The bipolar lead which provides the combination of greatest display of ST depression and minimal noise level and baseline shift is lead CM5; electrodes are located over the manubrium and the V5 position. The main disadvantage is that even the best single-lead system will miss approximately 10 percent of significant ST abnormalities. A lesser disadvantage is that P-waves, defining atrial depolarization, are not optimally displayed. This is important when arrhythmias occur and identification of P-waves is necessary for interpretation. Unfortunately, leads such as V1 which show P-waves best are poor for demonstrating ST segment changes. The problem may be resolved in single-lead recording systems by using electrodes for multiple types of ECG leads, and switching the leads as clinically indicated for rhythm or ST definition.

Orthogonal leads have theoretical advantages over single leads for exercise in the greater information content especially when recorded simultaneously. The Frank system [6], the most widely used for the resting ECG, was not designed for exercise applications. Noise in the vertical lead is the main problem.

Display of ECG Data

Display of exercise ECG data may be considered in these areas:

1. signal monitoring
2. paper recording
3. magnetic tape recording (for later display).

Monitoring should be performed continuously to ensure that the quality of the ECG signal is satisfactory and that the onset of significant ECG abnormalities is detected as soon as possible. An oscilloscope of the *bouncing ball* type is a minimal requirement. A memory oscilloscope is a useful refinement; the signal moves across the screen usually at 25 mm/sec and is visible for the time taken to traverse the screen. Monitoring is thus facilitated. A more complex display is a contourgram on the oscilloscope. Each ECG complex is stacked below its predecessors, so that the previous 20 cycles or more may be observed for morphology, rate, and rhythm.

A tachometer, which may be dial or digital, is a useful safeguard helping to ensure that target heart rates are not exceeded in testing and training situations.

Recording on 5-cm-wide heat-sensitive strip chart by a heated stylus is the conventional method of producing a record for later analysis and permanent storage. The calibration is usually 1 cm per mv, and the speed 25 or 50 mm/sec. This type of record is satisfactory for the great majority of clinical needs. Where precise measurements of ST segments are required, higher gain or speed is available in multichannel photographic recorders.

For recording on magnetic tape, reels or cassettes may be used. Both provide a convenient method of storing data, which in multistage tests with multichannel ECGs may be considerable. The tape may be played back to any desired display or to a computer system for analysis.

Portable tape recorders are available which record the ECG in subjects for up to 12 hrs during normal activities. Thus the effect of real-life stresses, physical and psychological, on the ECG may be documented. Another means of recording ECG data other than by direct wire connection in a fixed location is by telemetry. Such a method is well-suited to patients recovering from acute myocardial infarction (MI) who are still at risk for arrhythmias but who are fully ambulant. Another application is to document ECG changes in work, play, or other stressful situations where direct wire connection is impractical.

Analysis of Exercise ECG Data

Visual measurement of exercise ECG data is satisfactory for most clinical diagnostic purposes. Changes of rate, rhythm, ST segment, and conduction are the major areas of attention. The most frequent problem in analysis of exercise ECGs is that of motion artifacts and noise which adds to the inaccuracy of visual measurements. While it is normally possible to select, for gross analysis, a portion of the exercise ECG record which is sufficiently free of artifacts, accurate measurements may not be possible.

Computer technology has been applied to at least two main areas: the reduction of exercise artifacts and measurement of the ECG morphology. Sheffield and associates [7] reported a method of on-line analysis which performed computer averaging of a bipolar lead to obtain a noise-free record, and measured the area of the depressed ST segment. The findings in subjects without disease and those with angina were correlated. It was found that -7.5 μv sec provided a satisfactory criterion for the limit of normality. A similar procedure on a bipolar lead was followed by McHenry and associates [8], who measured ST segment change by the depression and slope between defined points, and by Hornsten and Bruce [9] who measured the ST depression at a series of points.

Another approach reported by Rautaharju and associates [10] and by Blomqvist [11] analyzed the Frank orthogonal lead system during exercise by computer techniques. The advantages, in addition to improved measurement, include comparability with the resting orthogonal ECG analysis programs and potentially greater ECG information intrinsic in simultaneously recorded orthogonal leads. The main disadvantages are the high noise levels, especially in the vertical lead, and the increased dependence on engineering support.

Recording Technique

To insure a satisfactory display of the ECG during exercise, the skin must be meticulously prepared for electrode attachment. Chest hair should be shaved, skin oils removed by an alcohol or, preferably, acetone-soaked gauze. Abrasion of the skin by rubbing with dry gauze until erythema is produced removes the high impedance epidermal layer. An electrode paste is applied to the skin and small electrode discs attached. Various types of electrodes are available. *Floating electrodes*, consisting of small cuplike discs, are filled with electroconductive paste and attached to the skin. An inadequate amount of paste causes a break in the skin-electrode contact and loss of the ECG signal. Electrodes are pre-packaged commercially in disposable sets. Not infrequently, defective electrode wires are encountered which result in loss of the ECG signal, or in artifacts on any movement of the wires; replacement is required.

Another electrode type consists of silver chloride (AgCl)-coated lead (Pb) discs. The lead (Pb) affords flexibility so that the electrode can be molded to the contour of the chest wall thereby providing better contact. In whichever system is used, the small electrode discs are attached to the skin by adhesive rings or by one of several perspiration-resistant, short, adhesive tapes. Adhesive tapes which are too long may cause electrode motion during exercise resulting in ECG artifact.

Excess electrode paste causes loss of adhesiveness of the rings and tape with consequent electrode motion and/or loss of contact. Problems occurring during exercise ECG recording include baseline artifact due to respiratory excursions, electrode motion in *flabby* subjects, and improper electrode positioning. Somatic muscle tremor artifact is seen in muscular individuals, particularly when an electrode overlies a large muscle. Electrode positions which overlie the sternum or ribs such as CM5 minimize this problem. Isometric hand-squeezing (holding on to the treadmill bar) during exercise also may produce somatic muscle tremor artifact. A loose electrode results in loss of contact and loss of the ECG signal. Women should wear snug fitting brassieres to minimize breast motion during exercise and thus avoid ECG motion artifact. A brief rest at the end of the warmup period provides an opportunity to make adjustments if any of these problems appear.

Preexercise ECG Evaluation

Prior to exercise testing, a resting 12-lead ECG should be recorded to exclude the presence of an acute process that otherwise may not be apparent. Evidence of an acute or recent MI contraindicates exercise testing. Repolarization changes due to subendocardial ischemia, left bundle branch block, left ventricular hypertrophy, Wolff-Parkinson-White syndrome, ventricular aneurysm, pericarditis, and electrolyte disturbances particularly involving potassium and drug effects (digitalis, quinidine, procainamide, diuretics) should be noted, since they may complicate or obscure exercise-induced ST changes [12, 13]. Failure to recognize these changes in the resting tracing may result in erroneous interpretation of the exercise ECG. Third-degree heart block with a slow ventricular rate and relatively fixed cardiac output are contraindications to exercise testing. Cardiac arrhythmias, whether supraventricular, AV junctional, or ventricular, although not a contraindication, may be a harbinger of more serious arrhythmias during exercise or in the post exercise period.

Responses to Exercise: Rate

With increasing exercise levels in the steady state there is a direct linear relation between heart rate, workload, cardiac output, and O_2 intake provided pulmonary function and ambient O_2 concentration are normal. This relation exists until maximal O_2 intake is achieved [14]. By monitoring heart rate during exercise and noting its increase, the approximate level of myocardial work can be inferred. Tables of age-adjusted predicted heart rates have been formulated for 100 percent, 85 percent, and 70 percent of predicted maximum [15]. By utilizing these tables, patients can be exercised to maximal or submaximal levels in a standardized fashion.

Responses to Exercise: ST Segment

Exercise produces an increase in heart rate and causes rate-related changes in the repolarization events of the ECG. More specifically, these changes are reflected in the ST segment and T-wave. An inverse relation exists between heart rate and QT duration. A normal ECG response to increasing heart rate includes a shortened QT interval, a shortened but isoelectric ST segment, and no change or a diminution in T-wave amplitude. Although some debate exists as to what ECG changes constitute an abnormal exercise response, it is generally agreed that nonspecific and nondiagnostic rate-related ST changes include 0.05 mv or less ST segment depression, *J* junctional depression with upward sloping of the R-ST segment, and *coving* of the R-ST segment due to atrial repolarization phenomena (Tp changes).

A widely accepted criterion for an abnormal response consistent with ischemia is 0.1 mv or more depression with flat or down-sloping ST segment of 80 msec or more in duration. Exercise-induced ST segment elevation strongly suggests ventricular aneurysm and has been described in 48 percent of patients with that entity by Manvi and Ellestad [16]. They reported no false positive results; however, 54 percent of their subjects with ventricular aneurysms, demonstrated by left ventriculography, did not demonstrate this change. Other investigators reported that exercise-induced ST segment elevation may occur infrequently as a manifestation of myocardial ischemia [17]. T-wave peaking during exercise when an anterior positive electrode is employed (V5) may signal localized posterior wall ischemia.

Friesinger and associates described a number of subjects without ischemic heart disease (IHD) who developed ECG alterations on standing and with exercise [18]. These changes consisted of T-wave inversion or 0.1 mv ST segment depression in either the inferior or lateral chest leads, or both, during the early phases of exercise. These changes disappear as exercise progresses and may reappear in the postexercise period. Their heart rates accelerated unduly on standing. It was concluded that these changes were due to abnormal autonomic responses to ordinary cardiovascular stress and did not reflect IHD. The condition has been termed *vasoregulatory abnormality*.

Responses to Exercise: Arrhythmias

Emergency treatment of exercise-induced arrhythmias. Arrhythmias which occur during exercise always require careful and continuous observation. Some necessitate termination of the test. Premature ventricular contractions (PVCs) present at rest are often abolished, or decreased in frequency, by exercise. Exercise-induced isolated PVCs may occur in subjects who have no clinical evidence of heart disease [19]. Exercise should be terminated with the occurrence of multifocal PVCs, increasingly frequent unifocal PVCs, or PVCs occurring in consecutive bursts of three or more (ventricular tachycardia). Exercise-induced vetricular bigeminy is most frequently seen in patients with organic heart disease [20].

Atrial arrhythmias occur during and after exercise in normal as well as diseased patients. Sinus arrhythmia, changes in the P-wave morphology, wandering atrial pacemaker, and ectopic atrial beats occur commonly in the postexercise period. Not infrequently during exercise, paroxysms of atrial and junctional tachyarrhythmias occur but tend to be brief. Most revert spontaneously; however, some may be sustained requiring carotid sinus pressure for reversioi.

Atrial fibrillation present at rest responds to exercise with an increase in ventricular rate in a variable and unpredictable manner. By monitoring the ventricular response to exercise, the adequacy of digitalization in a patient who appears well-digitalized at rest can be assessed. Exercise can unmask arrhythmias suggesting digitalis intoxication (premature beats, junctional arrhythmias, and paroxysms of ventricular tachycardia) in digitalized patients who are in atrial fibrillation. Paroxysmal atrial fibrillation rarely occurs during exercise. The few instances reported have been of brief duration and have terminated spontaneously [21]. Atrial flutter at rest responds to exercise with enhanced AV conduction and an increase in ventricular rate. When atrial flutter occurs during exercise, the episodes are transient and almost always in patients with rheumatic heart disease and chronic atrial fibrillation.

Paroxysmal ventricular tachycardia during exercise usually is preceded by PVCs; commonly, it is of brief duration; and it rarely produces symptoms [21]. Should ventricular tachycardia persist after termination of the test, intravenous lidocaine by bolus injection or direct current cardioversion may be necessary.

Fortunately, ventricular fibrillation rarely is associated with exercise testing [22]. However, should it occur, immediate cardiopulmonary resuscitative measures must be instituted.

Complete right or left bundle branch block may occur in relation to an exercise stress test. The block usually is rate-related since it occurs at a predictable and reproducible heart rate and disappears as the rate slows. Bundle branch block present prior to exercise usually persists.

AV block responds unpredictably to exercise [21]. With exercise, first-degree AV block may improve, but occasionally more advanced block is induced. Second-degree heart block may show transient improvement, no change, or an increase in the degree of block with increasing exercise levels. Third-degree heart block with slow ventricular rate and fixed cardiac output precludes strenuous exercise testing.

Correlation of Exercise Electrocardiography with Coronary Arteriography

The exercise ECG is one of the most useful noninvasive tools in evaluating coronary heart disease (CHD). It is important, therefore, that the diagnostic accuracy of the various testing procedures, such as the Master's test and submaximal tests, be measured against a standard.

Coronary arteriography is a definitive method of demonstrating the presence and extent of anatomic lesions in the evaluation of patients with coronary artery disease [23]. This is an essential step in the selection of patients for coronary artery bypass surgery. Left ventriculography, usually performed at the same time as coronary arteriography, provides important information about abnormal movement of the left ventricle (hypokinesia, akinesia, or dyskinesia) and thus gives some information concerning the functional status of the myocardium [24]. While coronary arteriography can usually define the site and extent of obstruction, it can give no indication whether the blood supply available through the affected coronary arteries or collateral channels is adequate for myocardial perfusion requirements. There are many reports of patients without hypertension or aortic valve disease with angina pectoris (AP) whose coronary arteriograms appeared normal [25-27]. Coronary arteriography is not, therefore, an infallible method of diagnosing either CAD (an anatomic abnormality) or IHD (a physiologic abnormality) and it seems possible that some patients judged to have false-positive responses to stress testing may indeed have vascular disease which is not detectable by current arteriographic methods.

Disorders of myocardial microcirculation may be related to AP and to ECG abnormalities during exercise, even though the gross coronary vasculature seen on arteriograms is within normal limits. The exercise ECG, while providing indirect evidence of insufficient myocardial perfusion during physical stress, does not permit precise localization of the site of coronary arterial obstruction. Thus, exercise electrocardiography and coronary arteriography are complementary: one provides indirect physiological data, the other provides information about the anatomic site and extent of obstructive lesions.

Study of the correlation between the Master's test and arteriographic findings has led to some criticism of this form of exercise test and its interpretation. Varied opinions have been expressed in regard to its reliability. In one report [28], comparison of the Master's test finding with those of coronary arteriography revealed a 16 percent false positive response in subjects with no angiographic evidence of coronary artery disease, and a 33 percent false negative response in patients with severe obstructive coronary atherosclerosis. It was concluded that the Master's test yielded an unacceptable number of false-positive results and that in view of the high proportion of false-negative results, reliance on the test as a means of excluding significant coronary disease was unwarranted. In another study where the two-step postexercise electrocardiogram was compared with the results of coronary arteriography [29], similar findings were obtained. The values for false negatives and false positives were 22 percent and 27 percent respectively. It was concluded that the two-step test should be retained as a screening procedure because of its safety and convenience, despite its limitations.

It has been recommended that more strenuous exertion may be used selectively when the Master's test is either negative or equivocal, particularly in patients who do not develop chest pain or tachycardia during or after the test. Multistage treadmill or bicycle ergometric exercise is now a widely used method of achieving adequate exercise levels.

The diagnostic accuracy of exercise electrocardiography in submaximal tests is greater than in two-step tests because higher exercise levels are achieved. In a report by Roitman and associates [30] the results in a group of 46 patients were analyzed. This group not only achieved a satisfactory level of exercise tachycardia but was free of recognized causes of false-positive exercise ECGs such as left ventricular hypertrophy and intraventricular conduction defects. The proportion of false-negatives was 20 percent and that of false-positives 12 percent. Another study by McHenry and associates [8] reported 18 percent false-negatives. It was found that the majority of patients who showed negative responses had disease limited to a single artery which, with one exception, was either the right coronary or the left circumflex artery. It was thought that the use of the bipolar V5 type lead system, which is more sensitive to ischemia arising in the myocardium supplied by the left anterior descending artery, might explain the inability to detect ischemia arising from disease of the other arteries. A report by Kaplan and associates [31] similarly demonstrated that a disproportionate number of patients with single vessel disease had negative exercise tests and the stress test findings were of no value in predicting the specific coronary artery involved.

The use of multiple leads for recording the exercise ECG and computer techniques for its measurement will further increase its diagnostic value.

REFERENCES

1. Master, A.M., and Rosenfeld, I. Exercise electrocardiography as an estimation of cardiac function. *Dis. Chest* 51:347, 1967.

2. Blackburn, H. The exercise electrocardiogram. *In*, Blackburn, H., Ed. *Measurement in Exercise Electrocardiography*, pp. 220-258. Springfield, Ill., Thomas, 1969.

3. Master, A.M., and Rosenfeld, I. Two-step exercise test: current status after 25 years. *Mod. Concepts Cardiovasc. Dis.* 36:19, 1967.

4. Robb, G.P., and Marks, H.H. Latent coronary artery disease. Determination of its presence and severity by the exercise electrocardiogram. *Am. J. Cardiol.* 13:603, 1964.

5. Mason, R.E., Likar, I., Biern, R.O., and Ross, R.S. Multiple lead exercise electrocardiography. *Circulation* 36:517, 1967.

6. Frank, E. An accurate, clinically practical system for spatial vectorcardiography. *Circulation* 13:737, 1956.

7. Sheffield, L.T., Holt, J.H., Lester, F.M., Conroy, D.V., and Reeves, T.J. On-line analysis of the exercise electrocardiogram. *Circulation* 40:935, 1969.

8. McHenry, P.L., Phillips, J.F., and Knoebel, S.B. Correlation of computer-quantitated treadmill exercise electrocardiograms with arteriographic location of coronary disease. *Am. J. Cardiol.* 20:747, 1972.

9. Hornsten, T.R., and Bruce, R.A. Computed ST forces of Frank and bipolar exercise electrocardiograms. *Am. Heart J.* 78:346, 1969.

10. Rautaharju, P.M., Friedrich, H., and Wolf, H.K. Measurement and interpretation of exercise electrocardiograms. *In*, Shephard, R.J., Ed. *Frontiers of Fitness*, pp. 295-315. Springfield, Ill., Thomas, 1971.

11. Blomqvist, G. The Frank lead exercise electrocardiogram. *Acta Med. Scand.* 178 (Suppl. 440):1, 1965.

12. Hurst, J.W., and Logue, R.B. *The Heart,* pp. 310, 315, 954-955, 1257, 1361-1364. New York, McGraw-Hill, 1966.

13. Dubnow, M.H., Burchell, H.B., Titus, J.L. Postinfarction ventricular aneurysm: A clinicomorphologic and electrocardiographic study of 80 cases. *Am. Heart J.* 70:753, 1965.

14. Mitchell, J.H., and Blomqvist, G. Maximal oxygen uptake. *N. Engl. J. Med.* 284, 1018, 1971.

15. Fox, S.M., and Haskell, W.L. The exercise stress test: needs for standardization. *Proceedings, Fourth Asian-Pacific Congress of Cardiology*, Tel-Aviv, September 1-7, 1968.

16. Manvi, K., and Ellestad, M. Elevated ST segment with exercise in ventricular aneurysm. *J. Electrocardiol.* 5:317, 1972.

17. Fortuin, N.J., and Friesinger, G.C. Exercise-induced ST segment elevation. *Am. J. Med.* 49:459, 1970.

18. Friesinger, G.C., Biern, R.D., Likar, I., and Mason, R.E. Exercise electrocardiography and vasoregulatory abnormalities. *Am. J. Cardiol.* 30:733, 1972.

19. Lamb, L.E., and Hiss, R.G. Influence of exercise on premature contractions. *Am. J. Cardiol.* 10:209, 1962.

20. Gooch, A.S., and McConnell, D. Analysis of transient arrhythmias and conduction disturbances occurring during submaximal treadmill exercise testing. *Prog. Cardiovasc. Dis.* 13:293, 1970.

21. Gooch, A.S. Exercise testing for detecting changes in cardiac rhythm and conduction. *Am. J. Cardiol.* 30:741, 1972.

22. Bruce, R.A., and Kluge, W. Defibrillatory treatment of exertional cardiac arrest in coronary disease. *J.A.M.A.* 216:653, 1971.

23. Sones, F.M. Cinecardioangiography. *In*, Gordon, B.I., Ed. *Clinical Cardiopulmonary Physiology*, 2nd ed., pp. 130-144. New York, Grune & Stratton, 1960.

24. Carlsten, A., Forsberg, S.A., Paulin, S., et al. Coronary angiography in the clinical analysis of suspected coronary disease. *Am. J. Cardiol.* 19:509, 1967.

25. Likoff, W., Segal, B., and Dreifus, L. Myocardial infarction patterns in young subjects with normal coronary arteriograms. *Circulation* 26:373, 1962.

26. Likoff, W., Segal, B.L., Kasparian, H. Paradox of normal selective coronary arteriograms in patients considered to have unmistakable coronary heart disease. *N. Engl. J. Med.* 276:1063, 1967.

27. Kemp, H.G., Elliott, W.C., Gorlin, R. The anginal syndrome with normal coronary arteriography. *Trans. Assoc. Am. Physicians* 80:59, 1967.

28. Fitzgibbon, G.M., Burggraf, G.W., Groves, T.D., Parker, J.O. A double Master's two-step test: clinical, angiographic and hemodynamic correlations. *Ann. Intern. Med.* 74:509, 1971.

29. Cohn, P.F., Vokonas, P.S., Most, A.S., Herman, M.V., and Gorlin, R. Diagnostic accuracy of two-step post-exercise ECG. Results in 305 subjects studied by coronary arteriography. *J.A.M.A.* 220:501, 1972.

30. Roitman, D., Jones, W.B., and Sheffield, L.T. Comparison of submaximal exercise ECG test with coronary cineangiocardiogram. *Ann. Intern. Med.* 72:641, 1970.

31. Kaplan, M.A., Harris, C.N., Aronow, W.S., Parker, D.P., and Ellestad, M.H. Inability of the submaximal treadmill stress test to predict the location of coronary disease. *Circulation* 47:250, 1972.

8

PHYSIOLOGIC APPROACH TO THE MEDICAL AND SURGICAL TREATMENT OF ANGINA PECTORIS

Ezra A. Amsterdam, M.D., *James L. Hughes*, III, M.D.,
Richard R. Miller, M.D., *Rashid A. Massumi*, M.D.,
Robert Zelis, M.D., and *Dean T. Mason*, M.D.

Ischemic heart disease (IHD), i.e., disease resulting from inadequate oxygen supply to the myocardium, may be manifested clinically in several fundamental forms. These include angina pectoris (AP), myocardial infarction (MI), cardiac arrhythmias, and congestive heart failure. Significant advances have been made in the past decade in the understanding and treatment of all aspects of IHD. These are typified by innovations along a broad therapeutic front in the management of AP, with which this discussion is concerned.

The treatment of AP can be considered most meaningfully in terms of the pathophysiology of the disorder. AP is the clinical expression of a disparity between myocardial oxygen requirements and the supply of oxygen to the myocardium [1]. The most common etiology of AP is obstructive coronary artery disease (CAD) due to atherosclerosis. However, less common disorders of the coronary arteries [2], severe aortic stenosis with left ventricular hypertrophy in the absence of coronary disease [3], and idiopathic hypertrophy of the myocardium may also result in an unfavorable balance between myocardial oxygen supply and demand and thereby produce AP.

Myocardial oxygen supply is primarily dependent on coronary blood flow and the structure and patency of the coronary arteries. On the other hand, the major determinants of myocardial oxygen demand are intramyocardial tension (directly related to both ventricular systolic pressure and volume), heart rate, and the contractile state of the myocardium [4] (Fig. 1). The interplay of these hemodynamic factors as affected by neural and humoral stimuli determines overall myocardial oxygen requirements. When oxygen needs surpass the delivery capacity of the coronary circulation, myocardial ischemia ensues, producing the symptoms and circulatory abnormalities of AP [5].

The therapy of AP is directed toward restoring a more favorable balance between myocardial oxygen supply and demand. This can be accomplished by decreasing myocardial oxygen requirements or increasing supply [6, 7]. Pharmacologic therapy in AP acts chiefly through reduction of myocardial oxygen requirements. Although not pharmacologic, the carotid sinus nerve stimulator

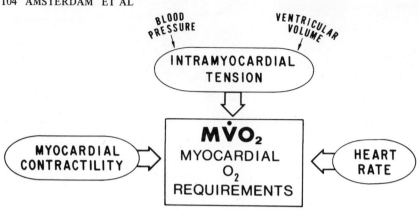

Fig. 1.   The major determinants of myocardial oxygen consumption ($M\dot{V}O_2$).

also utilizes this therapeutic mechanism. Certain surgical procedures such as aneurysmectomy may result in decreased myocardial oxygen demand. The surgical techniques of direct myocardial revascularization enhance myocardial blood flow and thereby oxygen supply.

Reduction of Myocardial Oxygen Requirements

Pharmacologic Therapy

Nitrites. Although the efficacy of nitroglycerin in AP has been demonstrated for more than a century, the precise mechanism of action of the nitrites has not been completely clarified. Recent studies of the effects of these agents on the peripheral circulation have provided increased understanding of their effectiveness in AP.

The nitrites produce direct relaxation of vascular smooth muscle and thereby coronary vasodilation in normal man. Although it has been suggested that blood flow to regional areas of myocardial ischemia is enhanced after nitroglycerin [8], these drugs do not consistently increase coronary blood flow in patients with CAD [9, 10, 11]. Factors tending to nullify coronary vasodilating effects of the nitrites in CAD patients are the mechanical obstructions in the vessels and myocardial hypoxia which may, itself, produce maximal coronary vasodilation [12].

Evaluation of the effects of the nitrites on the peripheral circulation has provided evidence that their efficacy in AP derives largely from these actions. Thus, the altered peripheral circulatory dynamics produced by nitroglycerin result in a decrease in myocardial oxygen requirements. Nitroglycerin administered sublingually reduces venous tone causing pooling of blood in peripheral veins and lowers peripheral arterial resistance resulting in a decline in blood pressure [13] (Fig. 2). Both end-diastolic and end-systolic dimensions of the left

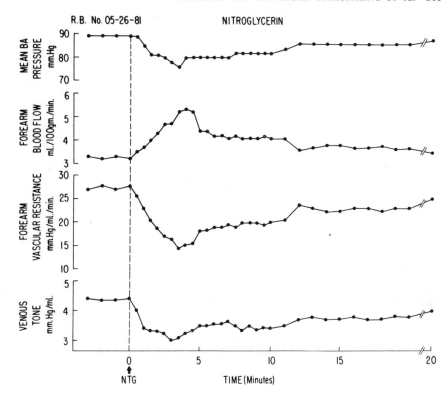

Fig. 2.   Changes in brachial artery (BA) pressure, forearm blood flow, forearm vascular resistance and venous tone before and after sublingual nitroglycerine in a normal subject.

ventricle are reduced [14], venous pooling producing the former effect and decreased peripheral vascular resistance the latter. End-diastolic volume is reduced more than end-systolic volume [14] and cardiac output and stroke volume decrease [14, 15], indicating that the predominant effect of nitroglycerin is on the peripheral veins. Myocardial oxygen needs are decreased primarily by reduction of intramyocardial tension (ventricular volume and pressure) (TABLE I), accounting for the rapid, salutary effects of the drug in AP. It is possible that when the coronary vessels are capable of dilating, the clinical effectiveness of nitroglycerin may be related to its dilatory action on the coronary arteries, as well as on the peripheral vasculature [8, 10, 16].

Nitroglycerin not only diminishes myocardial oxygen consumption by its direct actions on the peripheral circulation, but also produces opposite, indirect effects on the myocardium. Thus, reduction of systemic blood pressure results in baroreceptor stimulation and increased reflex sympathetic outflow to the heart with consequent rise in heart rate and myocardial contractility (TABLE I). However, these actions, which augment myocardial oxygen needs, are more than

TABLE I

Effects of antianginal therapy on the major determinants
of myocardial oxygen consumption

	NITRITES	BETA ADRENERGIC BLOCKADE	PHYSICAL TRAINING	CAROTID SINUS NERVE STIMULATION
INTRAMYOCARDIAL SYSTOLIC TENSION	↓↓	variable	↓	↓↓
HEART RATE	↑*	↓	↓	↓
MYOCARDIAL CONTRACTILITY	↑*	↓	?	↓

*Indⁱ ect Effect

offset by the reduction in oxygen demand produced by the drug. The net effect is thus improvement in the balance between myocardial oxygen supply and demand with resultant symptomatic benefit in angina pectoris.

Isosorbide dinitrate (ISDN) administered sublingually is another effective form of nitrite therapy. Objective evaluation of its efficacy has been documented by enhanced exercise capacity and delay in the onset of ischemic ECG changes after its use [17, 18]. These beneficial effects were associated with a reduction in the exercise-associated rise in blood pressure, heart rate, and left ventricular ejection time in addition to a small decrease in heart size [18, 19]. The duration of effective action of sublingual ISDN was less than 1 hour in most patients, and thus, in this respect, the drug is virtually the same as nitroglycerin. The so-called *long-acting*, orally administered nitrates, on the other hand, are of little proven benefit [19, 20, 21].

Amyl nitrite administered by inhalation also may provide effective treatment in AP. Its actions differ from the sublingually absorbed nitrites chiefly as a function of its very rapid entrance into the circulation and the specific hemodynamic effects resulting therefrom. Thus, the predominant effect of amyl nitrite is marked, direct arteriolar dilatation and a considerable decrease in arterial pressure accompanied by potent reflex sympathetic activity induced by baroreceptor stimulation and hyperventilation [22, 23]. There is marked reflex venous constriction which overrides the direct venodilating effect of the nitrite [22, 23]. Cardiac output is elevated because of the combined effects of decreased arterial resistance or afterload, enhanced venous emptying with augmentation of preload, and increased myocardial contractility; both of the latter result from reflex sympathetic stimulation. The predominant action, with regard to myocardial oxygen consumption, is the large decrease in systemic vascular resistance which causes a reduction in blood pressure and a decrease in ventricular volume consequent to reduced resistance to cardiac emptying. Intramyocardial tension is reduced significantly, overriding the opposite effect on myocardial oxygen consumption of reflexly augmented contractility and ventricular preload. It is conceivable, with the striking effects of inhaled amyl nitrite on peripheral resistance, that if perfusion pressure were excessively reduced in the presence of CAD, myocardial ischemia could be intensified despite the opposing actions of the drug to reduce myocardial oxygen consumption.

In evaluating the effects of the nitrites in AP, it is clear that their pharmacological actions as well as route of administration must be considered. Each of the nitrite drugs directly relaxes vascular smooth muscle in all the regional circulatory beds when entrance into the circulation is relatively slow, as with sublingual nitroglycerin, and dilation of both the systemic and venous beds occurs [23]. Arterial blood pressure decreases slightly and central venous pressure is reduced, resulting in peripheral venous pooling and reduction in stroke volume and cardiac output. In contrast, the rapid introduction of the nitrite (or intravenous administration of nitroglycerin) [23] results in profound arteriolar dilatation and thereby marked fall in systemic arterial blood pressure. This marked depressor effect produces carotid baroreceptor stimulation and heightened sympathetic activity resulting in enhanced myocardial contractility and some attenuation of the intense, direct, peripheral arteriolar dilation. The hyperventilation and anxiety which accompany the inhalation of amyl nitrite are largely responsible for the reflex venoconstriction [24]. Cardiac output is elevated as a consequence of the marked decline in resistance to ventricular emptying coupled with both reflex venoconstriction, elevated preload, and reflex augmentation of myocardial contractility. Reflex venoconstriction is usually not produced with sublingual nitroglycerin, and thus the predominant effect is venodilation. The principal direct action of sublingual nitroglycerin in man appears to be on the veins and that of inhaled amyl nitrite on the arterial bed.

Beta adrenergic blockade. It has been postulated that the actions of the adrenergic division of the autonomic nervous system are mediated by two types of receptors located in the organs which it ennervates [25]. They are termed alpha and beta adrenergic receptors and it is through them that adrenergic stimuli, whether neural or those of circulating catecholamines, act on end organs. The myocardium has only beta receptors while blood vessels, including the coronary arteries, have both alpha and beta receptors. Activation of alpha adrenergic receptors results in arteriolar constriction. Stimulation of beta adrenergic receptors produces arteriolar dilation and augments myocardial mechanical effort (contractility and rate of contraction) and electrical and metabolic activity. Thus, adrenergic stimulation may be intimately related to the production of AP by increasing myocardial oxygen demand. The therapeutic basis for the recently developed beta adrenergic blocking drugs is attenuation of adrenergic stimuli to the myocardium, thereby reducing myocardial mechanical effort and decreasing myocardial oxygen needs.

Although a large number of beta blocking drugs have been produced, propranolol has been the agent most widely utilized and current knowledge of the clinical uses of beta adrenergic blockade pertains largely to this agent. Propranolol has been used successfully in the treatment of patients with AP, as demonstrated by double blind trials [26-36] and objective tests of exercise performance [32, 37]. The primary actions of beta adrenergic blockade by propranolol in reducing myocardial oxygen requirements are attenuation of the rise in heart rate and myocardial contractility to a given stress such as exercise [38-43] (TABLE I). The blood pressure response may also be altered by reduction of cardiac output. This effect is less predictable since systemic vascular resistance is increased by propranolol through its removal of the vasodilating action of intrinsic beta adrenergic stimulation of peripheral arterioles [39-44].

Reduction of myocardial oxygen consumption has been demonstrated after beta blockade in experimental preparations [44] and in man during both exercise and catecholamine stimulation [26, 43]. Because of the decrease in myocardial oxygen needs effected by propranolol, the onset of myocardial ischemia in response to a given level of stress is delayed and effort tolerance is improved. Exercise capacity in the AP patient is thus enhanced, both intensity and duration increasing. This is demonstrated in Fig. 3 where beta blockade is achieved with practolol (a drug to be discussed subsequently). The onset of AP may thus be delayed or the end point to a particular stress be altered to, for example, fatigue. In either instance when therapy is successful, exercise tolerance is augmented.

Propranolol also may have the undersirable effect of increasing myocardial oxygen demand by prolonging systolic ejection period [41, 45] and increasing ventricular dimensions [46, 47]. These actions tend to be less prominent than those reducing oxygen requirements and the net effect is a favorable one on the balance between oxygen demand and supply of the heart. When, however, exercise capacity is reduced after propranolol, which may occur in some patients, it is inferred that myocardial oxygen consumption has been excessively increased. This may especially pertain to patients in overt or latent cardiac decompensation in whom the loss of sympathetic neural and humoral support of the failing myocardium results in an inordinate increase in ventricular volume and thereby myocardial tension. It is noteworthy that, in our experience, this occurrence has been unusual, and, while side effects to propranolol have been rather frequent, they usually have not involved the cardiovascular system [35]. This has been achieved by careful patient selection and prophylactic treatment of latent or overt cardiac failure [35].

It is to be emphasized that the successful use of propranolol in AP is predicated on adequate and individualized dosage [35]. This became apparent early in the use of the drug when equivocal results were obtained with uniform, predetermined doses [27, 29, 48] which, in the light of later experience [26, 32, 34] were shown to be inadequate for many patients. Similar results were obtained from a more recent study involving a fixed dose of propranolol [49].

Since propranolol and the nitrites act by different mechanisms in diminishing the needs of the heart for oxygen (TABLE I), combined use of these agents presents obvious advantages. The reflex tachycardia induced by the nitrites is opposed by propranolol and the latter agent's direct action of increasing peripheral vascular resistance is overcome by the more potent dilating effect of the nitrites. Thus, simultaneous use of both propranolol and short-acting nitrites has been more effective in AP than either drug alone [17, 50, 51].

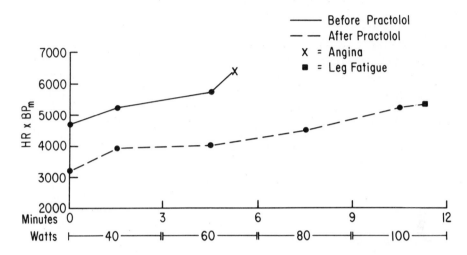

Fig. 3.   Effect of beta adrenergic blockade on exercise performance in CHD

Exercise performance on the upright bicycle ergometer in a patient with coronary heart disease (CHD) before and after cardioselective beta adrenergic blockage with practolol. The response to exercise of the product of heart rate and mean intra-arterial blood pressure, shown as their product (HR X BP$_m$), is attenuated after the drug resulting in increased duration and intensity (watts) of exercise. The end point becomes leg fatigue as opposed to angina during control exercise.

A further advance in the therapeutic application of beta adrenergic blockade has been the recent development of pharmacologic beta blockade of greater tissue selectivity. This has been achieved with practolol, which effectively antagonizes myocardial beta receptors while possessing relatively little opposition to beta receptors in the peripheral arterioles and bronchial smooth muscle [52]. This drug does not possess the local anesthetic or quinidine-like properties of propranolol [52] and is reported to have very little myocardial depressant action in doses that are effective in lowering heart rate in man [53, 54, 55]. Our studies (Fig. 3) [56], as well as those of other investigators, have demonstrated the clinical effectiveness of practolol in the treatment of patients with AP [57-61]. The drug may be especially useful in patients with obstructive pulmonary disease in whom the use of propranolol is frequently contraindicated because of resultant exacerbation of airway obstruction.

Exercise Reconditioning

It is now established that physical reconditioning programs are effective in the treatment of AP in many patients. This subject is considered in detail elsewhere in this volume, and will receive only brief commentary here in order to place it in perspective with the other forms of therapy. Exercise capacity in patients with AP can be augmented by physical training [62, 63, 64, 65]. This improvement is associated with a reduction in those measurable hemodynamic variables determining myocardial oxygen consumption so that with any level of submaximal exercise, the oxygen cost to the heart is reduced, compared with pretraining performance (TABLE I) [62, 63, 64, 75]. Thus, the onset of myocardial ischemia is delayed and the basic mechanism of therapeutic efficacy is similar to that discussed previously for the medical treatment of AP. Recent studies [65] suggest, however, that enhanced myocardial oxygen delivery may also play a role in the salutary effect of physical training in patients with symptomatic IHD.

Carotid Sinus Nerve Stimulation

An innovation in the treatment of refractory AP is electrical stimulation of the carotid sinus nerves [6, 66, 67]. This is achieved with a radio-frequency stimulator consisting of three separate parts. Implanted in the subcutaneous tissue of the anterior chest is a receiving unit to which are connected two bipolar electrodes, each of which is also surgically attached to a corresponding carotid sinus nerve. An induction coil is fixed on the skin above the internal receiving unit and attached to an externally placed, battery-powered signal generator that can be activated by the patient during an episode of AP or prophylactically before engaging in activity that is known to provoke AP. Carotid sinus nerve stimulation produces an increase in afferent impulse traffic to central autonomic centers and results in reflex diminution of adrenergic outflow to the entire cardiovascular system. Thus, arteriolar dilatation is produced, myocardial contractility is decreased, and heart rate is lowered [6, 66, 67], all of which reduce myocardial oxygen requirements (TABLE I). This method produces a potent combination of favorable actions for the alleviation of myocardial ischemia by its effects on both the heart and peripheral arterioles, but reduction of arterial pressure appears to be the most prominent action in reducing myocardial oxygen needs.

Electrical stimulation of carotid sinus nerves requires surgery under general anesthesia and thus has a predictable risk. At present, this mode of therapy is reserved for patients in whom pharmacologic treatment and exercise training have been unsuccessful in controlling AP.

Increasing Myocardial Oxygen Supply

Coronary Bypass Graft

Direct coronary artery surgery to achieve revascularization of the myocardium is a therapeutic innovation with monumental potential in the treatment of IHD. It differs fundamentally from the foregoing methods of treatment since its goal is increased myocardial oxygen supply. This procedure usually entails bypass of one or more obstructed coronary arteries by direct saphenous vein graft from the aorta to the coronary vessel distal to the lesion [68, 69]. Less commonly, an internal mammary artery is directly anastomosed to the coronary artery [70].

Direct coronary surgery has already been applied widely in the treatment of AP and a high degree of subjective success on AP symptomatology is reported [68, 69a]. Objective evidence of increased oxygen supply to previously ischemic myocardium, although not extensive, has also been demonstrated. Thus, early [71] and late [72] studies after direct coronary surgery have indicated enhanced blood flow directed to the myocardium via aortocoronary saphenous vein grafts. We have documented objective improvement in exercise performance on the upright bicycle ergometer 6 to 10 weeks after coronary artery bypass surgery [73]. Further, the maximum product of heart rate and intra-arterial blood pressure during exercise in these patients rose following operation, suggesting enhanced myocardial oxygen delivery (Fig. 4). Augmented tolerance to exercise [74] and atrial pacing stress [75] have also been reported by Johnson and colleagues following myocardial revascularization. Further evidence of the efficacy of this technique is the demonstration of its improvement of parameters of ventricular function such as left ventricular end-diastolic pressure [74, 76], cardiac index [7, 76], and left ventricular ejection fraction [76, 77, 78].

As promising as this approach is, however, certain reservations are indicated. Of prime importance is the long-term function of the grafts. While high early patency rates have been reported, these are 70-85 percent at 1 to 2 years after surgery [79]. Closure has been related to surgical technique, as well as to progressive obliterative disease of the grafts [71]. Although surgical mortality is low [79, 80], it is not negligible and intra-operative MI is a problem of concern [79, 80]. Further, deterioration of ventricular function has been documented in patients in whom graft closure has occurred [77, 78]. It has also been suggested that clinical improvement following aortocoronary bypass surgery may be variably related to graft patency, infarction of ischemic myocardium, or both [81].

Preliminary studies suggest that a high percentage of patients with coronary artery disease are suitable candidates for coronary bypass grafts on the basis of their coronary artery anatomy [82, 83]. However, it would appear prudent, at present, to limit this operation to patients with AP unresponsive to vigorous medical measures or with extent and distribution of coronary lesions thus far demonstrated to have a clearly unfavorable influence on prognosis [84, 85, 86, 87].

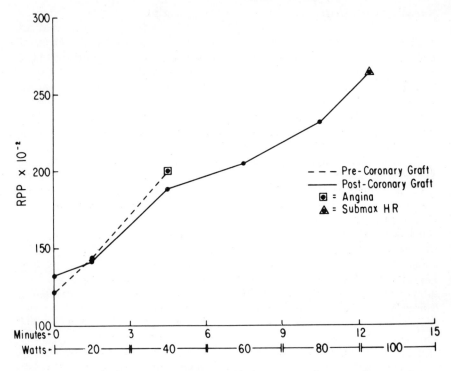

Fig. 4. Exercise capacity before and after coronary bypass graft

Exercise performance on the upright bicycle ergometer in a patient with coronary heart disease before and after aortocoronary saphenous vein bypass graft. There is a marked increase in duration and intensity (watts) of exercise in association with a corresponding elevation in the product of heart rate and blood pressure (RPP). The end point after surgery was achievement of 85% of predicted maximal heart rate (Submax HR) as opposed to angina prior to surgery.

Summary

The treatment of AP is viewed most rationally in terms of the pathophysiology of the disorder, the basis of which is an imbalance between the oxygen supply and demand of the heart resulting in myocardial ischemia. This can be alleviated by reduction of myocardial oxygen demands or augmentation of oxygen supply. The first approach is achieved through medical or related therapy: nitrites, beta adrenergic blockade, physical training, and carotid sinus nerve stimulation—by their inhibition of the major determinants of myocardial oxygen consumption, i.e., heart rate, myocardial contractility, and intramyocardial tension. Increase in myocardial oxygen supply is clearly demonstrated only by coronary artery bypass graft surgery which has proved capable not only of alleviating AP but also, in some instances, of enhancing myocardial function. At present, medical therapy comprises the initial approach to the treatment of AP. Surgical revascularization is indicated for carefully selected patients in whom AP is refractory to more conventional forms of treatment.

REFERENCES

1. Amsterdam, E.A., Zelis, R., Miller, R.R., Hughes, J.L., Bonanno, J.A., Massumi, R.A., and Mason, D.T. Pathophysiology of angina pectoris. *In*, Likoff, W., Moyer, J.H., and Segal, B.L., Eds., *Athersclerosis and Coronary Heart Disease*, pp. 178-189. New York, Grune & Stratton, 1972.

2. Wenger, N.K. Rare causes of coronary artery disease. *In*, Hurst, J.W., and Logue, R.B., Eds., *The Heart*, 2nd ed., pp. 1038-1050. New York, McGraw-Hill, 1970.

3. Fallen, E.L., Elliott, W.C., and Gorlin, R. Mechanisms of angina in aortic stenosis. *Circulation* 36:480, 1967.

4. Sonnenblick, E.H., Ross, J., Jr., and Braunwald, E. Oxygen consumption of the heart. Newer concepts of its multifactorial determination. *Am. J. Cardiol.* 22:328, 1968.

5. Amsterdam, E.A., Manchester, J.H., Kemp, H.G., and Gorlin, R. Spontaneous angina pectoris (SAP): Hemodynamic and metabolic changes. *Clin. Res.* 17:225, 1969.

6. Mason, D.T., Spann, J.R., Jr., Zelis, R., and Amsterdam, E.A. Physiologic approach to the treatment of angina pectoris. *N. Engl. J. Med.* 281:1225, 1969.

7. Mason, D.T., Amsterdam, E.A., Miller, R.R., Salel, A.F., and Zelis, R. Physiological basis of antianginal therapy: The nitrites, beta adrenergic receptor blockade, carotid sinus nerve stimulation, and coronary bypass graft. *In*, Russek, H., and Zohman, B.L., Eds., *Changing Concepts in Cardiovascular Disease*, p. 215. Baltimore, Williams & Wilkins, 1972.

8. Horwitz, L., Gorlin, R., Taylor, W.J., and Kemp, H.G. Effects of nitroglycerin on regional myocardial blood flow in coronary artery disease. *Clin. Res.* 18:312, 1970.

9. Gorlin, R., Brachfeld, N., MacLeod, C., and Bopp, P. Effect of nitroglycerin on the coronary circulation in patients with coronary artery disease or increased left ventricular work. *Circulation* 19:705, 1959.

10. Bernstein, L., Briesinger, G.C., Lichtlen, P.R., and Ross, R.S. The effect of nitroglycerin on the systemic and coronary circulation in man and dogs: Myocardial blood flow measured with xenon. *Circulation* 33:107, 1966.

11. Carson, R.P., Wilson, W.S., Nemiroff, M.J., and Weber, W.J. The effects of sublingual nitroglycerin on myocardial blood flow in patients with coronary artery disease or myocardial hypertrophy. *Am. Heart J.* 77:579, 1969.

12. Berne, R.M. Regulation of coronary blood flow. *Physiol. Rev.* 44:1, 1964.

13. Mason, D.T., and Braunwald, E. The effects of nitroglycerin and amyl nitrite on arteriolar and venous tone in the human forearm. *Circulation* 32:755, 1965.

14. Williams, J.F., Jr., Glick, G., and Braunwald, E. Studies on cardiac dimensions in intact unanesthetized man. V. Effects of nitroglycerin. *Circulation* 32:767, 1965.

15. Braunwald, E., Oldham, H.N., Jr., Ross, J., Jr., Linhart, J.W., Mason, D.T., and Fort, L., III. The circulatory response of patients with idiopathic hypertrophic subaortic stenosis to nitroglycerin and to the Valsalva maneuver. *Circulation* 29:422, 1964.

16. Fam, W.M., and McGregor, M. Effect of coronary vasodilator drugs on retrograde flow in areas of chronic myocardial ischemia. *Circ. Res.* 15: 355, 1964.

17. Epstein, S.E., Redwood, D.R., Goldstein, R.E., Beiser, G.D., Rosing, D.R., Glancy, D.L., Reis, R.L., and Stinson, E.B. Angina pectoris: Pathophysiology, evaluation, and treatment. *Ann. Int. Med.* 75:263, 1971.

18. Goldstein, R.E., Rosing, D.R., Redwood, D.R., Beiser, G.D., and Epstein, S.E. Clinical and circulatory effects of isosorbide dinitrate: Comparison with nitroglycerin. *Circulation* 43:629, 1971.

19. Russek, H.I. Therapeutic role of coronary vasodilators: Glyceryl trinitrate, isosorbide dinitrate, and pentaerythritol tetranitrate. *Am. J. Med. Sci.* 252:9, 1966.

20. Goldbarg, A.N., Morgan, J.F., Butterfield, T.R., Nemickas, R., and Bermudez, G.A. Therapy of angina pectoris with propranolol and long-acting nitrates. *Circulation* 40:847, 1969.

21. Battock, D.J., Alvarez, H., and Chidsey, C.A. Effects of propranolol and isosorbide dinitrate on exercise performance and adrenergic activity in patients with angina pectoris. *Circulation* 39:157, 1969.

22. Johnson, J.B., Gross, J.F., and Hole, E. Effects of sublingual nitroglycerin on pulmonary artery pressure in patients with failure of the left ventricle. *N. Engl. J. Med.* 257:1114, 1957.

23. Mason, D.T., and Braunwald, E. The effects of nitroglycerin and amyl nitrite on arteriolar and venous tone in the human forearm. *Circulation* 32:755, 1965.

24. Mason, D.T., and Braunwald, E. Mechanisms of action and therapeutic uses of cardiac drugs. *In*, Fulton, W.F., Ed., *Modern Trends in Pharmacology and Therapeutics*, p. 112. New York, Appleton, 1967.

25. Ahlquist, R.P. A study of the adrenotropic receptors. *Am. J. Physiol.* 153:586, 1948.

26. Wolfson, S., Heinle, R.A., Herman, M.V., Kemp, H.G., Sullivan, J.M., and Gorlin, R. Propranolol and angina pectoris. *Am. J. Cardiol.* 18:345, 1966.

27. Grant, R.H.E., Keelan, P., Kernohan, R.J., Leonard, J.C., Nancekievill, L., and Sinclair, K. Multicenter trial of propranolol in angina pectoris. *Am. J. Cardiol.* 18:361, 1966.

28. Gillam, P.M.S., and Prichard, B.N.C. Propranolol in the therapy of angina pectoris. *Am. J. Cardiol.* 18:366, 1966.

29. Rablin, R., Stables, D.P., Levin, N.W., and Suzman, M.M. The prophylactic value of propranolol in angina pectoris. *Am. J. Cardiol.* 18:370, 1966.

30. Ginn, W.M., and Orgain, E.S. Propranolol hydrochloride in the treatment of angina pectoris. *J.A.M.A.* 198:1214, 1966.

31. Nestel, P.J. Evaluation of propranolol (Inderal) in the treatment of angina pectoris. *Med. J. Aust.* 2:1274, 1966.

32. Gianelly, R.E., Goldman, R., Treister, B., and Harrison, D.C. Propranolol in patients with angina pectoris. *Ann. Intern. Med.* 67:1216, 1967.

33. Keelan, P. Double-blind trial of propranolol (Inderal) in angina pectoris. *Br. Med. J.* 1:897, 1965.

34. Hebb, A.R., Godwin, T.F., and Gunton, R.W. New beta adrenergic blocking agent, propranolol, in treatment of angina pectoris. *Can. Med. Assoc. J.* 98:246, 1968.

35. Amsterdam, E.A., Gorlin, R., and Wolfson, S. Evaluation of long-term use of propranolol in angina pectoris. *J.A.M.A.* 210:103, 1969.

36. Prichard, B.N.C. β-Receptor antagonists in angina pectoris. *Ann. Clin. Res.* 3:344, 1971.

37. Hamer, J., and Sowton, E. Effects of propranolol on exercise tolerance in angina pectoris. *Am. J. Cardiol.* 18:354, 1966.

38. Dwyer, E.M., Jr., Wiener, L., and Cox, J.W. Effects of beta-adrenergic blockade (propranolol) on left ventricular hemodynamics and the electrocardiogram during exercise-induced angina pectoris. *Circulation* 38:250, 1968.

39. Epstein, SE., Robinson, B.F., Kahler, R.L., and Braunwald, E. Effect of beta-adrenergic blockade on the cardiac response to maximal and submaximal exercise in man. *J. Clin. Invest.* 44:1745, 1965.

40. Sonnenblick, E.H., Braunwald, E., Williams, J.F., Jr., and Glick, G. Effects of exercise on myocardial force-velocity relations in intact unanesthetized man: Relative role of changes in heart rate, sympathetic activity, and ventricular dimensions. *J. Clin. Invest.* 44:2051, 1965.

41. Robin, E., Cowan, C., Puri, P., Ganguly, S., De Boyrie, E., Martinez, M., Stock, T., and Bing, R.J. A comparative study of nitroglycerin and propranolol. *Circulation* 36:175, 1967.

42. Wiener, L., Dwyer, E.M., Jr., and Cox, J.W. Hemodynamic effects of nitroglycerin, propranolol and their combination in coronary heart disease. *Circulation* 39:623, 1969.

43. Wolfson, S., and Gorlin, R. Cardiovascular pharmacology of propranolol in man. *Circulation* 40:501, 1969.

44. Naylor, W.G., McInnes, I., Swann, J.B., Carson, V., and Lowe, T.E. Effect of propranolol, a beta-adrenergic antagonist on blood flow in the coronary and other vascular fields. *Am. Heart J.* 73:207, 1967.

45. Sowton, E., and Hamer, J. Hemodynamic changes after beta adrenergic blockade. *Am. J. Cardiol.* 18:317, 1966.

46. Chamberlain, D.A. Effects of beta-adrenergic blockade on heart size. *Am. J. Cardiol.* 18:317, 1966.

47. Williams, J.R., Jr., Glick, G., and Braunwald, E. Studies on cardiac dimensions in intact unanesthetized man. V. Effects of nitroglycerin. *Circulation* 32:767, 1965.

48. Srivastava, A.C., Dewar, H.A., and Newell, D.J. Double-blind trial of propranolol (Inderal) in angina of effort. *Br. Med. J.* 2:724, 1964.

49. Aronow, W.S., and Kaplan, M.A. Propranolol with isosorbide dinitrate versus placebo in angina pectoris. *N. Engl. J. Med.* 280:847, 1969.

50. MacAlpin, R.N., Kattus, A.A., and Wenfield, M.E. The effect of β-adrenergic-blocking agent (Nethalide) and nitroglycerin on exercise tolerance in angina pectoris. *Circulation* 31:869, 1965.

51. Wiener, L., Dwyer, E.M., Jr., and Cox, J.W. Hemodynamic effects of nitroglycerin, propranolol and their combination in coronary heart disease. *Circulation* 39:623, 1969.

52. Dunlop, D., and Shakes, R.G. Selective blockade of adrenoceptive beta receptors in the heart. *Br. J. Pharmacol.* 32:201, 1968.

53. Sowton, E., Balcon, R., Cross, D., and Frick, H. Hemodynamic effects of I.C.I. 50172 in patients with ischemic heart disease. *Br. Med. J.* 1:215, 1968.

54. Gibson, D., and Sowton, E. Effects of I.C.I. 50172 in man during erect exercise. *Br. Med. J.* 1:213, 1968.

55. Banas, J.S., Jr., Gaasch, W.H., Oboler, A.A., and Levine, H.J. Chronotropic adrenergic blockade without intrinsic myocardial depression. *Circulation* 42(suppl.):133, 1970.

56. Amsterdam, E.A., Hughes, J.L., Mansour, E., Salel, A.F., Bonanno, J.A., Zelis, R., and Mason, D.T. Circulatory effects of practolol: Selective cardiac beta adrenergic blockade in arrhythmias and angina pectoris. *Clin. Res.* 19:109, 1971.

57. Areskog, N-H., and Adolfsson, L. Effects of a cardio-selective beta-adrenergic blocker (I.E.I. 50172) at exercise in angina pectoris. *Br. Med. J.* 2:601, 1969.

58. Frick, M.H., and Katila, M. Cardio-selective beta-adrenergic inhibition by practolol in angina pectoris. *Ann. Clin. Res.* 2:96, 1970.

59. George, C.F., Nagle, R.E., and Pentecost, B.L. Practolol in treatment of angina pectoris in a double-blind trial. *Br. Med. J.* 2:402, 1970.

60. Sandler, G., and Clayton, G.A. Clinical evaluation of practolol, a new cardio-selective beta-blocking agent in angina pectoris. *Br. Med. J.* 2:399, 1970.

61. Sowton, E., Smithen, C., Leaver, D., and Barr, I. Effect of practolol on exercise tolerance in patients with angina pectoris. *Am. J. Med.* 51:63, 1971.

62. Varnauskas, E., Bergman, H., Houk, P., and Bjorntorp, P. Hemodynamic effects of physical training in coronary patients. *Lancet* 2:8, 1966.

63. Hellerstein, H.K. Exercise therapy in coronary disease. *Bull. N.Y. Acad. Med.* 44:2, 1968.

64. Clausen, J.P., Larsen, O.A., and Trap-Jensen, J. Physical training in the management of coronary artery disease. *Circulation* 40:143, 1969.

65. Redwood, D.R., Rosing, D.R., and Epstein, S.E. Circulatory and symptomatic effects of physical training in patients with coronary-artery disease and angina pectoris. *N. Engl. J. Med.* 286:959, 1972.

66. Braunwald, E., Epstein, S.E., Glick, G., Wechsler, A.S., and Braunwald, N.S. Relief of angina pectoris by electrical stimulation of the carotid-sinus nerves. *N. Engl. J. Med.* 277:1279, 1967.

67. Epstein, S.E., Beiser, G.D., Goldstein, R.E., Redwood, D., Rosing, D.R., Glick, G., Wechsler, A.S., Stampfer, M., Cohen, L.S., Reis, R.L., Braunwald, N.S., and Braunwald, E. Treatment of angina pectoris by electrical stimulation of the carotid-sinus nerves: Results in 17 patients with severe angina. *N. Engl. J. Med.* 280:971, 1969.

68. Sheldon, W.C., Sones, F.M., Jr., Shirey, E.K., Fergusson, D.J.G., Favaloro, R.G., and Effler, D.B. Reconstructive coronary artery surgery: Postoperative assessment. *Circulation* 39:61, 1969.

69. Johnson, W.E., Flemma, R.J., Lepley, D., Jr., and Ellison, E.H. Extended treatment of severe coronary artery disease: A total surgical approach. *Ann. Surg.* 170:460, 1969.

69a. Alderman, E.L., Matlof, H.J., Wexler, L., Shumway, N.E., and Harrison, D.C. Results of direct coronary artery surgery for the treatment of angina pectoris. *N. Engl. J. Med.* 288:535, 1973.

70. Spencer, F.C., Green, G.E., Tice, D.A., and Glassman, E. Bypass grafting for occlusive disease of the coronary arteries: Report of experience with 195 patients. *Ann. Surg.* 173:1029, 1971.

71. Walker, J.A., Friedberg, H.D., Flemma, R.J., and Johnson, W.D. Determinants of angiographic patency of aortocoronary vein bypass grafts. *In, Cardiovascular Surgery 1971.* AHA Monograph No. 35, 1972.

72. Greene, D.G., Klochke, F.J., Schimert, G.L., Bunnell, I.L., Wittenbert, S.M., and Lajos, T. Evaluation of venous bypass grafts from aorta to coronary artery by inert gas desaturation and direct flowmeter techniques. *J. Clin. Invest.* 51:191, 1972.

73. Amsterdam, E.A., Iben, A., Hurley, E.J., Mansour, E., Hughes, J.L., Salel, A.F., Zelis, R., and Mason, D.T. Saphenous vein bypass graft for refractory angina pectoris: Physiologic evidence for enhanced blood flow to the ischemic myocardium (Abstr.) *Am. J. Cardiol.* 26:623, 1970.

74. Johnson, W.D., Flemma, R.J., Manley, J.C., and Leply, D., Jr. Physiologic parameters of ventricular function as affected by direct coronary surgery. *J. Thorac. Cardiovasc. Surg.* 60:483, 1970.

75. Manley, J.C., Johnson, W.D., Flemma, R.J., and Lepley, D., Jr. Objective evaluation of the effects of direct myocardial revascularization on ventricular function utilizing ergometer exercise testing. (Abstr.) *Am. J. Cardiol.* 26:648, 1970.

76. Chatterjee, K., Swan, H.J.C., Parmley, W.W., Sustaita, H., Marcus, H., and Matloff, J. Depression of left ventricular function due to acute myocardial ischemia and its reversal after aortocoronary spahenous-vein bypass. *N. Engl. J. Med.* 286:1117, 1972.

77. Reis, G., Bristow, J.D., Kremkau, E.L., Green, G.S., Herr, R.H., Griswold, H.E., and Starr, A. Influence of aortocoronary bypass surgery on left ventricular performance. *N. Engl. J. Med.* 284:1116, 1971.

78. Bourassa, M.G., Lesperance, J., Campeau, L., and Saltiel, J. Fate of left ventricular contraction following aortocoronary venous grafts. *Circulation* 46:724, 1972.

79. Kouchoukos, N.T., and Kirklin, J.W. Coronary bypass operations for ischemic heart disease. *Mod. Conc. Cardiovasc. Dis.* 41:47, 1972.

80. Williams, D., Iben, A., Hurley, E.J., Bonanno, J.A., Miller, R.R., Massumi, R.A., Zelis, R., Mason, D.T., and Amsterdam, E.A. Myocardial infarction during coronary artery bypass surgery. *Am. J. Cardiol.* (in press).

81. Achuff, S., Griffith, L., Humphries, J.O., Conti, C.R., Brawley, R., Gott, V., and Ross, R. Myocardial damage after aorto-coronary vein bypass surgery. (Abstr.) *J. Clin. Invest.* 51:1a, 1972.

82. Glassman, E., Spencer, F.C., Tice, D.A., Weisinger, B., and Green, G.E. What percentage of patients with angina pectoris are candidates for bypass grafts? *Circulation* (Suppl.) 43:I-101, 1971.

83. Miller, R.R., Mason, D.T., Massumi, R.A., Zelis, R., Amsterdam, E.A. Precatheterization evaluation for aortocoronary saphenous vein bypass graft: Relation of clinical factors to vessel operatiblity. *Clin. Res.* (in press).

84. Selzer, A., and Kerth, W.J. Surgical treatment of coronary artery disease: Too fast, too soon? *Am. J. Cardiol.* 28:490, 1971.

85. Amsterdam, E.A., Most, A.S., Wolfson, S., Kemp, H.G., and Gorlin, R. Relation of degree of angiographically documented coronary artery disease to mortality. *Ann. Intern. Med.* 72:780, 1970.

86. Friesinger, G.C., Page, E.E., and Ross, R.S. Prognostic significance of coronary arteriography. *Trans. Assoc. Am. Physicians* 83:78, 1970.

87. Cohen, M.V., Cohn, P.F., Herman, M.V., and Gorlin, R. Diagnosis and prognosis of main left coronary artery obstruction. *In, Cardiovascular Surgery 1971.* AHA Monograph No. 35., 1972.

9

THE EFFECTS OF PHARMACOLOGICAL AGENTS ON HUMAN PERFORMANCE

Alberto N. Goldbarg, M.D.

The effects of commonly used pharmacological agents on exercise performance and the exercise electrocardiogram (ECG) in normal subjects and in patients with cardiac disease will be reviewed in this chapter. The agents to be discussed include digitalis, nitroglycerin, the so-called *long acting nitrates*, and beta blockers.

The topic is important since exercise tests are being used with increasing frequency in the evaluation of drugs in coronary heart disease. Moreover, proper exercise evaluation will be enhanced by knowledge of the actions of these agents, commonly used in the daily practice of medicine.

Digitalis

A common problem in clinical practice is the interpretation of the exercise ECG in those patients who are taking cardiac glycosides. An example of a *false positive* response is shown in Fig. 1. The 42-year-old male complained of atypical chest pain and was placed on digoxin by his referring physician. Notice that the resting ECG shows no signs of digitalis effect, but during and after a multistage treadmill exercise test significant ST segment depression occurred. Further investigations disclosed a normal coronary arteriogram and a normal hemodynamic study.

It was reported by Zwillinger in 1935 [1] that normal young adults developed positive ECG exercise tests after digitalization. Other reports [2-6] confirmed and amplified those initial observations. These studies demonstrated that 50 to 60 percent of healthy young subjects will develop abnormal ST-T wave changes during exercise after digitalization. If the resting ECG shows shortening of the QT interval and either sagging or depression of the ST segment, the exercise ECG will definitely be abnormal. On the other hand, if the resting ECG does not show digitalis effect, it is impossible to predict whether the ST segment response will be abnormal or normal during effort.

P.R. 42 y-o Male on Digitalis

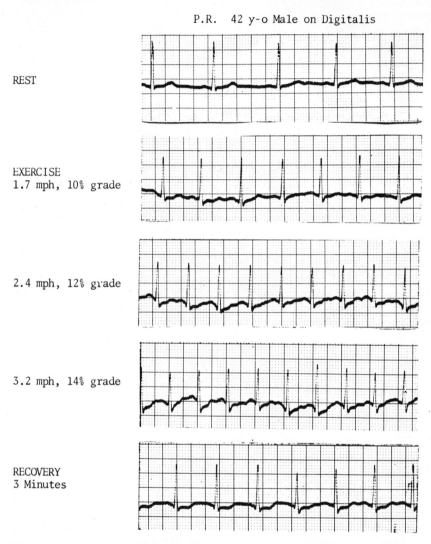

REST

EXERCISE
1.7 mph, 10% grade

2.4 mph, 12% grade

3.2 mph, 14% grade

RECOVERY
3 Minutes

Fig. 1. False positive response multistage treadmill exercise produced by digoxin in a 42-year-old man with normal coronary arteriograms. The ST segment changes induced by digitalis are indistinguishable from those found in coronary patients.

The ST-T changes found in digitalized healthy subjects during exercise are unaffected by previous administration of nitroglycerin or atropine. However, the exercise ST segment changes (which resemble exactly those found in patients with angina pectoris (AP)) are lessened or sometimes abolished by the administration of 100 percent oxygen or by previous administration of potassium salts (particularly with insulin). Conversely, the ST segment changes are worsened by induced hypoxia. Since ST segment depression during exercise is exaggerated by digitalis in ischemic patients, finding a normal ECG response to effort in a digitalized subject is strong evidence to rule out ischemia. It is important to point out that the manifestations of digitalis toxicity, particularly dysrhythmias, are exacerbated by exercise, even when of minimal intensity [7]. Therefore, exercise testing should not be carried out in subjects suspected of toxicity from digitalis.

The characteristic action of digitalis shortens the action potential of ventricular myocardium [8]. Similarly, increased heart rate also shortens the ventricular myocardial action potential [9]. However, these facts alone will not explain the changes observed in the exercise ECG. It is possible that digitalis may affect the epicardium differently, compared with the endocardium, and may in that manner induce abnormal ST segmental changes. However, this explanation is obviously speculative and there is not adequate explanation for the exercise ST changes after digitalization in healthy subjects.

When atrial pacing was used for electrophysiological studies, we observed in some patients taking digitalis that the ST segment changes appeared to be strictly rate-related [10]. An example of a patient with rate-related ST segment changes due to digitalis and the increased rate is shown in Fig. 2. We were impressed by the rapidity with which the ST segment changes occur. Note that the heart is paced at the rate of 130 beats/min and the ST segment is depressed after only 3 beats. Moreover, in the first sinus beat following the cessation of atrial pacing, the ST segment returned to its normal positions. If the ST segment changes were due to a metabolic state as they are in myocardial ischemia, it is improbable that these changes would develop or regress in such a short period of time. Thus, the study of the time course of ST segment changes induced by atrial pacing may be of significant value in differentiating truly ischemic changes from those induced by cardiac glycosides. Further studies are planned to resolve this apparent clinical dilemma.

Nitroglycerin

For over 100 years, nitroglycerin has been (and still is in my opinion) the preferred drug for the treatment of AP. The mode of action of nitroglycerin in patients with AP has received considerable attention from investigators in recent years [11-15]. Nitroglycerin, a potent smooth muscle relaxant, affects both the systemic and coronary circulations. The systemic effects are due primarily to arteriolar and venous dilatation which leads to a decrease in systemic arterial pressure and a decrease in venous return to the heart. A decrease in heart volume and a reduction in ventricular filling pressures also occurs. Therefore, wall tension in the heart is reduced, which in turn reduces the myocardial demands for oxygen. In addition, ejection time decreases and there is a compensatory tachycardia. These effects have been demonstrated at rest and during exercise. The coronary effects are more controversial and probably are not the cause for

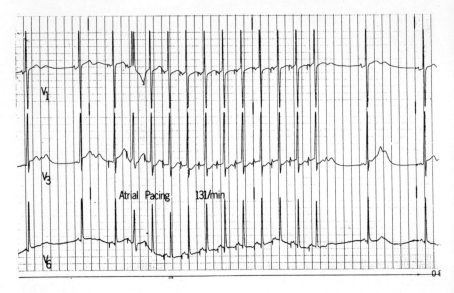

Fig. 2. Effects of increasing the heart rate by atrial pacing on ST segment changes in a digitalized patient. (Discussed in text)

the salutory effects of the drug. Although nitroglycerin is a coronary vasodilator, it is doubtful that the diameters of diseased and rigid coronary vessels would be increased as a result. In normal subjects, total coronary blood flow increases after administration of sublingual nitroglycerin. However, nitroglycerin does not increase total coronary blood flow in patients [16, 17] with AP. The complexity of flow dynamics in the diseased coronary arterial tree explains the difficulties in demonstrating a possible redistribution of flow in the ischemic myocardium. Ganz and Marcus [18] reported that the intracoronary injection of nitroglycerin was ineffective in relieving AP induced by atrial pacing, in contrast to the systemic administration of nitroglycerin which was effective. These observations, therefore, further substantiate the concept that the improvement after nitroglycerin is due to its systemic effects of decreasing myocardial oxygen needs, rather than an increase in oxygen delivery to ischemic areas of the heart.

An example of the improvement in exercise capacity and ischemic ST changes in a coronary patient is shown in Fig. 3. The patient was able to exercise twice as long after nitroglycerin and the ischemic ST changes were almost totally abolished. Horwitz and associates [19] correlated the clinical response to nitroglycerin with coronary angiography. These authors concluded that a failure to respond to nitroglycerin or a delayed response (more than 3 minutes) in alleviating symptoms occurred in patients in whom coronary arteriography demonstrated either no coronary obstructive disease or very severe coronary obstructions. Similarly, my associates and I have been impressed by the consistency with which exercise performance and ECG are improved following the administration of nitroglycerin. We have found that patients in whom the exercise performance and exercise ECG do not improve after nitroglycerin have either no coronary disease or very severe disease, as demonstrated by coronary arteriograms. Therefore, the specificity of the exercise ECG may be enhanced by the use of nitroglycerin as a diagnostic tool.

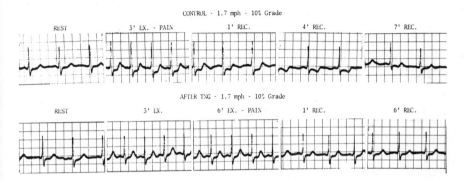

Fig. 3.   Effects of sublingual nitroglycerin (TNG) on exercise performance and ECG in a 55-year-old male with AP. Before TNG he experienced pain at the 3rd minute of exercise (EX). The ST segment changes persist until the 7th minute of recovery (REC). After TNG, he was able to exercise for 6 min at the same workload. The ST segment changes are of less magnitude and less duration.

Long-Acting Nitrates

The efficacy of the long-acting nitrates in the treatment of angina patients, although widely used, remains controversial [20-27]. The oral preparation of isosorbide dinitrate, pentaerythrityl tetranitrate, erythrityl tetranitrate, trolnitrate, and others are considered to be of no significant value by a number of investigators, in either preventing ischemic attacks, or more importantly, to be ineffective in improving exercise performance and the exercise ECG in coronary patients.

Our study [23] demonstrated that isosorbide dinitrate, given orally (10 mg 4 times daily), was no better than placebo in reducing the number of anginal episodes and nitroglycerin consumption, or to improve the exercise capacity in a group of 21 patients with AP. On the other hand, sublingual isosorbide dinitrate [26] and chewable erythrityl tetranitrate [27] are reported to be effective by demonstrating, with objective exercise testing, an improvement in exercise capacity of coronary patients. Goldstein and associates [26] concluded that sublingual isosorbide dinitrate closely resembles nitroglycerin in its alteration of circulatory responses to exercise and in the duration of improvement in exercise capacity. The oral preparations of these agents are, at the most, of questionable value; the sublingual and chewable preparations appear not to have longer action compared with nitroglycerin.

Earlier claims were made [20] indicating a synergistic action between long-acting nitrates and beta blocking agents. However, properly controlled studies from different laboratories [21-23, 25] have all failed to show a synergistic effect.

Beta Blocking Agents

The cardiovascular effects of propranolol, a beta adrenergic blocking agent, have been studied extensively at rest and during exercise [28-32]. In our studies [31], seven healthy subjects performed submaximal and maximal bicycle exercise before and after intravenous injection of 10 mg of propranolol (Inderal®). At rest, the heart rate decreased from 62 to 53 beats/min following administration of propranolol. During work, the reduction of heart rate after beta adrenergic blockade became progressively greater with increasing workloads, i.e., 17 beats/min at 25 percent of maximal oxygen intake ($\dot{V}_{0_2}$ max) and 36 beats/min at maximum. Although $\dot{V}_{0_2}$ max was not influenced by adrenergic blockade, the time the subjects could tolerate maximal work was reduced approximately 25 percent from the control values. These findings support the assumption that under normal conditions, sympathetic activity is gradually more pronounced as the exercise becomes severe. Thus it is not surprising that maximal physical performance decreases after beta adrenergic blockade due to impairment of sympathetic stimulation to the heart which plays an important role in the cardiovascular response during severe effort.

Cardiac output and systemic arterial pressure were found to decrease after beta adrenergic blockade during rest, submaximal and maximal exercise. In addition, there is a prolongation in the ejection time and ventricular volumes (dimensions) increase. Therefore, one of the compensatory mechanisms during heavy exercise after propranolol appears to be an increase in stroke volumes due to the higher diastolic filling pressures in the ventricles associated with progressive increases in the diastolic volume of the heart, which, by the Frank-Starling mechanism, would increase the force of myocardial contraction as a consequence of the greater initial length of the muscle fiber. Another compensatory mechanism takes place—the widening of the arteriovenous oxygen difference in order to secure the oxygen supply to the working skeletal muscles.

Since beta blocking agents decrease heart rate, blood pressure, and velocity of contraction, the myocardial oxygen demands are reduced. Thus, it would be anticipated that these agents are effective in the treatment of angina patients. It has been reported that propranolol is effective in alleviating symptoms in patients limited by coronary disease [20, 22, 23, 25, 27, 33]. Although most investigators have demonstrated improvement in exercise capacity, this has not been a universal finding [21, 23].

In marked contrast to nitroglycerin, which improves both exercise performance and the ischemic (ST changes) manifestations on the exercise ECG, propranolol appears to have no significant effect on the ST segment depression in the exercise ECG [22, 33, 34]. This is illustrated in Fig. 4, showing some

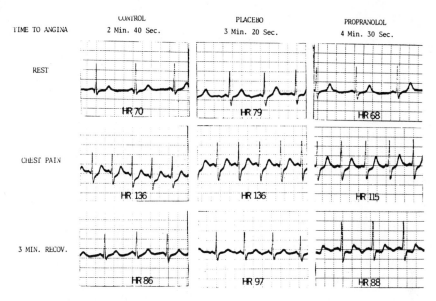

Fig. 4.   Effects of placebo and propranolol on exercise performance and ECG in a 49-year-old male with AP. Exercise capacity increases with both agents. In spite of significant reduction in heart rate (HR) at rest and during exercise there is little improvement in the ST segment changes.

improvement in the exercise capacity of an angina patient, but the ischemic manifestations in the exercise ECG are not reduced and remain for longer duration in spite of a significant reduction in heart rate. Based on similar observations, Furburg [34] has suggested the use of propranolol to distinguish between coronary and functional ST-T changes. The ST changes, for example, in neurocirculatory asthenia are improved after propranolol, while the ST changes in coronary patients are not affected by propranolol. A potentially harmful effect of propranolol is that it may precipitate or exacerbate congestive heart failure by removing sympathetic support from a diseased myocardium.

Based on these considerations, and that propranolol has not improved longevity in angina patients [35], my personal view is that propranolol is a useful adjunct to our armamentarium in the management of angina patients, but is far from the ideal anti-anginal agent and is probably not the drug of choice for the treatment of AP. As a matter of fact, we may conclude that at present, drug management of AP is definitely unsatisfactory.

Newer beta blocking agents (practalol, alprenolol, sotalol, oxyprenolol) are currently being investigated with the hope that these newer agents produce less myocardial depressant effects and that they may be used in patients with chronic obstructive lung disease and asthma (cardioselective agents).

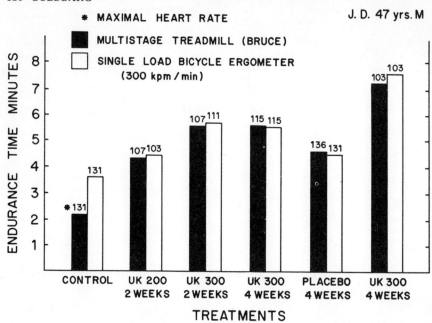

Fig. 5. Effects of a new beta blocking agent (UK 6558-01) on exercise capacity in a 47-year-old coronary patient. (Discussed in text)

In our laboratory we are investigating the anti-anginal effects of a new beta blocker, UK 6558-01, developed by Chas. Pfizer & Co. Fig. 5 shows the effect of this new beta blocker on exercise performance and maximal heart rate in an angina patient which was attained on the bicycle ergometer (single load, 300 kpm/min) and on the treadmill (multistage Bruce Test) [36]. After control data were obtained, the patient was placed on different dosages for 2 weeks (UK 200 and UK 300 refers to 200 mg and 300 mg daily of the oral preparation of UK 6558-01), administered in a single blind fashion. Subsequently, the patient participated in a double blind, crossover evaluation and exercise testing was performed every 2 weeks. Excellent correlation was found between the exercise capacity on the bicycle and on the treadmill. The heart rate was identical in both types of exercise testing.

It should be emphasized that the placebo effects should be taken into consideration in the evaluation of drugs for the management of patients with AP. The studies have just begun, and we hope to be able to document, in the near future, the effects of this new drug in the therapy of patients with AP.

Summary

The effects of commonly used pharmacological agents on exercise performance and the exercise ECG have been described. Knowledge of the pharmacological actions of each is essential for proper interpretation of exercise tests. Furthermore, this knowledge will enhance the specificity of the exercise ECG for the diagnosis of coronary heart disease. Drug evaluation in patients with AP is difficult. Therefore, objective exercise data are necessary to determine the usefulness of a particular agent.

Acknowledgments

The studies on the new beta blocking agent are being performed with the collaboration of Drs. Pablo Denes and Roberto Anastacio. The technical assistance of Mr. Robert Schuessler and the excellent secretarial work of Mrs. Geraldine Irby are gratefully acknowledged.

REFERENCES

1. Zwillinger, L. Die Digitalis Enwirkung auf das Arbeits—Elektrokardiogramm. *Med. Klin.* 30:977, 1935.

2. Liebow, I.M., and Feil, H. Digitalis and the normal work electrocardiogram. *Am. Heart J.* 22:683, 1941.

3. Nördstrom-Öhrberg, G. Effects of digitalis glycosides on electrocardiogram and exercise test in healthy subjects. *Acta Med. Scand.* 176(Suppl. 420):3, 1964.

4. Kawai, C., and Hultgren, H.N. The effects of digitalis upon the exercise electrocardiogram. *Am. Heart J.* 68:409, 1964.

5. Hirsch, E.Z. The effects of digoxin on the electrocardiogram after strenuous exercise in normal men. *Am. Heart J.* 70:196, 1965.

6. Hirsch, E.Z. The effects of digoxin on the electrocardiogram after strenuous exercise in normal men. II. Effect of potassium chloride with and without insulin on the exercise electrocardiogram of digitalized subjects. *Am. Heart J.* 70:204, 1965.

7. Natarajan, G., and Gooch, A.S. Arrhythmia behavior during exercise in digitoxic patients. *Clin. Res.* 20:390, 1972.

8. Hoffman, B.F. Effects of digitalis on electrical activity of cardiac fibers. *In*, Fisch, C., and Surawicz, B., Eds. *Digitalis*, p. 93. New York, Grune & Stratton, 1969.

9. Hoffman, B.F., and Suckling, E.E. Effect of heart rate on cardiac membrane potentials and the unipolar electrogram. *Am. J. Physiol.* 179:123, 1954.

10. Childers, R.W., Goldbarg, A.N., Gambetta, M., and de la Fuente, D. Unpublished data.

11. Fam, W.M., and McGregor, M. Effects of coronary vasodilator drugs on retrograde flow in areas of chronic myocardial ischemia. *Circ. Res.* 15:355, 1964.

12. Parker, J.O., Di Giorgi, S., and West, R.O. A hemodynamic study of acute coronary insufficiency precipitated by exercise. With observations on the effects of nitroglycerin. *Am. J. Cardiol.* 17:470, 1966.

13. Robinson, B.F. Mode of action of nitroglycerin in angina pectoris. *Br. Heart J.* 30:295, 1968.

14. Arborelius, M., Jr., Lecerof, H., Malm, A., and Malmborg, R.O. Acute effect of nitroglycerin on haemodynamics of angina pectoris. *Br. Heart J.* 30:407, 1968.

15. Weisse, A.B., and Regan, T.J. The current status of nitrites in the treatment.of coronary artery disease. *Progr. Cardiovasc. Dis.* 12:72, 1969.

16. Brachfeld, N., Bozer, J., and Gorlin, R. Action of nitroglycerin on the coronary circulation in normal and in mild cardiac subjects. *Circulation* 19:697, 1959.

17. Gorlin, R., Brachfeld, N., MacLeod, C., and Bopp, P. Effects of nitroglycerin on coronary circulation in patients with coronary artery disease or increased left ventricular work. *Circulation* 19:705, 1959.

18. Ganz, W., and Marcus, H.S. Failure of intracoronary nitroglycerin to alleviate pacing-induced angina. *Am. J. Cardiol.* 29:265, 1972.

19. Horwitz, L.D., Herman, M.W., and Gorlin, R. Clinical response to nitroglycerin as a diagnostic test for coronary artery disease. *Am. J. Cardiol.* 29:149, 1972.

20. Russek, H.I. Propranolol and isosorbide dinitrate synergism in angina pectoris. *Am. J. Cardiol.* 21:44, 1968.

21. Aronow, W.S., and Kaplan, M.H. Propranolol combined with isosorbide dinitrate versus placebo in angina pectoris. *N. Engl. J. Med.* 280:847, 1969.

22. Battock, D.J., Alvarez, H., and Chidsey, C.A. Effects of propranolol and isosorbide dinitrate on exercise performance and adrenergic activity in patients with angina pectoris. *Circulation* 39:157, 1969.

23. Goldbarg, A.N., Moran, J.F., Butterfield, T.K., Nemickas, R., and Bermudez, G.A. Therapy of angina pectoris with propranolol and long-acting nitrates. *Circulation* 40:847, 1969.

24. Goldbarg, A.N., Paxinos, J., and Miller, R.R. Current survey—anti-anginal drugs. *Postgrad. Med. J.* 26:84, 1970.

25. Dagenais, G.R., Pitt, B., and Ross, R.S. Exercise tolerance in patients with angina pectoris. *Am. J. Cardiol.* 28:10, 1971.

26. Goldstein, R.E., Rosing, D.R., Redwood, D.R., Beiser, G.D., and Epstein, S.E. Clinical and circulatory effects of isosorbide dinitrate. Comparison with nitroglycerin. *Circulation* 43:629, 1971.

27. Goldstein, R.E., and Epstein, S.E. Medical management of patients with angina pectoris. *Progr. Cardiovasc. Dis.* 14:360, 1972.

28. Bishop, J.M., and Segel, N. The circulatory effects of intravenous pronethalol in man at rest and during exercise in the supine and upright positions. *J. Physiol.* 169:112, 1963.

29. Epstein, S.E., Robinson, B.F., Kahler, R.L., and Braunwald, E. Effects of beta-adrenergic blockade on the cardiac response to maximal and submaximal exercise in man. *J. Clin. Invest.* 44:1745, 1965.

30. Cumming, R.G., and Carr, W. Hemodynamic response to exercise after propranolol in normal subjects. *Can. J. Physiol. Pharmacol.* 44:465, 1966.

31. Goldbarg, A.N., Ekblom, B., and Astrand, P-O. Effects of blócking the autonomic nervous system during exercise. *Circulation* 44(Suppl. II):118, 1971.

32. Parker, J.O., West, R.O. and Di Giorgi, S. Hemodynamic effects of propranolol in coronary heart disease. *Am. J. Cardiol.* 21:11, 1968.

33. Gianelly, R.E., Goldman, R., Treister, B.L., and Harrison, D.C. Propranolol in patients with angina pectoris. *Ann. Int. Med.* 67:1216, 1967.

34. Furburg, C. Adrenergic beta-blockade and electrocardiographical ST-T changes. *Acta Med. Scand.* 181:21, 1967.

35. Zeft, H.J., Patterson, S.D., and Orgain, E.S. Propranolol in the long-treatment of angina pectoris. *Ann. Int. Med.* 70:1082, 1969.

36. Doan, A.E., Peterson, D.R., Blakmon, J.R., and Bruce, R.A. Myocardial ischemia after maximal exercise in healthy man: A method for detecting potential coronary heart disease. *Am. Heart J.* 69:11, 1965.

10

PRINCIPLES OF EXERCISE PRESCRIPTION
For Normals and Cardiac Subjects

Herman K. Hellerstein, M.D., *Eugene Z. Hirsch*, M.D., *Richard Ader,*
Ned Greenblott, M.D., and *Martin Siegel*, M.D.

As soon as the state of physical fitness of the cardiac patient has been assessed, the physician and his fellow health professionals should formulate a program to enhance the patient's fitness. Physical reconditioning should be part of a comprehensive treatment program which includes supervision; periodic reevaluation; diet to improve nutrition and attain normal body weight and serum lipids; abstinence from the use of tobacco; continuation of gainful employment and customary social mode of life; and medication when indicated; as well as attention to psychologic and social adjustment.

At present a pharmacopoeia of physical activity is gradually being accumulated (but not yet fully developed), which makes allowances for special abnormalities in various biological parameters, hypertension, myocardial infarction (MI), cardiac enlargement, obesity, and the like. However, enough knowledge has accumulated so that principles of sound conditioning and exercise prescription have been developed and can be applied beneficially at all ages and in all states of health (TABLE I). Common sense, clinical judgment, and empiricism of past reports [1] can be supplemented and, at times, supplanted by quantitative recommendations, based on factual information gained about the individual subject.

Parameters of a Physical Activity Program

Pleasure principle. Participation in a long-term program of enhanced physical activity must be gratifying and pleasurable, or at least not distasteful. By no

This study was supported in part by grants from the American Heart Association (Northeastern Ohio Chapter), Mr. & Mrs. Edgar Weil, Mr. & Mrs. William H. Loveman, the Stanley Feil Fund, and the United States Public Health Service, Research Grant HE 06304, National Heart Institute, Bethesda, Maryland.

TABLE I

Principles of exercise prescription

Determine functional capacity, to highest safe level, including steady state, non-steady state, exercise of upper and lower extremities and torso
Exclude the ineligible
Determine the exercise load to induce the desired training effects
    Intensity, Frequency, Duration

Formulate individual targets for training
    Heart rate, blood pressure
    Heart rate X systolic blood pressure product
    ECG changes: ST-T, rhythm, intraventricular, atrioventricular conduction
    Clinical signs and symptoms
Education and active involvement of participants
Individualized prescription of activities
    Caloric equivalents of a variety of activities to attain target levels
    Pleasurable and acceptable to the individual and family

Program design
    Supervision
    Safety: precautions, monitor, trained personnel, equipment. Cardiopulmonary
        resuscitation certification
    Format of training sessions
            Warmup, interval design, dynamic isotonic activities, taper off
    Revision of prescription
    Scheduled reevaluations

means should the pursuit of *music and the arts* be slighted meanwhile. The activities should involve a substantial and sustained increment in metabolic, cardiovascular, respiratory, and neuromuscular functions. All exercise must be beneficial and build strength and muscular endurance. The magnitude of the physical activities should be prescribed, supervised, and changed progressively (gradually and only after reevaluation), to constitute a safe overload—more than customary use—of the muscles (skeletal: upper and lower extremities and torso, and of the heart). A multitude of activities can produce the desired effects. The fundamental prerequisite is that the activities involve rhythmical contraction of large groups of muscles, preferably the antigravity muscles. The desired effects can be produced by a variety of activities including vigorous walking, stationary and mobile cycling, swimming, jogging, running, bench-stepping, rope-jumping, graded rhythmical calisthenics, and selected noncompetitive sports.

The key for appropriate exercise prescription obviously is the assessment of the individual's physical fitness made from the relationships between cardiovascular and work parameters.

Pretraining evaluation. The purpose of the preliminary pretraining evaluations is not only to exclude the ineligible (TABLE II) but also to evaluate the cardiovascular system and function in order to provide guidelines (target levels) for training at a given time (TABLE III). In followup evaluations the target levels may be increased or reduced, if improvement or deterioration occurs

TABLE II

Indications and contraindications for participation in
programs planned to enhance physical fitness

INDICATIONS	CONTRAINDICATIONS	
	Cardiovascular	*Others*
Normal subjects, especially highly coronary prone, general deconditioning, neurocirculatory asthenia, before and after surgery*	Severe (80-90%) stenosis of three major coronary arteries	Uncontrolled diabetes mellitus, thyrotoxicosis
	Rapidly progressing angina	Marked obesity
	Impending infarction	Deforming arthritis*
	Massive ventricular aneurysm	Disabling skeletal-muscle disorders
Arteriosclerotic heart disease*	Congestive failure, uncontrolled	Psychosis
Intermittent claudication*	Arrhythmias	Recent pulmonary embolism
Pulmonary disease*	ventricular tachycardia 2nd, 3rd AV block	Severe pulmonary hypertension
	fixed ventricular rate pacemaker	Severe electrolyte imbalance
CAUTION:	untreated atrial fibrillation	Severe varicose veins with thrombophlebitis, phlebothrombosis
DRUGS: reserpine, propanolol, guanethidine, ganglionic blockers, procaine amide, quinidine, digitalis	ventricular premature beats at rest which increase with exercise	Anemia
	Valvular disease moderate to severe aortic valvular or subvalvular outflow obstruction	Central nervous system disease*
	Uncontrolled hypertension	Acute infections disease
	Acute myocarditis	Dissecting aneurysm

*Selected cases.

respectively The expectation is that the pretraining evaluations by stress testing will provide precise information in order to determine the intensity of training of musculature of the upper as well as lower extremities and torso. The evaluation must be multilevel, steady state (also ideally nonsteady state), on a calibrated ergometer (bicycle, treadmill, steps). The magnitude and duration should be sufficient to tax the individual's capacity, safely, to his highest safe level, or to elicit evidence of *strain* if at a lower level, as assessed by continuous measurements of cardiovascular functions (heart rate, blood pressure, electrocardiogram) and by clinical signs and symptoms (TABLE III).

The criteria to terminate the procedure determine the appropriate designation of the test:

Maximal Tolerated Workload (Symptom Limited Workload)—level at which symptoms appear

TABLE III
Target levels for training

A.   In Absence of "STRAIN" (disproportionate response to stress)

OXYGEN UPTAKE
57 & 78% Highest Aerobic Power (HAP) for Average & Peak Loads
        Maximal O_2 Intake ($\dot{V}O_2$ max)
        O_2 Intake of Highest Workload Performed (HWLP)

HEART RATE (HR)
70 & 85% Highest HR attained
70 & 85% Age Predicted Maximal HR (if HR of HWLP is within 10% APMHR)

EQUIVALENT HEART RATES*
Equivalent to Respiratory Exchange Ratio, R, = 0.95 to 1.0 +
Equivalent to 57 & 78 % HAP
Equivalent to Systolic Blood Pressure (SBP) mm Hg = 225 or less

SYSTOLIC BLOOD PRESSURE
Maximal value 225 mm Hg
Workload where SBP falls or fails to rise 9 to 12 mm Hg per increase of 10%
      $\dot{V}O_2$ max or of O_2 intake of HWLP (usually 0.8 to 1.2 METS)

B.   In SYMPTOMATIC SUBJECTS

OXYGEN INTAKE
57 & 78 % O_2 Intake of Highest Workload Performed

HEART RATE
70 & 85 % Highest HR Attained for Average & Peak Loads
EQUIVALENT HEART RATES (ALWAYS LESS THAN that which occurs with
        Any of the Following)
        ECG CHANGES
                Ventricular ectopic activity—frequent vpbs, salvos,
                    tachycardia
                Intraventricular and atrioventricular block
                ST-T displacement 4 to 5 mm +
        Blood pressure—inappropriate responses*
        Signs and symptoms

SIGNS AND SYMPTOMS
Cardiovascular
        Chest pain, discomfort, angina, with or without radiation
        New murmurs, gallops, marked venous distension
Respiratory
        Excessive dyspnea, rales
Central Nervous System
        Incoordination, light-headedness, faintness, syncope, glazed gaze
Other
        Cold sweat

SYMPTOMS AFTER EFFORT (immediately, delayed 2 to 24 hours)*
Insomnia, excessive excitement, exhilaration
Weakness, fatigue, muscular cramps, skeletal pain
Gastrointestinal disturbances, diarrhea, nausea, vomiting

---

*applies to A and B

Maximal Safe Workload—appearance of clinical signs and symptoms and especially ventricular ectopic activity in salvos or tachycardia, high degrees of AV or intraventricular block

Near Maximal Workload—in which neither symptoms nor signs appear, and 85 to 90 percent of age-predicted maximal heart rate is attained, from which data-predicted maximal O_2 intake may be obtained by extrapolation

Maximal oxygen intake ($\dot{V}O_2$ max)—when O_2 consumption does not increase with increasing workloads

Supermaximal—when increasing work is performed without an increase or with an actual decrease of O_2 intake (Fig. 1).

Regardless of which type of performance test is employed, the workload and its oxygen cost, and the physiologic responses can be used in prescribing the intensity of training. Needless to say, the prescribed effort for training should not exceed that of the exercise testing.

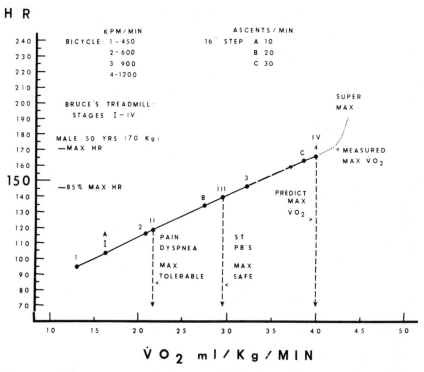

Fig. 1. Relationships among various types of highest performance tests: Maximal Tolerable, Maximal Safe, Predicted Maximal from high Submaximal, Maximal Oxygen Intake, and Supermaximal exercise tests (multilevel bicycle ergometer, Bruce's treadmill and step tests). Value of such tests in obtaining target levels for exercise prescription discussed in text.

In utilizing the results of exercise stress tests to formulate an exercise prescription, it must be ascertained that the tests were performed under standardized conditions of test protocol, environment, and preparation of the subject for the tests.

The performance of an individual may be underestimated and the exercise prescription geared at an unnecessarily low intensity because of the anxiety and unfamiliarity associated with the initial ergometric evaluation, especially if submaximal. Furthermore, the interpretation of the training responses may be clouded by the effects of lessening anxiety and the learning of the test procedure. For this reason, several tests (at least two) should be performed several days apart and the average of the tests, or the top value, used as a pretraining baseline [2].

Although the maximal performance ($\dot{V}O_2$ max) on the treadmill ergometer usually exceeds that on the steps or bicycle ergometer (3 and 6 percent respectively), the formulation of an exercise prescription, particularly in regard to the intensity of training, rarely will be influenced. However, the personal preference, dislike, or physical intolerance may determine the proper instrument for testing and/or training. For example, walking or jogging on a treadmill may be poorly tolerated by subjects with arthritic changes in the knees, hips, or spine. The bicycle seat may be discomfiting for subjects with sparse gluteal adipose tissue, varicocele, or prostatic difficulties.

Target levels for training. The target level for training is that parameter or the parameters which indicate that a desired workload has been imposed and that biochemical and physiological responses have been obtained, sufficient to produce a favorable effect on aerobic metabolism and physical fitness. The targets obviously will be determined by the parameters measured during the exercise tests. Heart rate, electrocardiograms (ECG), blood pressure, clinical signs, and symptoms are the most common end points because of the ease of their measurements. O_2 intake, cardiac output, systolic intervals, respiratory exchange ratio, serum lactates, and enzymatic determinations are probably equally desirable, but not yet practicable clinically.

Fortunately, there are interrelationships among these variables so that the quantitative evaluation of the heart rate, ECG, blood pressure, and symptoms provides a rational approach to exercise prescription. In general, the targets should indicate that a substantial load has been placed on the various functions of the muscle groups and of the heart being stressed. Because the threshold of the various functions of the heart differ, their perturbations can serve equally well as target levels: heart rate, alteration of repolarization (ST-T displacement), ectopic activity, delayed intraventricular or atrioventricular conduction, and disturbance of regulation of blood pressure.

Thus, evidence of *strain* includes the appearance of frequent ventricular ectopic beats or tachycardia, atrioventricular, intraventricular conduction defects, marked ST-T displacement (3 mm or more) or less if associated with severe angina pectoris (AP) or equivalents, disproportionate blood pressure responses (too high or too low—failure to increase blood pressure with higher work levels), chest pain with increasing radiation and severity, and excessive dyspnea. Central nervous system symptoms of confusion and incoordination occasionally serve as an important end point [3]

The energy cost of the exercise test level which is associated with the appearance of *strain*, or in its absence, a significant submaximal load serves as a guideline in prescribing other activities with equivalent or lesser aerobic demands in the subject with *strain*.

In this discussion, we will present the rationale for the use of heart rate, blood pressure, their products as an indirect measure of myocardial O_2 intake ($\dot{V}O_2$ max), and the external work performed as indices to prescribe the intensity of the exercise and the matching with activities of equivalent aerobic demands.

Essential Features of Workloads Which Influence Effectiveness of Training Programs

INTENSITY

The main factor that influences the response to a training regime is the intensity of effort relative to the individual subject's initial aerobic power. Training is also influenced by the frequency of exercise, and (marginally) by its duration [2].

In exercise testing and exercise prescription, it is highly desirable to select a known workload which places the same relative cardiovascular load upon individuals of different ages and fitness, or on the same individual at different times.

Oxygen intake has been used as a direct index of the intensity of training and other parameters (heart rate, blood pressure, electrocardiographic changes, lactates, respiratory exchange ratio-R, and other metabolites) as indirect indices.

The Body's Oxygen Intake During Training

The changes in cardiovascular and skeletal muscular fitness are directly related to the relative and absolute intensity of the training load [4]. Although enhancement of aerobic capacity is greatest with loads of 90-100 percent of the individual's capacity (usually in young healthy athletes) [5], significant improvement occurs at lower levels (50, 60, 70 percent), and less striking even at 25 percent [4-13] (Fig. 2). Cardiovascular function of middle-aged men improves equally at the intensities of 80 and 92 percent maximum heart rate, equal to 70 and 87 percent maximal oxygen intake [4]. Training loads of 50-70 percent of aerobic capacity are applicable to middle-aged and older normal subjects and selected postcoronary patients, and are preferred over potentially dangerous maximal levels. The latter should be restricted to healthy, untrained subjects and athletes.

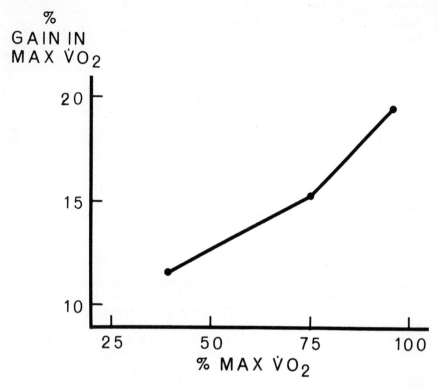

Fig. 2.   Relationship between the gain in aerobic power and intensity of exercise conditioning program which is standardized for all variables (frequency, duration, type of effort) except for intensity of training. Training at 38, 75, and 96 percent of initial maximal O_2 intake (abscissa) produced 11.8, 15.3, and 19.5 percent gain in aerobic power, respectively. For more fit subjects, the curve shifts to the right, indicating a greater improvement in less fit subjects than for more fit subjects when trained at the same relative intensity. (Modified after R.J. Shephard)

Åstrand and most other physiologists generally agree that enhancement of physical fitness of normal subjects requires the imposition of a moderate submaximal load (approximately 60 to 70 percent of the individual's maximal aerobic capacity) during training periods [14]. At this relative load, many physiological and biochemical changes [15] transpire: respiratory exchange ratio (R) approaches unity (Fig. 3), increases in blood lactate, fibrinolytic activity, urinary catecholamine excretion, capacity to oxidize fatty acids, release of fatty acids from adipose tissue, capacity to regenerate ATP by oxidative phosphorylation, protein content of mitochondrial fraction of skeletal muscle, etc., desirable changes which are associated with favorable adaptation and improvement [15-20]. Only recently has the question been raised whether the same training intensity can be applied to cardiacs and older normal subjects with limited performance.

Similar changes transpire in the myocardium when high submaximal loads are placed upon the circulation. When the oxygen demands exceed the available oxygen supply, metabolic myocardial acidosis occurs, R exceeds unity, coronary venous lactate rises, left ventricular end-diastolic pressure rises, and ectopic activity and displacement of the ST-T complex of the electrocardiogram (ECG) appear.

Estimation of oxygen intake in training. The routine direct measurement of oxygen intake during training is not feasible presently. For this reason, the body's oxygen intake during training is usually estimated from indirect measures, i.e., heart rate, and from activities whose energy costs are known.

Heart Rate

Since heart rate and body oxygen intake have a linear relationship at high submaximal and maximal levels of effort under standardized conditions, the heart rate during exercise can be used as a measure of the body's oxygen intake for the individual. Since heart rate and oxygen intake change with age, deconditioning, and disease, a specific heart rate may represent a wide range of oxygen intake. Arbitrary heart rates should not be used for testing, and especially not for training.

As age increases, the maximal heart rate decreases so that a particular heart rate represents a different percent of the maximal heart rate and of the maximal oxygen intake of subjects of different ages. Thus a heart rate of 150 represents 77, 81, 86, and 91 percent of the age-predicted maximal heart rate for men age 24, 35, 45, and 55 respectively. Effort tests which determine the workload

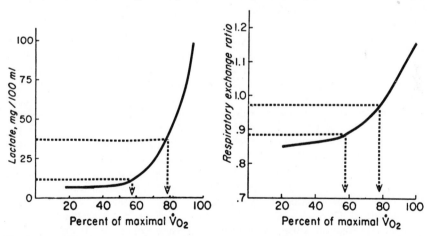

Fig. 3.   Relationship between intensity of exercise expressed as percent of maximal oxygen intake and changes in respiratory exchange ratio (R) and serum lactate. Between the range of 57 to 78 percent of maximal oxygen intake which corresponds to 70 and 85 percent of maximal heart rate, significant increase occurs in lactate and R approaches unity.

necessary to produce preset heart responses (150 or 170) fail to impose the same relative cardiovascular load, mainly because the target heart rates represent different percentages of the maximal heart rates for subjects of different ages. Obviously, to obtain a target level of effort to impose a desired metabolic load, one must either measure the individual's maximal oxygen intake and the oxygen intake of specific activities, or have an equivalent index thereof in the form of heart rate, blood pressure, ECG changes, or signs or symptoms.

Our recent investigations have shown that the relative workloads can be estimated with greater accuracy from heart rates expressed as fractions of maximum in men of varying ages, with widely divergent maximal oxygen intake in the presence or absence of coronary artery disease [21]. The heart rate expressed as percent of maximal heart rate bears significant relationships with coronary blood flow, myocardial oxygen intake, oxygen consumption as percent of maximal oxygen consumption, respiratory exchange ratio, lactate production, and catecholamine excretion [17, 18, 20] (Fig. 4).

Relationship Between Percent Maximal Oxygen Intake and Percent Maximal Heart Rate. Rationale for Target Heart Rates as Fractions of Maximal Pulse Rate in Submaximal or Near-Maximal Exercise Tests and in Exercise Training

Steady state exercise (Figs. 5 and 6). Fig. 5 presents the relationship between oxygen intake as percent of maximal oxygen intake and of heart rate as percent of heart rate at maximal oxygen intake, at rest, and during submaximal, near-maximal and maximal steady-state bicycle ergometer lower extremity exercise by 164 male subjects. Group I, 65 younger males, average age 27.1, S.D. 9.02; Group II, 63 older males (firemen), average age 40.2, S.D. 7.7; and Group III, 36 males with clinical coronary arteriosclerotic heart disease (ASHD), confirmed by coronary arteriograms in 26 subjects [21, 24]. The average age of Group III was 50.6, S.D. 1.00. True maximal oxygen intake was measured directly in 16 subjects of Group III, and indirectly by extrapolation to the age-predicted maximal heart rate in the remainder. The extrapolation was made from three near-maximal steady state work levels, the last of which elicited an average of 174 S.D. 19.1, 171.2, S.D. 12.7, and 153, S.D., 12.6 in Groups I, II, and III respectively, equivalent to 89, 95, and 91 percent of their age-predicted maximal heart rates of Groups I, II, and III respectively. The younger and older normals (Groups I and II) had an average functional aerobic impairment (FAI) of 9.0 and 14.0 percent, and the ASHD group 25.9 percent, calculated from Bruce's formula for maximal oxygen intake for normal sedentary subjects tested on a treadmill (Y = 55.8 - 0.41 age in years, where Y = functional aerobic impairment). Since maximal oxygen intake measured on a bicycle ergometer is consistently 5 to 6 percent lower than on a treadmill, the FAI of groups I, II, III can be estimated to be nearer to 3, 8, and 19 percent.

Our normal populations seem to be representative of the general urban, white, male, middle-class population, in that the quartiles based on functional

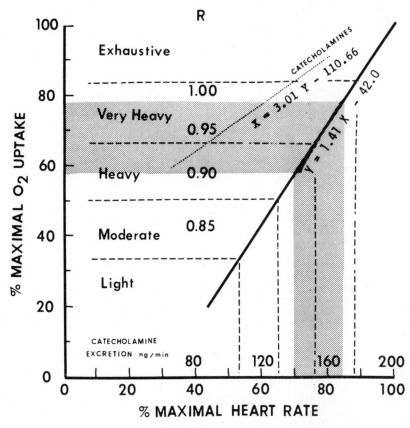

Fig. 4. Relationship between percent maximal O_2 intake (Y) and percent maximal heart rate (X) for normal and cardiac subjects. $Y = 1.41 \ X - 42.0$. Shaded area represents 70 to 85 percent of maximal heart rate equal to 57 and 78 percent of maximal O_2 intake, respectively. The favorable physiologic, biochemical, and anatomic adaptive responses to training within these intensities are considered to be related to the evoked changes in catecholamine excretion, respiratory exchange ratio (R), perceptive rating of the effort (light to exhaustive), and (not shown) significant elevations of lactate, renin, fibrinolysins, etc. (Discussed in text)

aerobic impairment (FAI) ranged from 32 percent impairment to a highly fit group with -16% impairment, i.e., 16 percent above normal fitness. The coronary subjects are representative of those who could attain a high submaximal heart rate.

The relationship between percent of age-predicted or attained maximal heart rate and percent of maximal oxygen intake was determined for each subject, for each age group, for the normal populations and its quartiles of functional aerobic impairment and for the total ASHD group (TABLE I). Regression lines were calculated on an Olivetti Programma 101. The formula for the regression

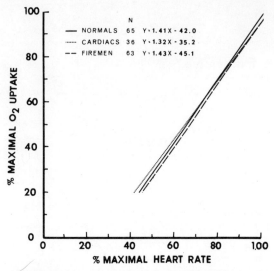

Fig. 5. The regression lines of two groups of normals and one of CHD subjects show similar relationship between submaximal oxygen intake expressed as percent of maximum and heart rates as percent of maximal heart rate. In the formula Y = percent maximal oxygen intake, and X = percent maximal heart rate.

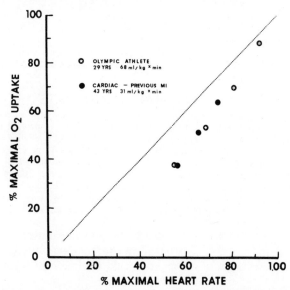

Fig. 6. A 29-year-old Olympic athlete and a 43-year-old man with a previous myocardial infarct showed similar relationship between their submaximal oxygen intake expressed as percent of maximum and percent maximal heart rate. Their data fall upon the regression lines for young and old normal subjects and for cardiacs (Figs. 3 & 4).

lines for the younger normal population (Group I) was $Y = 1.41 X - 42.0$, for the older normal population (Group II) $Y = 1.43 X - 45.1$ and for the ASHD subjects (Group III), $Y = 1.32X - 35.2$, where Y equals percent maximal oxygen intake ($\dot{V}O_2$ max) X = percent maximal heart rate (MHR). 't' was not significant between the upper and lower quartiles of the normals even at the 45 percent maximal oxygen level. The regression line of the ASHD group was not significantly different from our normal populations at any level.

Data collected on several age groups of normal subjects by Robinson who used treadmill techniques and by the Åstrands who used bicycle procedures were plotted by Taylor et al [14] on a graph of percent $\dot{V}O_2$ max against percent max heart rate. The agreement was ". . . excellent regardless of techniques, country in which the work was done, or the uncertainties of sample selection." Their data fell directly on the regression lines of our study populations which included normals and cardiacs. This agreement indicates that the relative oxygen cost of steady-state work can be predicted with remarkable precision from the heart rate, and that the relationship pertains in young and old, in the extremes of fitness, fit and unfit, and in normals and cardiacs (Fig. 6).

Limitations of the Use of Restricted Highest Heart Rate as Indices of Maximal Oxygen Intake and of Training Intensity

When the highest tolerated workload is significantly reduced, a degree of uncertainty may be expected in the use of the heart rate as an index of oxygen intake and of training intensity. This did not apply in Group III where the maximal heart rate was not reduced significantly; these ASHD subjects either attained their maximal heart rate or 90 percent of the age-predicted maximal heart rate and extrapolation to age-predicted maximal heart rate would not introduce a significant error. However, in a large number of ASHD subjects, the limiting factor may be the highest attained heart rate, which is often significantly reduced even in the absence of ischemic ST-T changes and would vitiate estimation of $\dot{V}O_2$ max. Thus in middle-aged normals, the average predicted maximal heart rate is 165 to 170, and in similar aged ASHD it may be 140 or less. Even though *strain* does not appear, the reduced ceiling on the heart rate may determine the level of training. An extreme example is the ASHD subject who has marked sinus bradycardia at rest (36/min) and at his tolerated work level attains a maximal heart rate of 96 to 100/min.

The restriction in the rise of the heart rate may be due to intrinsic disease of the sino-atrial or AV nodes, or due to the appearance of signs and symptoms which preclude exercising at a higher work level, which are: exertional hypertension, hypotension, ventricular ectopic activity in salvos or paroxysms, S-A or high degrees of AV block, 3 or 4 mm of ST-T displacement, severe AP, or other severe symptoms. In these cases, the age-predicted maximal heart rate should be considered unrealistically high; extrapolation from low values is unwarranted and heart rate cannot be considered as a measure of the $\dot{V}O_2$ max.

Instead, the heart rate at which any of the above signs or symptoms cause the termination of the test can be designated as the Maximal Safe Heart Rate and an average of 70 and peaks of 85 percent of this value can be used as guidelines in training prescription [3].

Although the intensity of training would appear to be too modest in such cases, significant improvement has been obtained in such subjects. This method is realistic and safe, in contrast to one scheme in which the intensity of training is based on the heart rate expressed as percent of the heart rate in age-predicted maximal exercise. In Karvonen's formula, the training heart rate (THR) equals the maximum age-adjusted heart rate (Max AAHR) minus the resting heart rate (MHR) times 60 or 70 percent plus the resting heart rate [25]. THR = (Max AAHR - RHR) X 60 or 70 percent + RHR. For example, if a 45-year-old man with an age-predicted maximal heart rate of 175 and resting heart rate of 62 attains a highest heart rate of 120 beats/min at which time he developed 4 mm ST-T displacement and severe chest pain, and the test is terminated, the theoretical available maximal heart rate would be 113 and the training heart rate according to Karvonen's formula would be (175 - 62) X 60 percent + 62 equals 130. This would be an unrealistic and potentially dangerous workload. At no time should the training intensity and heart rate exceed those of the exercise test. Our recommendation for training this subject would be an average heart rate of 84 (70 percent X 120) and peak heart rate of 102 (85 percent X 120). These values would correspond to 38 and 69 percent respectively of his actual heart rate reserve plus his resting heart rate: i.e., $84 = (120 - 62) x + 62$; and $102 = (120 - 62) x + 62$, respectively where x = percent available maximum heart rate and would represent 19.4 and 35.4 percent of the theoretical maximal heart rate reserve $(84 - 62) \times 100/175 - 62$, and $(120 - 62) \times 100/175 - 62$. Gualtiere and associates have confirmed that ASHD subjects with restricted maximal heart rates and work capacity show significant improvement when trained at 16 to 43 percent of theoretical maximal available heart rates [26].

In our opinion, the Karvonen formula has limited application in normals and especially in cardiacs.

Non-steady state exercise (Figs. 7 and 8). The relationship between percent of maximal heart rate to percent of maximal oxygen intake during non-steady state exercise was studied in 10 college students [27]. Their average age was 19.3, average maximal oxygen intake was 41.0 ml O_2/kg X min. Continuous oxygen intake was measured with a Guyton oxygen analyzer computer as the subjects exercised on a Lifecycle Exercise Bicycle with a built-in interval exercise program (Fig. 8). The program consisted of 30-second stepwise increments in resistance to pedaling followed by a relative decrease in resistance, a 2.5-min *steady state* period, followed by four 30-sec levels of increasing exercise interspersed with 30 sec of relative rest levels. The complete 12-min cycle of interval exercise can be varied in intensity and may be set at one of several arbitrary levels designated on the Lifecycle as 30, 50, 70, and 90 percent of the maximal capacity of the bicycle. The last 30-sec peaks of the exercise correspond to 6.23, 10.25, 14.73, and 18.77 cal/min respectively at the above four intensity settings.

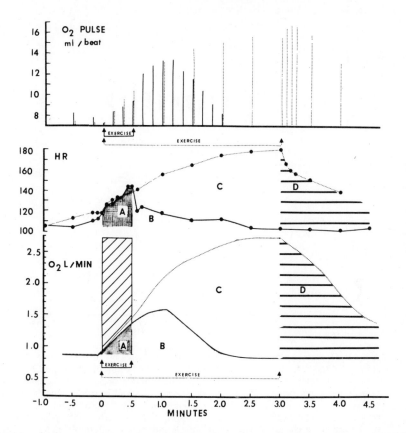

Fig. 7. Effects of duration of equal intensity bicycle ergometer exercise on O_2 intake, heart rate, and O_2 pulse. For the same intensity of effort (2.8 liters of O_2), in non-steady state exercise (NSS) for 30 seconds, the O_2 intake was less, the recovery O_2 intake and O_2 pulse were relatively greater than after steady state exercise (SS) for 3 minutes by the same subject. The ratio of the O_2 debt to O_2 consumed during effort was greater in NSS than in SS. The value of both types of effort in training and the relationship of the percent maximal heart rate and percent maximal O_2 intake during submaximal effort in NSS and SS are discussed in the text.

Total oxygen intake for the various work levels were obtained by integrating the total area under the oxygen intake curve for the particular level recorded on a Gilson Recorder. Regression lines were calculated for the relationship between the percent of the maximal heart rate during the last 10 seconds of the non-steady state exercise and the total oxygen intake during the 30 seconds of non-steady state exercise.

The oxygen intake during 30 seconds of exercise expressed as percent of maximal oxygen intake and showed a relationship to the heart rate during the

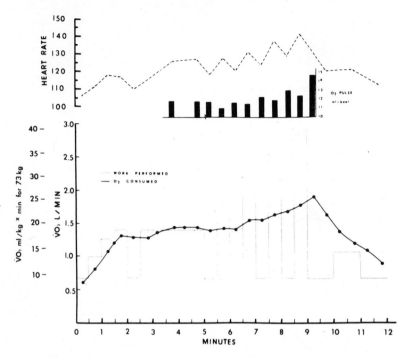

Fig. 8. Average O_2 intake, heart rate, and O_2 pulse responses of 10 men during steady-state (SS) and non-steady state (NSS) exercise on a 12-min programmed Lifecycle bicycle ergometer. The O_2 intake in the last half-minute of SS cycling equalled the rate of work performed. The O_2 intake during NSS and in subsequent 30 sec of recovery were equal and their sum was identical to the O_2 cost during SS of the same effort. The heart rate decreased during recovery after NSS while the O_2 intake remained elevated. As a result, the O_2 pulse increased, implying an increase of stroke volume and/or peripheral AV O_2 extraction. (Discussed in text)

last 10 seconds of 30 seconds of exercise expressed as percent of maximal heart rate. The formula for the regression line expressing the above relationship was ·y = 1.32 x - 34.6 where y = percent of maximal oxygen intake during 30 seconds exercise, and x = percent of maximal heart rate during the last 10 seconds of the 30 seconds of exercise. The regression lines for steady state and non-steady 30-second exercise are remarkably close to each other.

The heart rate when expressed as a percent of the individual's maximal heart rate (or maximal safe heart rate, or maximally tolerable heart rate) is valuable not only for steady·state exercise, but also for non-steady 30-seconds exercise. Furthermore, the relationship between cardiac output and O_2 intake has been shown to be similar during non-steady states of exercise to that of the steady state [28]. The heart rate reflects the actual O_2 intake during effort, brief or prolonged, but does not reflect as sensitively the RATE of work performed. In Fig. 8, during the hills of increasing magnitude, the oxygen intake, during the 30 seconds, constitutes approximately 50 percent of the oxygen intake during the fourth or fifth minute of sustained effort.

Oxygen pulse. Oxygen pulse (oxygen intake/heart beat) during the 30 seconds of exercise increased as the magnitude of each workload increased and showed an even greater oxygen pulse in the 30-second recovery period. At this time, the postexercise heart rate decreased and the oxygen intake increased slightly. The increase of oxygen pulse indicates that the stroke volume SV and/ or arterial-venous oxygen (AV O_2 difference) extraction increased during the recovery periods.

$$O_2 \text{ intake} = SV \times HR \times AV\ O_2 \text{ difference}$$

$$O_2 \text{ pulse} = \frac{O_2 \text{ intake}}{HR} = SV \times AV\ O_2 \text{ difference}$$

The enhancement of the latter two functions may be considered favorable from the standpoint of the myocardium and of the skeletal musculature. Since myocardial oxygen intake is influenced more by changes in heart rate [22] than in stroke volume, it is reasonable to believe that myocardial oxygen intake decreased as the oxygen pulse increased. The other possibility of an increased AV oxygen extraction by the peripheral tissues is one of the desirable major effects of training according to Detry and Bruce [29], and implies hypertrophy and/or hyperplasia of the skeletal muscular mitochondria and other favorable adaptive changes [15]. The implication can be made that 30 seconds of high-intensity work may have beneficial effects on aerobic capacity of the peripheral tissues.

Application of the Relationship Between Percent Maximal Heart Rate and Percent Maximal Oxygen Intake Application to Normal Subjects

The same relationship between percent maximal heart rate (MHR) and maximal oxygen intake pertains not only in cross-sectional but also in longitudinal studies, i.e., in individual subjects with changing aerobic capacity. We have demonstrated the value of this relationship in training a group of eight subjects, average age 24, who participated in an 8-week training program with three 30-minute sessions a week [27]. The intensity of training was designed to elicit 50 and 60 percent of MHR during 4 minutes of warmup, 70 percent for two periods, each 9 min in duration, interrupted by 4 min at 85 percent, followed by 4 min of tapering off for 2 min each at 60 and 50 percent of MHR respectively. Prior to entry into the study, true maximal oxygen intake was determined from the second test on a Monark bicycle ergometer. The workloads were adjusted (increased) during the training period to attain the prescribed heart rate. The average $\dot{V}O_2$ max increased from the initial pretraining value 46.6 to 53.5 ml O_2/kg B.W. x min, an improvement of 14.8 percent, $p < 0.005$. Similar improvement in aerobic capacity of other normal young, and of middle-aged subjects, and hypertensives has occurred in studies in which the intensity of the training program was based on a measured percent of the maximal heart rate [4, 5, 7, 10, 31-35]. Pollock and associates obtained an improvement of VO_2 max of 19 and 14 percent in 22 middle-aged men trained for 45 min 2 days per week at 92 and 80 percent of maximal heart rate, respectively. These authors stated that a training heart rate of approximately 85 percent of max is both desirable and comfortable for normal middle-aged men [4].

Shephard demonstrated that the main factor influencing the extent of training achieved was the intensity of the effort relative to the subject's initial aerobic power [2]. A group of 39 sedentary subjects was trained on the treadmill, using one of three graded intensities of effort equivalent to 39, 75, and 96 percent of maximal aerobic power and 57, 83, and 98 percent of maximal heart rate [2]. The sedentary subject with an initial aerobic power of 41.8 ml/kg x min trained at the highest intensity (96 percent) five times per week for 3 weeks and showed a 19.5 percent gain of aerobic power. In contrast, the same intensity produced a training response of only 5.8 percent in a subject with initial aerobic power of 51.8 ml/kg x min. In other words, the most unfit subjects showed the greatest improvement with the same intensity of training. Saltin and associates found a similar relationship between initial fitness and improvement in his study of five young subjects reconditioned after 3 weeks of bed rest [5].

Application to ASHD subjects. Our reported experiences in the training of 254 convalescent and postconvalescent ASHD subjects have been reevaluated in terms of the above relationships [32]. These subjects showed an average improvement of 24.6 percent of $\dot{V}O_2$ max (TABLE IV). In the CWRU-JCC study, following the evaluation of each subject, a program was formulated to enhance his overall fitness. The subject met with a study physician and a physical educator who reviewed with him the results of all tests performed, answered any questions, and prescribed for him a specific exercise program. The exercise program purposely was not restricted solely to running or calisthenics. It consisted of walking and running to build endurance and calisthenics for strength. The caloric expenditure of full participation at each training session totaled approximately 400 calories per hour (average 4.5 METS). Calisthenics required up to 200 calories (average 4.4 METS, maximal 6 METS) over a 30-min period; run-walk sequences, 120 calories (5.2 METS) over a 15-min period; and recreational exercise for fun, 80 calories (3.5 METS) over a 15-min period. Since the average subject on entry had an average maximal aerobic power of 6-7 METS, few were entered at full participation. Most individuals began by performing 1/2-2/3 of each series of calisthenic exercises, and slower paces of the run-walk sequences. The design of the calisthenic sequences purposely included a warmup period, work period, and a tapering-off period. Run-walk sequences were initially prescribed at low levels of work and were gradually increased until a subject could run a mile. Recreational activity, i.e., basketball, volleyball, swimming, bag-punching, etc., was advocated, but highly competitive games demanding sudden spurts of energy were proscribed. In addition, the subjects were advised to be active physically elsewhere, to climb stairs, to avoid

TABLE IV

Changes in cholesterol and hemodynamic parameters of 100 ASHD subjects after training [32]

Item	Initial	Followup	p
Cholesterol (mg/100 ml)	263.5	241.1	.01
Blood pressure (mm Hg)	s 129.9	121.7	.01
at rest	d 86.8	84.3	.05
during exercise	s 191.3	171.6	.001
Maximal O_2 intake (ml O_2/kg BW/min)	23.2	28.9	.01
Workload 150 (kpm/kg BW/min)	8.1	9.8	.01
SBP $\times$ HR $\times$ 10-^{2} during exercise	248.3	192.7	.001
SBP $\times$ HR 25 $\times$ 10-^{3} (kpm/min)	496	609	.001

the use of elevators, to walk instead of riding a bicycle, to park farther away from the parking lots, and similar.

Monitored heart rates during early training demonstrated that an average heart rate of 120 beats/min was attained during 30 min of calisthenics, equal to 73 percent of the predicted maximal heart rate for men 50-years-old, equivalent to 60 percent of maximal oxygen intake. The peak heart rate of 140/min during running sequences corresponded to approximately 80 percent of maximal heart rate and 70 percent of maximal oxygen intake (Figs. 9, 10).

The relationship between percent maximal oxygen intake and percent maximal heart rate could be applied to subjects as their physical fitness improved. Since improving fitness was accompanied by an increased maximal intake, the same percent of maximal oxygen intake represents an increasing workload. Thus, as the training subject improved, more work was required to achieve the same heart rate.

Sixty to 75 percent of the patients with MI, but without congestive heart failure and/or uncontrolled arrhythmias, responded favorably to the CWRU-JCC supervised, long-term reconditioning programs (TABLE IV). Beneficial effects include: (1) improvement of subjective well-being and decrease of psychological depression; (2) marked improvement of aerobic power and cardiovascular hemodynamics (increased stroke volume, decreased tension time index, and increased vigor of heart beat); (3) decreased lactate production for the same workload; (4) reduction of hypertensive blood pressure values during exercise, and of peripheral vascular resistance; (5) diminution of the heart rate at rest, during sleep, and during exercise; (6) quantitative lessening of the RS-T segment

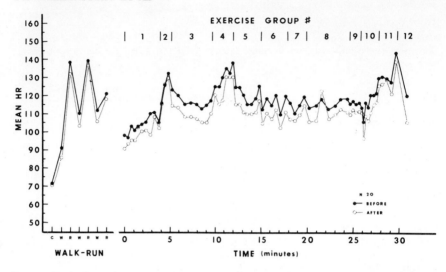

Fig. 9. Average heart rates of walk-run sequences (W = walk, R = run, C = control) and of consecutively performed calisthenics done routinely in the CWRU-JCC study. The ECGs of 20 subjects (average age 48) were telemetered before (solid lines) and several months after (dotted lines) participation in the training program. Note that the average heart rate was about 120 beats/min, representing 70 percent of their highest exercise test heart rate. Exercise numbers: (1) shoulder exercises, standing, warmup; (2) hops, walk steps; (3) arm sweeps, standing; (4) hops, sailor's horn-pipe; (5) body bends; (6) leg exercises, supine; (7) leg-arm-hip exercise, sitting on floor; (8) leg exercises, lying on side; (9) leg exercises, bicycle movements, supine; (10) situps; (11) pushups—not performed by all subjects; and (12) shoulder exercises, standing, cool off.

displacement during exercise; (7) lowering of serum lipid levels; (8) reduction of adipose tissue; (9) enhanced oxygen extraction by the peripheral tissues; (10) suggestive reduction in mortality; (11) enhancement of intercoronary collaterals rarely demonstrated by coronary angiograms; (12) partial or complete normalization of pretraining pathological ballistograms; and (13) enhancement of sexual activity [36, 37].

Indirect Estimation of Myocardial Oxygen Intake During Testing and Training

Heart Rate and Blood Pressure Guidelines

The intensity of an activity can be measured by the aerobic load placed upon the body, the working skeletal musculature, and on the myocardium. The ability to perform muscular effort depends in large part on the capacity of both the skeletal musculatures and the myocardium to extract and to utilize oxygen, from the peripheral and coronary arteries respectively. The magnitude of the oxygen consumption depends on the load placed on the myocardium as well as the integrity of the coronary arteries, the perfusion pressure and the status of the myocardium.

The myocardial oxygen consumption cannot be measured directly by noninvasive techniques. However, it may be estimated from its relationship to its major determinants: heart rate, intramyocardial tension (pressure X stress), and the contractile state of the heart. In practical terms, myocardial oxygen consumption in ml/min/100 gm left ventricle may be estimated from the relationship of the product of the heart rate (HR) and systolic blood pressure (SBP mm Hg), r = 0.88 [22] or the triple product of HR X SBP X left ventricular ejection time (LVET).

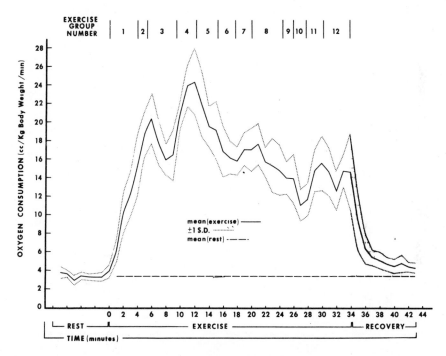

Fig. 10. O_2 cost of consecutively performed calisthenics performed routinely in the CWRU-JCC study. Exercise numbers 1-12 performed were described in Fig. 9 caption. Shaded area represented cooling-off period. Upon intake into the study most subjects performed one-half or one-third of the frequencies of the above exercises, depending upon their highest performance on the initial exercise pre-training tests. As capacity improved, their exercise prescriptions were evised until the full cadence and count of the exercises were attained. Pushups were not performed by subjects with hypersensitive carotid sinus reflexes or abnormal re sponses to the Flack (Valsalva) ECG test.

Fig. 11 presents the relationship of the HR × SBP product with the oxygen intake of 100 gm of left ventricle. From this product, the myocardial oxygen requirement can be estimated for any work level. Blood pressure response to multilevel exercise provides a measure of the intensity of the effort and a target for training. We have previously reported that for the same absolute workload, untrained normals and untrained ASHD subjects have higher systolic and diastolic pressures and heart rates and HR × SBP product than trained subjects (Fig. 12). In other words, the former have relative tachycardia and hypertension during effort.

The ratio of $M\dot{V}O_2$/100 gm LV to the body's $\dot{V}O_2$ is approximately 13 to 1 at rest in fit and unfit normotensive subjects, and is lower during submaximal

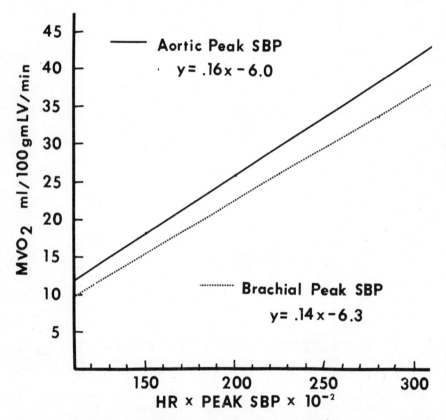

Fig. 11. Linear relationship between myocardial O_2 intake ($M\dot{V}O_2$) and heart rate × systolic blood pressure product (HR × SBP) obtained in normal young subjects during multilevel exercise, r = .92 (Kitamura, et al [22]). The HR × SBP product provides an indirect estimation of the $M\dot{V}O_2$, as expressed in terms of ml 02 per 100 gm left ventricle. For example, a product of 25,000 corresponds to 30 ml 02/100 gm LV/min, when the brachial cuff blood pressure is used, and 34 ml 02/100 gm LV/min when central aortic pressure is obtained.

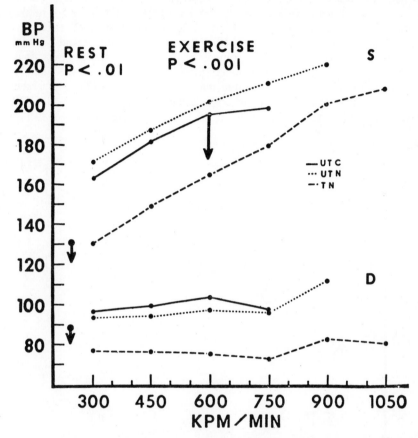

Fig. 12. Systolic and diastolic blood pressures during submaximal steady-state bicycle ergometer exercise are much lower in trained normal subjects (TN) than in untrained subjects (UTN = normals, UTC = cardiacs). Systolic blood pressure becomes comparable at the highest work levels. At any absolute work level the TNs have a lower systolic and lower diastolic blood pressure than the untrained subjects. However, the systolic blood pressure at submaximal and maximal effort is comparable in the above three groups when related to the percent of maximal heart rate and percent of maximal oxygen intake. (See Fig. 13) The arrow shows the improvement in blood pressure response of CHD subjects after participating in a training program. (Discussed in text)

and maximal effort in fit subjects than in unfit subjects, i.e., 14 to 1, and 18 to 1, respectively [24]. Stated otherwise, unfit normals and cardiacs have a disproportionately large myocardial oxygen consumption during effort, which may explain in part why coronary insufficiency occurs in ASHD, hypertensive subjects with normal coronary arteries, and subjects who have systemic hypertension or left ventricular hypertension due to aortic valvular stenosis.

When the systolic blood pressure is correlated with the percent of the maximal attained heart rate or with the percent of the maximal oxygen intake, differences disappear between fit and unfit subjects. The formula $Y = 1.15 X + 85.72$ expresses the relationship between systolic blood pressure during submaximal to maximal bicycle ergometer exercise testing and the percent of maximal heart rate. Y = systolic blood pressure in mm Hg, X = percent of maximal heart rate. Fig. 13 shows the relationship between SBP and percent max HR and $\dot{V}O_2$ max, in 63 firemen who attained maximal performance. The average maximal systolic blood pressure was 198.6 mm Hg S.E. 3.39, with 75

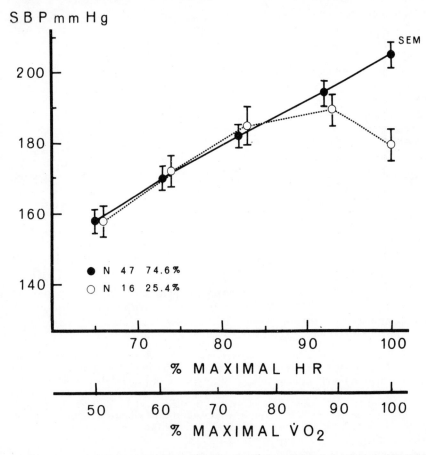

Fig. 13. Data from bicycle ergometer exercise of 63 firemen shows a linear relationship between submaximal O_2 intake and heart rate, expressed as percent of maximal, and simultaneously measured systolic blood pressure. This relationship is linear to maximal level in 74.6 percent and is linear in 25.4 percent up to 90 percent of the maximal heart rate and 85 percent of maximal O_2 intake, following which the systolic blood pressure decreases. The functional aerobic capacity, age, and health status were not significantly different in the type groups of responders.

percent of the subjects having an average of 205 mm Hg, S.E. and occurring at the highest workload, and 25 percent having their maximal SBP occurring at 85 to 90 percent of the MHR. There were no significant differences between the regression lines of the relationship between SBP and % MHR in the three age groups (25-34, 35-44, and 45 and older), or in the fit and unfit subjects [24].

The systolic blood pressure increases 12 to 15 mm Hg for each 10 percent increment of MHR and 9 to 12 for each increment of 10 percent $\dot{V}O_2$ max. Because of the differences in $\dot{V}O_2$ max of fit and unfit subjects, the increments of systolic blood pressure are expressed in terms of increments of $\dot{V}O_2$ max rather than in absolute terms of METS or ml O_2/kg B.W. X min. In the case of the firemen whose average $\dot{V}O_2$ max was 33.2 ml O_2/kg B.W. X min, S.D. 5.09, 10 percent of $\dot{V}O_2$ max equals 0.94 METS; for the average CHD subject with $\dot{V}O_2$ max of 25 ml O_2/kg B.W. X min, 10 percent of $\dot{V}O_2$ max would equal 0.71 MET.

The blood pressure response can be considered to be inappropriate if the blood pressure fails to rise appropriately with increasing workloads, at least to 90 percent MHR, or falls outside of 198.6 mm plus or minus one S.D, 26.9, i.e., 226 - 171, relative exertional hypertension or hypotension, respectively.

Thus the blood pressure itself, and the heart rate X systolic blood pressure product - a measure of myocardial O_2-correlate with the appearance of clinical and ECG evidence of coronary insufficiency (AP, ST-T changes, ectopic activity) and can be used as guidelines in exercise training. The ECG changes of the heart rate at which an excessive HR X SBP product or significant exertional hypertension occur also serve as valuable target indicators of the effective intensity of training.

Factors which Influence the Indirect Indices of Oxygen Intake by the Body and by the Myocardium

Arm exercise vs leg exercise. The heart rate is significantly higher in both the sitting and supine positions during arm work compared to leg work at a given oxygen intake or external workload [38]. A representative example shows that a heart rate of 186 beats occurred during 600 kpm/min arms bicycle ergometer work, with $\dot{V}O_2$ max 18.6 ml O_2/kg B.W. X min, and 190 beats during leg bicycling, with $\dot{V}O_2$ max 41.2 ml O_2/kg B.W. X min (Fig. 14). Thus the maximal $\dot{V}O_2$ of the body is significantly lower with arm work than with leg work.

O_2 intake during maximal arm work, including that involved in maximal swimming, does not reach the same level in most subjects as during maximal running or bicycling [39]. The reasons for this difference are not known. In swimming, the supine body position may favor capillary perfusion of the working muscle, because of lesser hydrostatic pressure compared to that in the legs in the upright working position. Also, swimming and arm exercise out of water both activate muscle groups of lesser total mass than in running and cycling. The O_2 intake and cardiac output during maximal arm cycling amounted to 66 and 80 percent respectively of the maximal values in leg cycling [39].

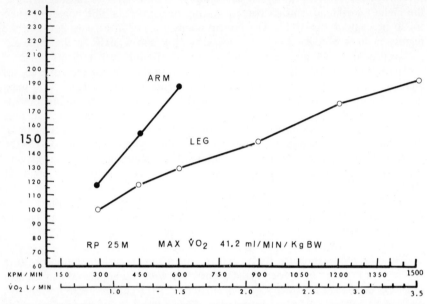

Fig. 14. Comparison of work performance of a normal 25-year-old man performing multi-level steady-state cycling using the arms and a day later the legs. His highest heart rate was 190/min during leg cycling at 1500 kpm/min. The heart rate was 186/min at 600 kpm/min during arm cycling. The maximal O_2 intake was 41.2 and 18.6 ml O_2/kg B.W. $\times$ min, respectively. (Discussed in text)

Because of the high cost in terms of energy expenditure and heart rate, even of floating and swimming at low speeds, swimming can be considered a good type of training of the oxygen transport system [39]. Since the breaststroke is the least efficient style in relation to swimming speed, Åstrand recommends it for training in preference to the front crawl or other stroke.

The relationship between % MHR and % $\dot{V}O_2$ max has not yet been calculated for arm exercise, although it is reasonable to estimate that the regression line will be located to the left of that for leg exercise. In exercise prescription, the differences in heart rate responses to arm and to leg exercises must be taken into account, and because of the lack of cross-adaptation, arm and torso exercises, as in calisthenics, should be included with walking, jogging, and bicycling. Clausen and Trap-Jensen have shown that training of arm muscles affected heart rate response only during arm exercise, and vice versa [40].

Environmental factors. Exercise stress tests are usually performed in a temperature-controlled environment, with the subject usually clad in light clothes or shorts. The heart rate and blood pressure responses during effort are affected by humidity, dusts, and particularly by external changes in temperature (heat and cold), and when the subject wears protective clothes, which interferes with the dissipation of heat (Fig. 15). The heart rate and blood pressure targets

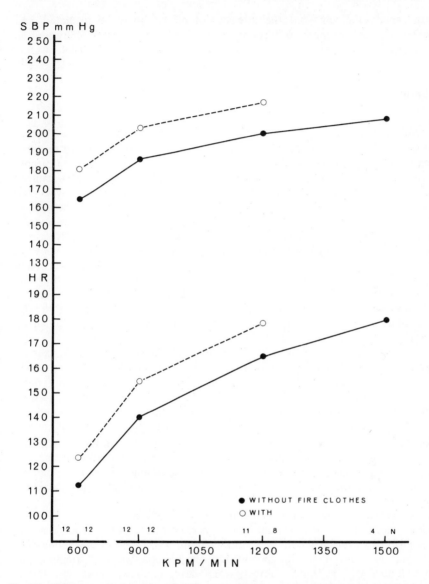

Fig. 15. Influence of protective clothing on exercise tolerance of 12 firemen, aged 40. Heart rate and systolic blood pressure responses to steady-state bicycle ergometer exercise were consistently higher when performed while wearing clothing which interfered with heat loss than while wearing shorts. The highest tolerated workload was reduced from 1500 to 1200 kpm/min. Thus for any given workload, the heart rate and systolic blood pressure were higher, causing the relationship between percent of maximal heart rate and percent maximal O_2 intake to shift to the left of the regression line shown in Fig. 4.

may remain the same but the intensity of effort should be regulated, i.e., decreased. Under these conditions, the myocardial oxygen consumption becomes disproportionately high compared to the body's oxygen intake.

FREQUENCY

Although many sports physiologists [31] believe that cardiorespiratory fitness is best improved and maintained by *vigorous* (70 to 85 percent maximal heart rate) exercise five times per week, convincing evidence has been offered recently that similar benefits can be attained by participating in organized training programs of approximately 30 to 45 minutes, three times a week and maintained by 2 to 2.5 sessions a week. Shephard reported that the gain in aerobic power decreased from 19.5 to 16.0 percent when subjects decreased the frequency of training from five to three times per week [2]. Recently, Brynteson and Sinning studied the effects of different weekly exercise exposures on retention of cardiovascular fitness of 21 subjects who were first conditioned by 5 weeks of bicycle ergometer exercise with work rates to accelerate the heart rate to 80 percent of its maximum. The subjects were divided into four groups which exercised one, two, three, or four times per week at the same work rate. $\dot{V}O_2$ max, recovery heart rate and O_2 pulse improvements were retained by exercising three times per week [41].

In our experience with over 350 ASHD subjects who were given an exercise prescription which required full participation of 1 hour three times a week, analysis of the daily record of attendance indicated that significantly more subjects who trained from 2.2 to 3 sessions per week or more showed improvement in aerobic capacity and ST-T responses to exercise tests and less significant improvement occurred in participants in 1.0 to 2.0 sessions per week. Surprisingly, the subjects who did attend from 3.5 to 5.0 sessions per week did not show more improvement than the 2.2-3.0 groups. Nevertheless, normal subjects have increased their aerobic capacity by attending twice a week, training at higher intensities than the cardiac subjects (80 and 92 percent of maximal heart rate [4]).

The detraining effects of reducing the frequency of training periods of 9 blind men demonstrated that approximately 50 percent of the gain in aerobic power was lost in 10 weeks if the subjects continued the same intensity of training once a week, in contrast to 50 percent lost in 5 weeks when all training was discontinued [34]. Other investigators have reported most circulatory parameters return to pretraining levels after 10 weeks of detraining [42].

DURATION

The main factor influencing the extent of training produced by a training program is the intensity of the training effort, with frequency and duration exerting lesser and marginal effects respectively [2]. A review of over 29 training programs of normal and cardiac subjects reveals a similarity of improvement, despite a considerable variation in the duration of the training sessions [1]. In general, high-intensity and short-duration training programs have been prescribed for normal subjects and the opposite (less intensity and longer duration) for older normal subjects, cardiacs, and hypertensives, or coronary-prone subjects. Hollmann and coworkers reported significant improvement in subjects trained by stationary running for only 10 min/day [43]. Siegel and associates trained blind subjects with four periods of bicycle ergometer exercise each lasting 3 min and followed by a 3-min rest period, totaling 21 minutes excluding time for warmup and cooling-off. The duration of training of larger groups of subjects generally is longer, with 3 to 15 minutes' warmup, 20 to 40 minutes' dynamic workout and often games, and 3 to 5 minutes for cooling-off. The longer training sessions with their greater diversity of activities undoubtedly favorably influence adherence to a training program, especially when conducted in groups. This may account for the superiority of group over individual training.

Hopefully, in the near future, studies will be made to determine if Shephard's sophisticated observations on the *Intensity, Duration, and Frequency of Exercise as Determinants of the Response to a Training Regime* [2] can be applied equally well to cardiac subjects. Meanwhile, on the basis of our experiences and others reported, we feel justified in recommending the optimal minimum to be 30 minutes, for 3 or 4 nonconsecutive sessions a week. This includes warmup, high-intensity, submaximal effort prescribed according to the principles described above, and cooling-off.

In other words, matching test performance with specific activities is validated by the dose-response relationship that prevails during or after the activities. The responses may vary from session to session because of differences in the vigor of performing the activity, intercurrent infection, changing cardiac emotional and health status, and the like. The tables of energy costs and other systems of estimating the intensity of activities (Cooper's point system [44]) have limited value unless related to the responses of the individual.

The intensity of the prescription should be revised downward as well as upward on the basis of test reevaluations and upon the response to the prescriptions. Resumption of training after an intercurrent illness or other absenteeism, should be set at a lower intensity than prior to the interruption. The subject should perform minimal exercise in the first resumed session and progress up the scale of his original exercise prescription, recapturing his former level in a time period relative to the period of inactivity.

Method of Equivalence in Exercise Prescription

(Matching Test Performance with Specific Activities)

Mode of training. Training effects are basically independent of the mode of isotonic muscular training when the frequency, duration, and intensity of training are held constant. Pollock and associates recently reported that improvement in cardiovascular function was similar in three groups of subjects who were trained for 30 minutes three times a week for 20 weeks, at 85 to 90 percent of their maximal heart rate. Maximal O_2 intake increased in the walkers, runners, and bicyclists, respectively, 37 to 41, 38 to 42, and 39 to 42 ml O_2/kg B.W. × min, with equal changes in resting heart rate, weight loss (3 pounds), skinfold fat and waist girth [35]. The major consideration should be the individual's personal preferences and feasibilities of the various types of activities.

It was mentioned in a previous section that since training of arm muscles affects heart responses only during arm exercises, and not during leg exercises, and vice versa, arm and torso exercises should be included in training programs, and not restricted to running and cycling, which is so often practiced.

Matching test performance with specific activities. In the pretraining evaluation, the energy cost of the level of the exercise test which elicited the targets for training is determined. This energy cost is best expressed in ml O_2/kg B.W. × min., or in METS, and while not measured directly, can be obtained from published data for all currently used standardized exercise test [45]. As soon as the O_2 cost of the desired training level has been determined, a pharmacopeia of activities (TABLE V, Fig. 16) and their oxygen costs can be

TABLE V

Approximate metabolic cost of activities*

(By permission of The American Heart Association, Inc. [45])

	Occupational	Recreational
1½–2 METs† 4–7 ml O₂/min/kg 2–2½ kcal/min (70 kg person)	Desk work Auto driving‡ Typing Electric calculating machine operation	Standing Walking (strolling 1.6 km or 1 mile/hr) Flying,‡ motorcycling‡ Playing cards‡ Sewing, knitting
2–3 METs 7–11 ml O₂/min/kg 2½–4 kcal/min (70 kg person)	Auto repair Radio, TV repair Janitorial work Typing, manual Bartending	Level walking (3¼ km or 2 miles/hr) Level bicycling (8 km or 5 miles/hr) Riding lawn mower Billiards, bowling Skeet,‡ shuffleboard Woodworking (light) Powerboat driving‡ Golf (power cart) Canoeing (4 km or 2½ miles/hr) Horseback riding (walk) Playing piano and many musical instruments
3–4 METs 11–14 ml O₂/min/kg 4–5 kcal/min (70 kg person)	Brick laying, plastering Wheelbarrow (220 kg or 100 lb load) Machine assembly Trailer-truck in traffic Welding (moderate load) Cleaning windows	Walking (5 km or 3 miles/hr) Cycling (10 km or 6 miles/hr) Horseshoe pitching Volleyball (6-man noncompetitive) Golf (pulling bag cart) Archery Sailing (handling small boat) Fly fishing (standing with waders) Horseback (sitting to trot) Badminton (social doubles) Pushing light power mower Energetic musician
4–5 METs 14–18 ml O₂/min/kg	Painting, masonry Paperhanging	Walking (5½ km or 3½ miles/hr) Cycling (13 km or 8 miles/hr)

TABLE V cont.

	Occupational	Recreational
5–6 kcal/min (70 kg person)	Light carpentry	Table tennis Golf (carrying clubs) Dancing (foxtrot) Badminton (singles) Tennis (doubles) Raking leaves Hoeing Many calisthenics
5–6 METs 18–21 ml O_2/min/kg 6–7 kcal/min . (70 kg person)	Digging garden Shoveling light earth	Walking (6½ km or 4 miles/hr) Cycling (16 km or 10 miles/hr) Canoeing (6½ km or 4 miles/hr) Horseback ("posting" to trot) Stream fishing (walking in light current in waders) Ice or roller skating (15 km or 9 miles/hr)
6–7 METs 21–25 ml O_2/min/kg 7–8 kcal/min (70 kg person)	Shoveling 10/min (22 kg or 10 lbs)	Walking (8 km or 5 miles/hr) Cycling (17½ km or 11 miles/hr) Badminton (competitive) Tennis (singles) Splitting wood Snow shoveling Hand lawn-mowing Folk (square) dancing Light downhill skiing Ski touring (4 km or 2½ miles/hr) (loose snow) Water skiing
7–8 METs 25–28 ml O_2/min/kg 8–10 kcal/min (70 kg person)	Digging ditches Carrying 175 kg or 80 lbs Sawing hardwood	Jogging (8 km or 5 miles/hr) Cycling (19 km or 12 miles/hr) Horseback (gallop) Vigorous downhill skiing Basketball Mountain climbing Ice hockey Canoeing (8 km or 5 miles/hr) Touch football Paddleball
8–9 METs 28–32 ml O_2/min/kg 10–11 kcal/min (70 kg person)	Shoveling 10/min (31 kg or 14 lbs)	Running (9 km or 5½ miles/hr) Cycling (21 km or 13 miles/hr) Ski touring (6½ km or 4 miles/hr) (loose snow) Squash racquets (social) Handball (social) Fencing Basketball (vigorous)

10 plus METs
32 plus ml O_2/min/kg
11 plus kcal/min
(70 kg person)
	Shoveling 10/min
	(35 kg or 16 lbs)
		Running: 6 mph = 10 METs
		         7 mph = 11½ METs
		         8 mph = 13½ METs
		         9 mph = 15 METs
		        10 mph = 17 METs
		Ski touring (8+ km or 5+ miles/hr)
		   (loose snow)
		Handball (competitive)
		Squash (competitive)

*Includes resting metabolic needs.

†1 MET is the energy expenditure at rest, equivalent to approximately 3.5 ml O_2/kg body weight/minute.

‡A major excess metabolic increase may occur due to excitement, anxiety, or impatience in some of these activities, and a physician must assess his patient's psychological reactivity.

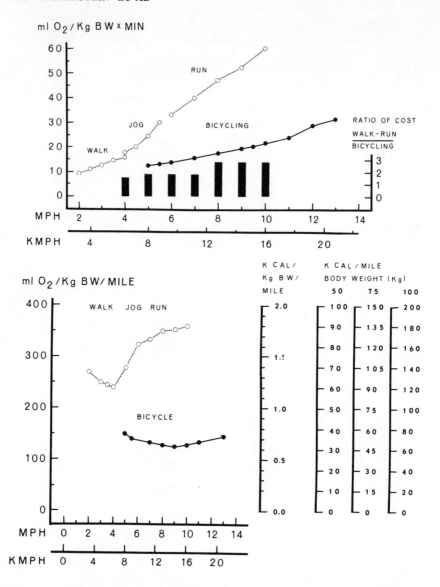

Fig. 16. Relationship between O_2 cost in ml O_2/kg body weight/min (Part A) and in ml O_2/kg body weight/mile (Part B), and speed of walking, jogging, running, and bicycling. The cost of walking, jogging, or running is approximately 2.5 to 3 times more costly than bicycling 4 to 10 mph. The most efficient rates of walking and of bicycling are between 3.5 to 4.0 and 9.0 mph, respectively, in terms of O_2 intake/kg/mile covered. For the individual whose aerobic capacity or whose O_2 cost of highest workload performed has been measured, the speed of locomotion by foot or by bicycling can be prescribed to produce a desired intensity and training effect.

consulted and a plan of activities formulated. For example, let us consider a subject who has a $\dot{V}O_2$ max of 28 ml O_2/kg B.W. × min and associated highest heart rate of 170 beats/min. His training intensity at an average, and peak expenditures during the training session have been recommended to be 16 and 22 ml O_2/kg B.W. × min and heart rates 120 and 144 respectively. Fig. 16 and TABLE V would provide a wide choice of activities for these energy levels: for the average expenditure, walking at 3.0 to 3.5 mph, cycling at 8 mph, table tennis, dancing foxtrot, raking leaves, etc.; for peak level activities—jogging at 4.5 to 5 mph, cycling at 11 mph, singles tennis, folk square dancing, etc.

Of course, each training session should include warmup, interval activities, and cooling down. Also, the subject would initially start somewhat below the prescribed level. The pace ordinarily would increase within several weeks to the intensity of the target levels. The propriety of the prescription can be determined by checking the heart rate, blood pressure, ECG, signs and symptoms, and from the retest evaluations of performance. Whenever the target levels are exceeded by a prescribed activity, the intensity of the activity should be decreased, or in some cases, the subject should be reevaluated if functional capacity seems to be deteriorating.

The individual subject should be instructed and urged to participate actively in evaluating his own responses, by recording his symptoms and heart rate. He should be able to determine whether his heart rate is within the range of his prescribed average and peaks. In the symptomatic subject, the relative magnitude of the training activity can be estimated from the time of appearance, type, intensity, progression, location, and radiation of pain or equivalent distress.

Fig. 17 presents a guide and form used by our symptomatic subjects to describe their responses to training [46]. When pain predictably recurs,

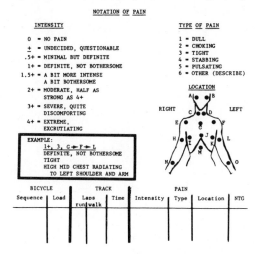

Fig. 17. Symptoms as target levels in exercise training of subjects with CHD. This method of coding and recording is valuable in assessing the response to training and in regulating its intensity.

sublingual nitroglycerin has been prescribed prior to and during each training session. Generally, nitroglycerin increases the subsequent effort by 1 to 1½ METS (Fig. 18). The apparent improvement of performance on medications

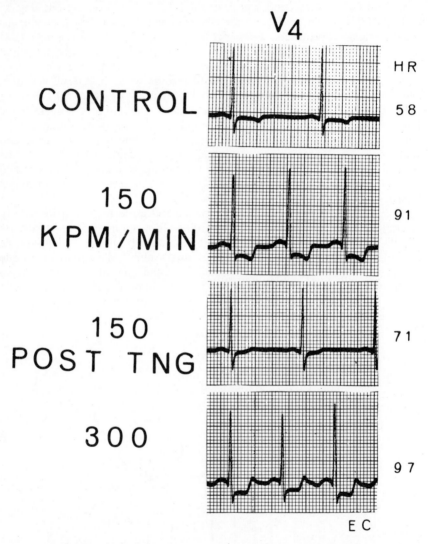

Fig. 18. Beneficial effects of nitroglycerin on ECG and heart rate responses to effort in subjects with severe CHD. Marked ischemic ST-T depression and heart rate of 91/min occurred during 150 kpm/min. Following sublingual nitroglycerin, the same intensity of effort produced a slower heart rate and no ST-T depression. The next workload, 300 kpm/min, produced ST-T depression and heart rate equal to those at 150 kpm/min, without nitroglycerin.

(nitroglycerin, isosorbide dinitrate, propanolol, etc.) may be misleading (Figs. 19 and 20). For this reason, reevaluation stress tests should be performed not only while the subject is taking his medications but also at a period of suitable length after their discontinuation (2 weeks after withdrawal of digitalis glycoside, 3 to 4 days after nitrites, propranolol, etc.).

Proscription of activities which modify training responses or are potentially hazardous [46]. Features or practices frequently associated with physical training sessions should be specifically prohibited and cautioned against, both for normal and coronary heart disease (CHD) subjects, which are:

1. Ingestion of large meals either less than 2 hours before or within 1 hour following active exercise.
2. The ingestion of coffee or other xanthine-containing beverages (tea, colas) before or after exercise.
3. Drinking iced or very hot drinks, or alcoholic beverages.
4. Tobacco smoking at all times, but particularly while dressing after exercise.

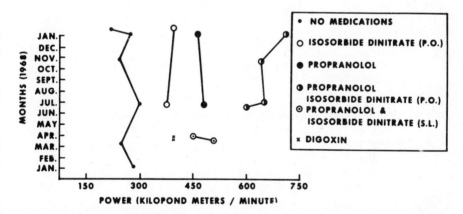

Fig. 19. Example of failure of 1 year's adherence to a training program to improve Maximal Safe Performance although while on various medications work performance improved promptly and reproducibly. This subject had complete occlusion of the proximal right and the left anterior descending coronary arteries and 70 percent stenosis of the left circumflex coronary artery. Workload 120 was calculated from multiple standardized multilevel bicycle ergometer exercise tests during 1 year of physical training. Medications indicated were administered for at least 2 days prior to testing; propanol and isosorbide dinitrate were discontinued 3 days prior to testing without medications and digoxin was discontinued at least 2 weeks prior to tests. Improvement of myocardial function as evidenced by lesser ST-T depression while on medications left no residual effects on work performance when discontinued.

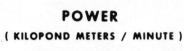

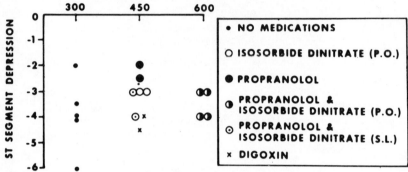

ECG CHANGES AT HIGHEST ATTAINABLE EFFORT LEVEL

Fig. 20. (Same subject as in Fig. 19) Improvement in myocardial function as evidenced by reduction of ST-T depression (initially 6 mm), and hemodynamic responses to exercise, namely stroke volume, mean systolic ejection rate, mean left ventricular systolic pressure, left ventricular minute work index, and left ventricular efficiency index (not shown in this Fig.). All ST-T segment measurements were made from the same ECG lead, during the last 5 seconds of the exercise periods of effort tests throughout a year of conditioning.

5. Wearing heavy clothes during high-level sustained effort.

6. Cold or very hot showers, before or immediately after training sessions.

7. Dry or wet "hot" rooms or towels.

8. Passing quickly from a warm locker room into cold winter weather while still perspiring.

The above proscriptions are important because they constitute additional stresses to the cardiovascular system. Also, items 1 to 5 modify the heart rate response to effort sufficiently to obscure the propriety of the intensity of the exercise prescription. It has been well-documented that marked thermal stress (extremes of hot or cold) can evoke considerable strain. Sudden death during snow shoveling is considered to be due to a combination of the effects of cold exposure on the blood pressure and heart rate to produce acute coronary insufficiency and arrhythmias, and the sudden severe effort in an unconditioned subject. Large meals tend to divert a greater portion of the cardiac output to mesenteric vascular beds and to produce marked shifts in serum electrolytes. Such meals can also cause significant ECG changes, such as arrhythmias and ischemic ST-T changes.

Summary

Appropriate prescription of exercise depends upon a comprehensive and quantitative assessment of the individual's functional capacity. The relationships among heart rate, blood pressure, O_2 intake by the body and by the heart have been quantitated in submaximal exercise and can be used in formulating guidelines of exercise prescription. Target levels for training can be formulated for the individual and related to his aerobic capacity and the energy costs of training activities.

The intensity (the primary determinant of training response), duration, and frequency of a training program can be prescribed on a scientific basis, supplementing common sense and past experiences.

REFERENCES

1. Merriman, J.E. Long-term activity programs for coronary patients. *In*, Naughton, J., and Hellerstein, H.K., Eds., *Exercise Testing and Exercise Training in Coronary Heart Disease.* New York, Academic, 1973.

2. Shephard, R.J. Intensity, duration and frequency of exercise as determinants of the response to a training regime. *Int. Z. Angew. Physiol.* 26:272, 1968.

3. Hellerstein, H.K. Techniques of exercise prescription and evaluation. *In*, Parmley, L.F., Jr., Ed. *Proceedings of the National Workshop on Exercise in the Prevention, and in the Evaluation, in the Treatment of Heart Disease,* 104 pp. *J.S.C. Med. Assoc.* Supplement to vol. 65, Dec., 1969.

4. Pollock, M.L., Broida, J., Kendrick, Z., Miller, H.S., Jr., Janeway, R., and Linnerud, A.C. Effects of training two days per week at different intensities on middle-aged men. *Med. Sci. Sports* 4:192, 1972.

5. Saltin, B., Blomqvist, G., Mitchell, J.H., Johnson, R.L., Wildenthal, K., and Chapman, C.B. Response to exercise after bedrest and after training. *Circulation* 38 (Suppl. 7):1-78, 1968.

6. Cureton, T. *The Physiological Effects of Exercise Programs on Adult Men*, pp. 6-23. Springfield, Ill., Thomas, 1969.

7. Faria, I.E. Cardiovascular response to exercise as influenced by training of various intensities. *Res. Q. Am. Assoc. Health Phys. Educ.* 41:44-50, 1970.

8. Kilbom, A., Hartley, L., Saltin, B., Bjure, J., Grimby, G., and Astrand, I. Physical training in sedentary middle-aged and older men. I. *Scand. J. Clin. Lab. Invest.* 24:315-322, 1969.

9. Pollock, M.L., Miller, H., Janeway, R., Linnerud, A.C., Robertson, B., and Valentino, R. Effects of walking on body composition and cardiovascular function of middle-aged men. *J. Appl. Physiol.* 30:126-30, 1971.

10. Sharkey, B.J., and Holleman, J.P. Cardiorespiratory adaptations to training at specified intensities. *Res. Q. Am. Assoc. Health Phys. Educ.* 38:398-404, 1967.

11. Sharkey, B.J. Intensity and duration of training and the development of cardiorespiratory endurance. *Med. Sci. Sports* 2:197-202, 1970.

12. Skinner, J., Holloszy, J., and Cureton, T. Effects of a program of endurance exercise on physical work capacity and anthropometric measurements of fifteen middle-aged men. *Am. J. Cardiol.* 14:747-752, 1964.

13. Wilmore, J.H., Royce, J., Girandola, R.N., Kasch, F., and Katch, V. Physiological alterations resulting from a 10-week program of jogging. *Med. Sci. Sports* 2:7-14, 1970.

14. Taylor, H.L., Haskell, W., Fox, S.M., III, and Blackburn, H. Exercise tests: A summary of procedures and concepts of stress testing for cardiovascular diagnosis and function

evaluation. *In*, Blackburn, H., Ed., *Measurement in Exercise Electrocardiography*, pp. 259-305. (The Ernst Simonson Conference) Springfield, Ill., Thomas, 1969.

15. Scheuer, J. Physical training and intrinsic cardiac adaptations. *Circulation* 47:677, 1973.

16. Holloszy, J.O. Effects of exercise on mitochondrial oxygen uptake and respiratory enzyme activity in skeletal muscle. *J. Biol. Chem.* 242:2278, 1967.

17. Howley, E.T., Skinner, J.S., Mendez, J., and Buskirk, E.R. Effect of different intensities of exercise on catecholamine excretion. *Med. Sci. Sports* 2:193, 1970.

18. Kotchen, T.A., Hartley, L.H., Rice, T.W., Mougey, E.H., Jones, L.G., and Mason, J.W. Renin, norepinephrine, and epinephrine responses to graded exercise. *J. Appl. Physiol.* 31:178, 1971.

19. Wilkerson, J.E., and Evonuk, E. Changes in cardiac and skeletal muscle myosin ATPase activities after exercise. *J. Appl. Physiol.* 30:328, 1971.

20. Astrup, T. The effects of physical activity on blood coagulation and fibrinolysis. *In*, Naughton, J., and Hellerstein, H.K., Eds., *Exercise Testing and Exercise Training in Coronary Heart Disease*. New York, Academic, 1973.

21. Hellerstein, H.K., and Ader, R. Relationship between percent maximal oxygen uptake (% MHR) in normals and cardiacs (ASHD). *Circulation* 43-44. Suppl. II. October 1971.

22. Kitamura, K., Jorgensen, C.R., Gobel, F.L., Taylor, H., Wang, Y. Hemodynamic correlates of coronary blood flow and myocardial oxygen consumption during upright exercise. *Am. J. Cardiol.* 26:643, 1970.

23. Jorgensen, C.R., Kitamura, K., Gobel, F.L., Taylor, H. L., and Wang, Y. Long-term precision of the N_2O method for coronary flow during heavy upright exercise. *J. Appl. Physiol.* 30:338, 1971.

24. Hellerstein, H.K., Studies of firefighters and firefighting. (Unpublished data)

25. Karvonen, J.J., Kentala, E., and Mustala, O. The effects of training on heart rate. A "longitudinal" study. *Ann. Med. Exp. Biol. Fenn.* 35:307, 1957.

26. Gualtiere, W.S., Zohman, L.R., Lopez, R.H., and Flores, A.M. Effects of physical training on cardiorespiratory capacity of patients with angina pectoris (In press).

27. Hellerstein, H.K. (Unpublished data)

28. Gilbert, R., and Auchincloss, J.H., Jr. Comparison of cardiovascular responses to steady- and unsteady-state exercise. *J. Appl. Physiol.* 30:388, 1971.

29. Detry, J-M.R., Rousseau, M., Vandenbrouchek, G., Kusumi, F., Brasseur, L.A., and Bruce, R.A. Increased arteriovenous oxygen difference after physical training in coronary heart disease. *Circulation* 44:109, 1971.

30. Fox, E.L., Bartels, R.L., Billings, C.E., Mathews, D.K., Bason, R., and Webb, W.M. Intensity and distance of interval training programs and changes in aerobic power. *Med. Sci. Sports* 5:18, 1972.

31. Roskamm, H. Optimum patterns of exercise for healthy adults. *Can. Med. Assoc. J.* 96:895, 1967.

32. Hellerstein, H.K. Exercise therapy in coronary disease. *Bull. N.Y. Acad. Med.* 44:1028, 1968.

33. Mann, G.V., Garret, H.L., Farhi, A., Murray, H., and Billings, F.T. Exercise to prevent coronary heart disease. *Am. J. Med.* 46:12, 1969.

34. Siegel, W., Blomqvist, G., and Mitchell, J. H. Effects of a quantitated physical training program on middle-aged sedentary males. *Circulation* 41:19, 1970.

35. Pollock, M.L., Dimmick, J., Millers, H.S., Jr., Kendrick, Z., and Linnerud, A.C. *Med. Trib.*, April 18, 1973.

36. Hellerstein, H.K., and Ford, A.B. Comprehensive care of the coronary patient. Optimal (intensive) care, recovery, and reconditioning. An opportunity for the physician. *In, Symposium on Coronary Heart Disease*, 2nd rev. ed. New York, Amer. Heart Assn., 1969. (Monograph No. 2)

37. Hellerstein, H.K., and Friedman, E.H. Sexual activity and the post coronary patient. *Med. Aspects Hum. Sex.* 3:70, 1969.

38. Stenberg, J., Astrand, P.O., Ekblom, B., Royce, J., and Saltin, B. Hemodynamic response to work with different muscle groups, sitting and supine. *J. Appl. Physiol.* 22:61, 1967.

39. Holmer, I., and Astrand, P.O. Swimming training and maximal oxygen uptake. *J. Appl. Physiol.* 33:510, 1972.

40. Clausen, J.P., Trap-Jensen, J., and Lassen, N.A. The effects of training on the heart rate during arm and leg exercise. *Scand. J. Clin. Lab. Invest.* 26:295, 1970.

41. Brynteson, P., and Sinning, W.E. The effects of training frequencies on the retention of cardiovascular fitness. *Med. Sci. Sports* 5:29, 1973.

42. Michael, E., Evert, J., and Jeffers, K. Physiological changes of teenage girls during months of detraining. *Med. Sci. Sports* 4:214, 1972.

43. Hollmann, W., und Venrath, H. Experimentelle Untersuchungen zur Bedeutung eines Trainings unterhalb und oberhalb der Dauerbelastungsgrenze. *In*, Korbs, W., u.a., *Carl Diem Festschrift*, Frankfurt a.M./Wein, 1962.

44. Cooper, K.H. *The New Aerobics*. New York, M. Evans, 1970.

45. Fox, S.M., III, Naughton, J.P., and Gorman, P.A. Physical activity and cardiovascular health. III. The exercise prescription; frequency and type of activity. *Mod. Concepts Cardiovasc. Dis.* 41:25, 1972.

46. Hirsch, E.Z., Hellerstein, H.K., and Macleod, C.A. Physical straining and coronary heart disease. *In*, Morse, R.L., Ed. *Exercise and the Heart. Guidelines for Exercise Programs* (Chap. 8), p. 106. Springfield, Ill., Thomas, 1972.

11

THE EFFECTS OF PHYSICAL ACTIVITY ON
BLOOD COAGULATION AND FIBRINOLYSIS

Tage Astrup, Ph.D.

Among the many effects of physical activity on the parameters of circulating blood, those involving coagulation and fibrinolysis have been investigated frequently because of their possible significance in influencing thrombotic disease and the development of vascular disorders. Only recently, following the establishment of the syndrome of disseminated intravascular coagulation (DIC) and the realization that this syndrome is part of many otherwise unrelated disease processes, have the wide implications of the processes of blood coagulation and fibrinolysis, beyond their simple function in hemostasis, become clear. Contributing to the present interest in the effects of exercise on blood coagulation and fibrinolysis, is the fact that physical exertion is one of the few known mechanisms by which these parameters can be influenced within the physiological limitations of presumably healthy individuals. Behavioral and, possibly dietary, influences are two other causes of change within the realm of normal physiology.

Influence of Exercise on Blood Coagulation

Several reports describe an enhancement of the spontaneous coagulation of blood following heavy exercise. Iatridis and Ferguson [1] tried to elucidate the cause of the measured hypercoagulability by determining the levels of coagulation factors in samples of post-exercise blood. It is of particular interest in the present context that Cannon [2, 3], in his studies of adrenalin as a defense hormone, reported in 1914, that pain and emotional excitement hastened blood coagulation.

The recognized factors in the mechanism of blood coagulation can be divided into three groups. The first comprises the factors causing activation of the *intrinsic* coagulation system resulting in the formation of plasma thromboplastin.

The preparation of this review was supported by USPHS Grant HL-05020 from the National Heart and Lung Institute.

They are: Factor VIII (AHF, antihemophilic factor); Factor IX (PTC, plasma thromboplastin compound, Christmas factor); Factor XI (PTA, plasma thromboplastin antecedent), Factor XII (Hageman factor), platelets, and calcium.

A second group, comprising Factor VII (proconvertin) and a cellular factor (tissue thromboplastin, Factor III), initiates *extrinsic* coagulation by the formation of an activating agent, convertin, which in its action is equivalent to plasma thromboplastin.

A third group consists of factors essential to the rapid conversion of prothrombin into thrombin by plasma thromboplastin or by convertin (tissue thromboplastin + Factor VII). These are Factor V (proaccelerin) and Factor X (Stuart-Prower factor). Following this, the thrombin acts on fibrinogen and forms fibrin. The fibrin-stabilizing factor (Factor XIII) does not affect the coagulability of blood although it determines the structure of the fibrin network formed.

Iatridis and Ferguson collected blood samples from 60 male subjects, aged 18 to 37, immediately before and after heavy exercise, using the silicone technique. Platelet-rich and platelet-poor plasma were prepared, kept at 4°C, and tested as soon as possible. No differences were observed between pre- and post-exercise levels of prothrombin, Factor VII (proconvertin), Factor V (proaccelerin) or Factor X (Stuart-Prower factor). A slight increase in fibrinogen level (8 percent) could be attributed to a slight hemoconcentration following exercise. One of their subjects was deficient in Hageman factor. Post-exercise samples from this subject showed neither a shortening of the spontaneous recalcification times nor the enhanced formation of thromboplastin in the screening test of Hicks and Pitney which was observed in the 59 other normal samples.

Confirming observations by others, Iatridis and Ferguson found assays of Factor VIII to indicate an approximate doubling in concentration. However, the increase was questionable or absent in 8 of 58 normal subjects and in the Hageman patient. Assays of the Hageman factor level in normal subjects showed a significant increase (3 times) in the post-exercise samples, while no detectable Hageman factor activity appeared in the sample from the Hageman patient. Additional experiments questioned the specificity of the Factor VIII assay. Hence, the failure of their Hageman patient to increase Factor VIII activity, together with the absence of a shortened spontaneous clotting time, in addition to the findings previously mentioned, made the authors suggest that the post-exercise hypercoagulability could be caused by an increase in Hageman factor activity.

Egeberg [4], in a systematic study of the influence of exercise on blood coagulation, reported unchanged levels of Factor VII (proconvertin), Factor V (proaccelerin), prothrombin and fibrinogen, as well as an unchanged thromboplastin time after Quick. Using a partial thromboplastin time test (cephalin test), a marked shortening of the clotting time occurred immediately after exercise, returning to normal within a few hours. Assayed by a cephalin time technique, the levels of Factor VIII increased more than 200 percent, slowly returning to the normal level within 24 hours. The increase was still marked after 8 hours of recovery. There were no significant changes in the levels of Factor IX (PTC) or

Factor XI (PTA). When patients with von Willebrand's disease were exercised, the same changes were observed as in normal persons. Also, patients deficient in Factor XI (PTA) reacted as did normal subjects [5]. Rizza [6] reported an increase in Factor VIII activity following exercise in patients partially deficient in Factor VIII. Interestingly, in mildly affected von Willebrand patients, the bleeding time returned to normal following exercise or with the infusion of fresh exercise plasma [7]. In patients with greatly diminished Factor VIII levels and greatly prolonged bleeding times, there was no post-exercise increase in Factor VIII levels, and the plasma cephalin time or the bleeding time did not decrease [8].

The absence, following exercise, of a shortening of the prothrombin time (thereby excluding an enhancement of the effects of prothrombin and Factors V, VII and X) reported by Egeberg [4] and Iatridis and Ferguson [1] confirms several earlier findings, beginning with Overman, Newman, and Wright [9]. However, other authors reported a shortening of the prothrombin time or an enhanced activity of prothrombin, Factor V, and Factor VII following exercise. The degree of shortening depended upon the severity of exercise (workload) and a subject's capacity for work [10, 11]. One study [12], unable to confirm the post-exercise hypercoagulability, should be mentioned. Whole blood clotting times and the thromboplastin generation were unchanged, despite a slightly enhanced thrombin generation test in 6 of 16 subjects. The authors suggest that the use of insensitive methods could explain their deviating observations.

While the increase in measured Factor VIII activity received repeated confirmation [11, 13], Hageman factor (Factor XII) was reported unchanged [4, 13]. A recent report mentions a lower increase in Factor VIII activity in Hageman patients and a small increase in Hageman factor activity in normal persons [14]. Interestingly, the administration of the beta blocker, propranolol, prevented the exercise-induced rise in Factor VIII activity [13, 15]. One report [16] documents a failure to increase in Factor VIII activity following exercise in horses; interestingly, horses are low in Hageman factor [16, 17].

Biggs et al [18] reported a moderate and transient increase in the number of circulating platelets following exercise, a finding confirmed by some investigators [19], but not by others [13]. Propranolol had no effect on the platelet increase following exercise [19]. The exercise-induced rise in platelet number and in Factor VIII was reported to be absent in splenectomized individuals [20] although others report a delayed rise [19]. A recent report adds to the confusion by describing a normal increase in Factor VIII in asplenic subjects [21]. Studies with Factor VIII antiserum suggest that the exercise-induced rise in Factor VIII activity represents a real increase in Factor VIII concentration [21, 21a]. Most authors have reported that the exercise-induced elevation in Factor VIII activity resembles that produced by adrenalin. This includes its prevention by propranolol and by other beta blockers, as well as its absence in asplenic persons. However, the similarity does not extend to the rise in platelet number, because beta blockers are reported to prevent the platelet increase following the administration of adrenalin [22] but not following exercise [19]. A recent study [22a] deals specifically with the role of the spleen in the exercise-induced increase in Factor VIII activity and platelet adhesiveness.

Exercise is also reported to increase the adhesiveness of platelets [23], resembling in this respect the effect of adrenalin [24]. A shortened one-stage prothrombin time and normal platelet count was observed in normal persons immediately after performing a Masters' two-step exercise test, while a decrease in the total platelet count and in the adhesive platelet count was observed in patients with angina pectoris (AP) exposed to the same test [25]. This decrease was prevented by administration of pyridinol carbamate. A similar difference between healthy volunteers and patients, following exercise, was observed in ADP-induced platelet aggregation [26].

Some of the discrepant reports on platelets may result from differences in methodology; others may be caused by the use of varying degrees and durations of exercise. Thus, following a very prolonged, moderate exertion (a 50-mile walk), the degree of platelet adhesiveness measured by two different methods (yielding different averages on normal samples) was reported as significantly decreased in two-thirds of the subjects while the total platelet count remained normal [27]. The latter result agrees with data obtained on subjects who performed a 10-mile march within 90 minutes, while more strenuous exercise of short duration gave a moderate increase in platelet count [28]. Sarajas et al suggested that the hypercoagulability following exercise is related to the rise in platelet count. It is now evident that this is a moderate rise, smaller than the fluctuation of normal platelet counts, and therefore, is unable to explain the marked shortening of the spontaneous clotting times repeatedly observed by several authors. In a study of brief, heavy exercise, a hypercoagulability is reported with no concomitant change in platelet count, but with enhancement of activity due to Factor V, Factor VIII, and *contact factor* [29]. The *contact factor* designates a combined determination of Factors XI and XII, and the observation may, therefore, be considered in agreement with the increase in Hageman factor activity reported by Iatridis and Ferguson [1]. An increased platelet adhesiveness with unchanged platelet agglutination has been reported [30].

In view of the possible physiological significance of an increase in measured Factor VIII activity, it is useful to remember that this increase may occur as a general phenomenon in many, apparently unrelated physiological and pathological states [20]. Egeberg, in particular, reported hypercoagulability related to thyrotoxicosis and delayed coagulation associated with hypothyroidism [31].

It is apparent that the effect of exercise on blood coagulation has given rise to many discordant reports which leave many observations in a state of confusion. Much work is needed to resolve these discrepancies. To attain this goal, carefully standardized exercise programs are required. Blood samples must be carefully collected and cautiously treated. Methods must be rigidly standardized and controlled, and they must be accurate and sensitive. Until this is accomplished, the available data cannot be compared and assessed accurately. It is obvious that many of the data currently available stem from the application of inadequate methods of assay and the use of insufficiently defined experimental designs. The nost reliable results, as far as currently determined, are briefly presented in TABLE I.

TABLE I

Exercise and blood coagulation

Enhanced spontaneous coagulation
Enhanced formation of plasma thromboplastin
Increase in measured Factor VIII activity
Moderate increase in platelets
Possible increase in measured Hageman factor activity
Measured Factor VIII activity increases in patients with moderate Factor
     VIII deficiency, but not in those with low Factor VIII levels
Factor VIII may not increase in Hageman patients
Increase in Factor VIII activity prevented by propranolol

Influence of Exercise on Blood Fibrinolysis

In contrast to the many discrepant reports on the effects of exercise on blood coagulation, studies of its influence on the blood fibrinolytic system have been rather consistent, despite the fact that the accuracy of several of the methods used leaves much to be desired. One reason for this general agreement is that the fibrinolytic system in blood comprises fewer factors and variables than the blood clotting system. Another reason is that the collection and assay of samples for determination of blood fibrinolysis is easier, because the separated plasma can be stored at -20°C without deterioration. Therefore, determinations need not be performed immediately on the freshly collected samples such as in assays of enhancement of coagulation.

Discovery of Exercise-Induced Fibrinolysis

The observation that heavy exercise enhances the fibrinolytic activity of blood was reported by Biggs et al in 1947 [17], and subsequently confirmed by many authors using different methods of assay. Biggs et al attempted to clarify several of the physiological problems related to the production of fibrinolytic activity in the circulating blood. In preliminary studies [32] a globulin precipitate was found to contain the fibrinolytic activity of the plasma sample with most of the plasma inhibitors remaining in the supernatant. The effect of inhibitors could also be decreased by dilution of the plasma, greatly simplifying the technique [33]. Plasma was diluted 1 in 16; 1 in 32; and 1 in 64; clotted with thrombin; and incubated for 24 hours at 37°C. A strongly fibrinolytic plasma produced lysis in all tubes within a few hours. A positive result was recorded if fibrin had disappeared from one or more tubes within 24 hours.

In 70 blood samples from 54 normal subjects, a weakly positive reaction was obtained in one subject on only one occasion. Samples from 137 pregnant women were all negative, nor was any activity observed in relation to the ovarian cycle. Fibrinolytic activity was observed in samples from about 50 percent of patients undergoing surgery, but was unrelated to the disease or the type of surgical intervention. It was present also in blood samples obtained immediately before the operation. In the absence of any other obvious explanation, it was thought that agitation and anxiety could be responsible for the active samples. This suggestion was put to trial in a study of normal individuals [18]. A subject who developed urticaria when exercising, provided some important clues. Swimming in cold water produced maximum fibrinolytic activity with no urticaria, while the opposite followed a 15-minute rest in hot water. This observation changed the attention from reactions of hypersensitivity to those caused by exercise. When a group of 20 normal subjects were studied while climbing a staircase, increased fibrinolytic activity was observed in 28 of 29 samples collected after 5 or more ascents. Interestingly, the single negative response was from a subject in very good physical condition and little incommoded by the exercise. The fibrinolytic activity decreased rapidly during rest, completely disappearing after 30 minutes. There was a marked increase in the lymphocyte count and moderate or small increases in numbers of neutrophils and platelets. Their increase was related to the duration of exercise and the counts rapidly returned to normal during the resting period. A causal relationship between the changes in the blood cells and the increase in plasma fibrinolytic activity was unlikely because the appearance of fibrinolytic activity preceded changes in the white blood count. Nor did addition to blood of excessive amounts of lymphocytes, leukocytes, or platelets produce fibrinolytic activity in the separated plasma. A positive response was observed in 5 of 6 subjects swimming for 15 minutes in cold water. The sixth person, a strong swimmer untired by the efforts, failed to respond.

The possible involvement of anxiety prompted a study of the effects of adrenalin as the fibrinolytic mechanism. Between 1 and 2 ml of adrenalin (1 in 1000) was injected subcutaneously in the upper arm at a rate of about 0.25 ml/min. In 22 experiments, samples of blood collected 10 to 20 minutes after injection showed positive fibrinolysis, the effect lasting longer than that observed following exercise. Injection of adrenalin in three splenectomized patients and in three hemophilic patients produced maximal fibrinolytic response. Adrenalin injection in two patients with Addison's disease also produced a normal fibrinolytic response [34], indicating that the pathway of activation of blood fibrinolysis does not involve the release of adrenocortical hormones.

The results obtained by Macfarlane and Biggs, although of a preliminary nature, solved some of the problems related to the physiological activation of the fibrinolytic system, and their most important findings have been confirmed by subsequent authors in more extensive and detailed investigations.

Identity of Exercise-Induced Fibrinolytic Activity

The agent responsible for the fibrinolytic activity in blood was not identified by Macfarlane and Biggs [34] though circumstantial evidence suggested that the active agent might be the blood protease, plasmin (fibrinolysin). However, differences in behavior were noticed between the active agent in blood and the reported properties of plasmin. Mole [35], who studied the fibrinolytic activity in blood following sudden death, related his *cadaver fibrinolysin* to the activity observed by Macfarlane and Biggs and suggested that it represented a blood proteinase different from plasmin. Fantl and Simon [36] reported that electroconvulsant therapy produced a transient fibrinolytic activity in blood resembling that observed to occur following exercise, the administration of adrenalin, or anxiety. The active agent differed from trypsin and they believed it to be plasmin in low concentrations. Later, Bidwell [37] compared *cadaver lysin* with plasmin prepared by chloroform activation. She reported a good recovery of the *cadaver lysin* in the euglobulin-precipitate in contrast to a negative finding by Mole. She confirmed its difference from plasmin and noticed a similarity with the active agent in exercise blood. The question of identity was eventually solved when Müllertz [38] reported that the activity in postmortem blood and following electroconvulsive treatment was caused by an activator of plasminogen. Increased lysis resulted when additional amounts of plasminogen were mixed with the active solutions. These findings were reviewed in 1956 [39]. While Bidwell [37] had failed to identify *cadaver lysin* as an activator of plasminogen, Fearnley, noticing that *plasma active fibrinolysin* differed from plasmin [40], reported the possibility that it could be an activator of plasminogen [41]. Sherry et al [42], using several different assay techniques, demonstrated that the fibrinolytic activity in blood following electroshock, pyrogen injection, severe exercise, injection of adrenalin or acetylcholine, or following local ischemia, could be traced to a plasminogen activator in all instances. The presence of an activator was demonstrated by following the activation of a plasminogen solution, as well as by determining the sensitivity to epsilonaminocaproic acid (EACA), a compound having greater inhibitory effect on plasminogen activators than on plasmin. Later, using a radioactive, preformed fibrin clot lysis method of assay, in which a plasminogen-enriched clot was incubated for 2 hours with samples of oxalate plasma, they found low concentrations of plasminogen activator in undisturbed plasma samples from normal persons [43].

Origin of the Plasminogen Activator in Blood

Truelove [44] observed that adrenalin produced a slight, transient rise in the number of eosinophils, followed after 1 to 2 hours by a brisk fall reaching a minimum between 3 to 5 hours, while fibrinolytic activity appeared from 1/2 to 1 hour following injection. In none of the six subjects exposed to strenuous exercise did a steep decline in number of eosinophils occur despite marked fibrinolysis in five of the subjects. Likewise, a patient with a severe anxiety state, inducible by suggestion, yielded markedly fibrinolytic samples during states of mental agitation while the eosinophil count remained unchanged. Following the injection of adrenalin, this patient exhibited delayed eosinopenia accompanied by a moderate degree of fibrinolysis. Also, according to Truelove's data, the patient showed the normal fibrinolytic response to exercise with no decrease in eosinophil count. These findings made Truelove reject the suggestion that exercise and mental stress produce fibrinolytic activity through a liberation of adrenalin. He substantiated his opinion by reporting that noradrenalin failed to induce fibrinolytic activity, but produced a marked eosinopenia, although not as large as that following adrenalin. In addition, an adrenolytic drug (Priscol, 2-benzyl-2-imidazoline hydrochloride) caused fibrinolysis but not eosinopenia. He also observed [45] that ACTH or cortisone had no effect on the fibrinolytic response to adrenalin or exercise, in good accordance with Macfarlane and Biggs' finding of a normal fibrinolytic response to adrenalin in patients with Addison's disease [34]. Furthermore, patients undergoing surgery developed fibrinolytic activity and eosinopenia independently [46]. These findings indicate again that adrenocortical activity is not involved in the activation of blood fibrinolysis.

In all the reports mentioned, the usual finding in normal healthy persons was an absence of measurable blood fibrinolytic activity. However, Fearnley et al [47] noticed that the fibrinolytic activity decreased with time in blood samples collected from healthy persons given adrenalin. This decline could be delayed if blood was drawn into ice-cold utensils under paraffin and the separated plasma kept under paraffin at $0°C$. The decrease occurring within the first 30 minutes then became negligible. The lability of the adrenalin-induced fibrinolytic activity in blood was simultaneously observed by Truelove [48].

Using the cold technique throughout and setting up the incubation of plasma dilutions at $37°C$ within 10 to 12 minutes after vein puncture, Fearnley and Tweed [40] reported the presence of fibrinolytic activity in the majority of samples from normal, unstressed persons. It is of interest in a later context to notice that most of their samples were collected between 2 and 5 P.M. In a reinvestigation of the effects of adrenalin and exercise using the cold technique [49], they collected the blood by silicone technique without anticoagulant. Samples were collected between 5 and 6 P.M. The final plasma dilutions were placed at $37°C$ and clotting occurred spontaneously within 5 to 10 minutes. At 10 percent plasma concentration lysis occurred spontaneously within 10 to 40 hours in the normal samples, and was shortened to less than 5 hours after the administration of adrenalin, and to 10 hours following moderate exercise.

Later, whole blood was collected, diluted with cold phosphate buffer, and thrombin was added [41]. The tubes were placed in a refrigerator for 1/2 to 1 hour and subsequently incubated at $37°C$. These changes facilitated the procedure, but some loss in activity occurred during the preincubation period. In samples collected during 24 hours at intervals of 4 to 5 hours, a minimum of activity was observed during the night (at 4 A.M.), and the activity was considerably lower at 8 A.M. than during the remainder of the day. A diurnal increase in activity occurred whether the subject was ambulant or at rest, indicating an independence from the degree of physical activity and suggesting a diurnal rhythm. This was confirmed in a study of day nurses and night nurses. In spite of the physical activity of the night nurses, their fibrinolytic activity was less at 4 A.M. than at 4 P.M. These results prompted Fearnley and his associates to do a comprehensive study, extending over many years, of the development of blood fibrinolytic activity; its relation to various diseases; and the effects of various hormones and other pharmacologic agents on it [50]. The pharmacology of fibrinolysis was also studied by von Kaulla [51]. Sherry et al [42], reporting euglobulin clot lysis times as short as 15 to 20 minutes after electroshock, noticed that strenuous exercise for 2 hours (basketball) produced a delayed rise in fibrinolytic activity, but found no clear evidence of a diurnal fluctuation using the preformed clot lysis method on normal persons [43]. A delayed response, reaching its maximum 2 hours after injection, also was seen in pyrogen-induced fibrinolysis, while that following injection of nicotinic acid was particularly abrupt returning to normal in less than 20 minutes. The physiologic significance of some of these findings has been reviewed elsewhere [52].

Several authors have suggested that the venous wall, either the vasa vasorum [53] or the intima [54], is a source of the blood activator. Venous occlusion makes the trapped blood fibrinolytic [42, 55, 56, 57, 58]. It is known from histochemical studies [59] and the assay of tissue extracts [60, 61] that the venous endothelium as well as the adventitia of veins and arteries are highly fibrinolytic. Aoki and von Kaulla [62] described the collection of solutions with high plasminogen activator content by postmortem flushing of the vascular tree with saline. Holemans [63] suggested that vasoactive drugs free stagnant fibrino-lytic blood from the vascular bed to enter into the circulation. Menon [64] reported evidence that exercise releases fibrinolytic activity from the muscles. It is tempting to relate these observations to the possible release of activator into the circulating blood, but the mechanisms are far from clarified. Thus, Sherry et al [42] reported that succinylcholine did not abolish the fibrinolytic response following electroshock indicating that the muscular component of the induced convulsions did not participate in the production of fibrinolytic blood. Further-more, the cellular activator belongs to a class of activators much more stable than reported for the blood activator [65]. However, some tissues also contain labile activators [66]. Hamberg [67] used gel filtration and density gradient distribution to distinguish between the activator in postmortem blood and the plasminogen activator produced in human blood by streptokinase.

Problems of Methodology

An accurate method of assay is an essential prerequisite for the elucidation of the physiology of the blood plasminogen activator. As discussed, several methods have been used. Apart from the provision of sufficient sensitivity, there are several additional obstacles to the quantitative determination. First, blood contains excessive amounts of inhibitory agents. The methods used by Macfarlane, and the various modifications proposed by Fearnley, try to diminish the effects of the inhibitors but essentially the assays are only approximate. In dilution methods, the fibrinogen, plasminogen, and active agents also are diluted. Originally, Macfarlane and Pilling [32] prepared the dilutions in a solution of human fibrinogen in order to keep the fibrinogen concentration constant, but this method was discontinued when it was found that simple dilution of the plasma sample gave a higher sensitivity. Sherry et al [42, 43] tried several different methods. They found the preformed clot lysis assay sensitive enough to observe the low activator concentrations in normal blood, but it did not record the diurnal fluctuations. The determination of the euglobulin clot lysis time has been used frequently but the method is not particularly sensitive and is influenced by the amounts of fibrinogen, plasminogen, or inhibitors precipitated with the euglobulin. The composition of the substrate is better stabilized in the fibrin plate method because of the constant concentrations of fibrinogen and plasminogen, but in its early design the method was not sensitive enough to respond to the small amounts of activator present in normal blood [68]. Improvements in the preparation of the bovine, plasminogen-rich fibrin substrate [69, 70], and the precipitation of the euglobulins at the optimum pH of 5.9 [71], increased the sensitivity and accuracy of the method so that solutions of euglobulin precipitates from resting, normal persons regularly produced lysed zones with diameter products from 50 to 200 mm^2 [72]. The presence of phosphate increased the sensitivity of the substrate to activators [69], but the results were erratic [73] and this modification was discontinued. Modifications of the fibrin plate method were used by Amery et al [58] in their study of blood fibrinolytic activity induced by venous occlusion, and by Blix [74] in a comparison with the euglobulin clot lysis time method. The latter author recommended a precipitation of the euglobulins at pH 6.4 for maximum recovery of the activator. He found that storage of the separated plasma samples at -20°C did not change the fibrinolytic activity of the euglobulin precipitates. This observation is in accordance with our findings [75] and it greatly facilitates the handling and assay of blood samples. Blix confirmed the increase in blood fibrinolytic activity following exercise and reported a diurnal pattern in 3 of 4 subjects with a maximum of activity around noontime.

The most accurate determinations of plasminogen activator activity in samples of blood are obtained by the fibrin plate method, standardized as described [69, 70, 72]. Data obtained by this method are reported below. One problem remains unsolved, namely, the conversion of the measured activities to arbitrary concentrations of activator. The variable slopes of the double logarithmic curves obtained with dilutions of the euglobulin precipitates [72] are suggestive of the presence of variable amounts of inhibitor and preclude an immediate conversion into units of concentration. Other methods are lacking in accuracy. Fearnley [76], using a sensitive dilution method, observed the diurnal fluctuation in only half of the group of nurses studied. Similarly, Iatridis and Ferguson [1], reporting a mean euglobulin lysis time of 379 minutes (range: 258-480 minutes) in 19 normal persons before exercise, and 70 minutes (range: 13-180 minutes) after exercise, found no activity in the pre-exercise euglobulin samples tested on their fibrin plates, and only 12 of 60 (20 percent) did so after exercise. Fearnley tried to standardize the euglobulin clot lysis time assay to yield results in accordance with those obtained by the plasma dilution methods [77]. Investigators who are uncertain about the meaning of data determined by dilution methods or by the assay of euglobulins might be consoled by the finding that undisturbed plasma also exerts fibrinolytic activity, even though the measurements are low because of the inhibitors present [43, 78, 79]

Production of Exercise-Induced Fibrinolysis

Current interest in the fibrinolytic response to exercise is related to the possibility that the production of fibrinolytic blood might be one of the alleged beneficial effects of physical activity. The enhanced fibrinolysis could increase the rate of resolution of minute deposits of fibrin in the blood vessels, thereby acting to prevent thrombosis and vascular disease, such as arteriosclerosis. This viewpoint is perhaps most clearly expressed in a brief presentation by Cash [80]. The effects of graded exercise and of prolonged physical activity are problems of particular significance. Several authors have studied brief periods of strenuous exercise, while others have used lower degrees of exercise for longer periods of time. Discrepancies between reported results could easily stem from a failure to use the same schedules or programs of physical activity. Likewise, differences between individual responses to the same exercise could be related to the observation already reported by Biggs et al [18], i.e., that persons who are well trained and are little affected by the exertion do not produce the same degree of fibrinolytic response as those who are exhausted by the exercise. When sufficiently sensitive methods of assay are used, other factors such as diurnal fluctuations or the presence of emotional stress might also influence the results. A relation to the age of the exercising subjects may also exist.

Menon et al [81] compared prolonged, strenuous exercise lasting 90 minutes (football, squash, hockey) or 30 minutes (squash), with a graded exercise of brief duration (Masters' standard two-step test lasting less than 8 minutes). The subjects were healthy young men and women of ages 18 to 29. The method of assay employed was a modified von Kaulla euglobulin clot lysis time test. A considerable shortening of the lysis times occurred in all 58 volunteers after their games, the means being 248 minutes before the game and 87 minutes after the game. Their tables show large individual differences. The 10 volunteers participating in the graded exercise study were not in athletic training. They all showed enhanced lysis after Masters' standard number of ascents (20-25). The mean lysis time was 429 minutes before exercise and 290 minutes after. Both values are considerably longer than those observed in the trained group. Additional ascents (until 100) did not reduce the lysis time any further and the enhancement persisted after an hour's rest. This observation does not agree with several reports describing the disappearance of the enhanced fibrinolysis within 30 minutes. However, the prolonged exercise (basketball) studied by Sherry et al [42] also produced a delayed response. The post-exercise activity in Menon's graded exercise group is in the same range as the pre-exercise activity in the group exposed to strenuous exercise, and it is of significance that all samples in the latter group were obtained in the afternoon when the diurnal increase would have added to the level of fibrinolytic activity. It is also quite possible that the mental strain associated with the games (before as well as after) added further to the activity level.

The authors speculate whether the raised body temperature during exercise causes the increase in fibrinolytic activity, and they mention a study by Bedrak [82] in which dogs exercised in a hot environment showed enhanced fibrinolysis, but had a reduced response when acclimatized. However, Biggs et al [18] had already excluded this possibility by their finding of enhanced fibrinolysis in subjects exercising in cold water, whereas there was no effect after a rest in hot water (43°C for 15 minutes). Bedrak et al [83], using a whole blood clot lysis assay in which the loss of hemoglobin is determined and a 50 percent lysis time calculated [84], also studied the effect of exercise in hot surroundings on acclimatized and unacclimatized persons. The subjects were exposed to a 2-hour exercise of stepping up and down. It was, therefore, of the prolonged type. In all instances a very marked shortening of the 50 percent whole blood clot lysis time occurred. In addition, when the unacclimatized subjects were brought to the hot environment, the resting value (after 2 hours of bed rest) was considerably shorter than the lysis time following rest in the temperate environment, and this difference disappeared after acclimatization. Bedrak et al suggested that acclimatization caused the disappearance of the difference, and that the hot environment gives rise to a shortening of the lysis time in the unacclimatized group by a mechanism of response similar to that producing an increase in blood fibrinolytic activity in heat stroke. However, the increased fibrinolysis in heat stroke is probably a pathological phenomenon related to DIC [85, 86, 87, 88]. It should not be compared with exercise-induced fibrinolysis or with the enhancements within reasonable physiological limits caused by various environmental influences. More likely, the first exposure of the subjects to the unfamiliar and uncomfortable hot environment produced an emotional response which did not arise when the experiment was repeated after the subjects had been accustomed to the heat exposure. This situation confuses the issue in many otherwise well-designed exercise experiments. It should also be recalled that the diurnal fluctuations will add to the problems of assessment. Some exercise studies run into this difficulty. Thus, elevated resting levels in the trained athletes reported by Menon et al [81] were probably caused, in part, by the diurnal increase, since the samples were collected during the afternoon, and in part, by a state of anticipation of the upcoming games. They should not be considered as normal resting values. In a study of the resting levels of fibrinolytic activity in samples of blood collected from a group of regularly exercising men and a similar group following a normal pattern of sedentary life, we found no significant difference between the early morning averages in the two groups [89]. Hence, the exercise effect is of a transient nature. Nor did observable differences exist between the plasma inhibitor levels in the two groups.

Menon et al [81] also reported that the trained athletes produced a higher fibrinolytic response to exercise than the untrained subjects. This disagrees with the observations by Biggs et al [18] and is probably explained by the effects of the diurnal increase and emotional response, as mentioned previously. Of seven highly trained subjects who performed an exercise test [89], five experienced a marked increase in fibrinolytic activity while two did not. In a comparison of untrained and highly trained subjects, Winckelmann et al [11] reported that the resting values were similar in the untrained group (euglobulin clot lysis times in six subjects: 130.5 ± 31.5 minutes) to the trained group (nine individuals: 124.4 ± 36.6 minutes). Following a standard exercise (bicycle ergometer) the lysis time was reduced considerably in the untrained group (77.5 ± 30.3 min) but not in the trained group (130.2 ± 27.2 min). When exposed to a maximal load, both groups responded comparably with a reduction of the lysis times to 58.3 ± 24.1 minutes in the untrained group and to 45.7 ± 20.6 in the trained group.

A detailed study of the response to graded workloads was performed in collaboration with Dr. Stephen E. Epstein and associates, Cardiology Branch, National Heart and Lung Institute [90]. Using standardized fibrin plate assays and exposing the subjects to brief periods of intensive exercise, a clear correlation between workload and levels of euglobulin fibrinolytic activity was observed. The subjects were 14 presumably healthy persons, age 19 to 30, in good physical condition but not trained as athletes. Control blood samples were collected from the subjects at 8 A.M. After the overnight fast, it was first observed that the diurnal increase occurred whether or not the subjects remained in bed, and that the increase remained the same whether the subjects were fasting (mean at 8 A.M.: $92mm^2$, recorded as diameter products of lysed zones; at 3 P.M.: 255 mm^2) or nonfasting (mean at 8 A.M.: 66 mm^2; at 5 P.M.: 266 mm^2). When the subjects were disturbed by sampling of blood at intervals of 3 hours, the activities did not decrease during the night to reach normal resting values.

Brief exposure (5 min) to a maximal workload on the treadmill produced an immediate fibrinolytic response. The average euglobulin fibrinolytic activity in 10 subjects was 90 mm^2 before exercise and reached 658 mm^2 immediately after exercise. The activity returned to normal within 30 minutes confirming previous reports. The fibrinolytic activity of arterial blood was exactly the same as that of the venous blood, demonstrating the absence of arteriovenous differences, and confirming a previous observation by Moser [91] made with the euglobulin clot lysis time assay. When 5-minute bouts of maximal exercise were repeated at hourly intervals for 4 hours the fibrinolytic response decreased only slightly.

When workload was fixed at 70 percent of the subjects' measured maximal exercise level, the 5-minute exercise period produced only a slight, statistically insignificant increase in fibrinolytic activity (from a mean of 129 mm^2 to 206 mm^2). However, after 15 minutes of exercise the activity had increased to a mean of 421 mm ^{2}, and after 30 minutes to 626 mm^2. It is apparent that the degree of response depends upon the exercise load as well as upon its duration. At a 40 percent maximal workload, 15 minutes of exercise increased the mean activity from 80 mm^2 to only 144 mm^2. After 30 minutes' exercise, the mean activity had increased to 173 mm^2, which is less than the diurnal increase in fibrinolytic activity. Significantly, when maximal exercise or exercise at 40 percent of the maximal load was performed in the afternoon (at 4 P.M.), a higher total fibrinolytic activity was obtained than following exercise in the morning. This indicates that the diurnal increase adds to and does not replace the activity produced by exercise.

Although this study describes the diurnal increase in fibrinolytic activity and the relationship between the levels of exercise-induced fibrinolysis and the individual workloads in more detail than was reported previously, it leaves several questions open to speculation and suggests lines of additional exploration. Among the most important are:

1. The possible independence of the diurnal rise in activity from the increase resulting from exercise;

2. The possibility that repeated heavy bouts of exercise yield approximately the same fibrinolytic response while the response to a number of drugs declines after repeated application (nicotinic acid and others [51]);

3. How does the limited increase in fibrinolytic activity following a workload of 40 percent of the maximal load compare with that produced by prolonged, low-grade exercise?

The latter question seems important, because it is related to the problem of whether average, non-strenuous exercise programs enhance blood fibrinolysis. It is quite possible that the physiologic mechanisms of fibrinolysis enhancement differ in brief exposures to strenuous exercise and in prolonged periods of low workloads. It is not surprising the the large transient increase in fibrinolytic activity following brief, exhausting exercise made Biggs et al [18] suggest a causative relationship to adrenalin release though this, as described, was later disproved [44]. Similarly, as mentioned, the effect of a rise in body temperature can be discounted. In this context it is of interest to mention that the fibrinolytic activity produced by pyrogens is reported to precede the rise in temperature, indicating an independence of the response [92, 93]. Administration of antipyretic compounds does not prevent the appearance of fibrinolytic activity. Inhalation of 7.5 percent carbon dioxide, but not voluntary hyperventilation, was reported to enhance blood fibrinolytic activity [91].

Several authors have compared the effects produced by various forms of exercise. Ogston and Fullerton [94], assessing the residual, undissolved fibrin after predetermined periods of incubation of the diluted plasma clot as described by Bidwell [37], assayed samples from subjects walking 2, 4, 8, and 12 miles. A marked increase in fibrinolytic activity was observed in the beginning, but beyond 2 hours (8 miles) a slight decrease occurred. The activity had not returned to normal after 1 hour of rest, even in subjects who had walked only 2 or 4 miles. The latter finding differs from the response to brief, strenuous exercise, where the activity disappears within 30 minutes, and may explain some earlier discrepant reports. Increased fibrinolytic activity was still present 3 hours after completion of walks of 5 to 6 hours duration in inconvenient country. Samples collected the next day showed a slight depression of fibrinolytic activity in all except one subject who was accustomed to long periods of physical exertion.

Plasminogen levels remained normal. The authors suggest that prolonged exercise may release an *antiactivator* which decreases the fibrinolytic activity [95]. In the latter study, a euglobulin clot lysis time assay was used to determine the fibrinolytic activity. The presence of antiactivator was investigated by a fibrin plate method using human fibrinogen (Kabi). However, in the fibrin plate technique weakly binding inhibitors present in the small volumes applied to the fibrin layer diffuse into the surrounding substrate so that only strongly binding inhibitors can be accurately assayed. The antiactivator was determined by its neutralizing effect on urokinase (the urinary plasminogen activator), which might not necessarily behave as the activator in blood. Newer observations indicate that separate inhibitors exist for different types of activators. The possible role of corticosteroids in the delayed response following prolonged exercise is confused by discrepant reports on the effects of ACTH and corticosteroids on blood fibrinolysis. Fearnley [50] reported an enhancement of blood fibrinolysis in a patient with Addison's disease treated with cortisone, but Macfarlane and Biggs [34] observed a normal fibrinolytic response to adrenalin in two Addison patients.

Cash and Allan [96] determined the fibrinolytic activity following moderate exercise and intravenous administration of adrenalin in the same subjects to see whether similar patterns of response occurred. In assessing their results, it should be recalled that Truelove [44] and others reported that the fibrinolytic response to exercise was not mediated through a release of adrenalin. Cash and Allan infused a weak solution of adrenalin and determined the lytic activity by a euglobulin lysis time assay using a cold technique with precipitation at pH 6.0. In a group of 25 normal, healthy subjects a reasonably good correlation was observed between the fibrinolytic response to exercise and to adrenalin. In spite of this correlation, recent studies by the same authors [97] indicate the possible existence of two independent mechanisms of plasminogen activator response. That elicited by adrenalin was reported to be partially blocked by propranolol. However, other authors found no decrease in fibrinolytic response to adrenalin following adrenergic blockade [98]. Exercise-induced fibrinolysis is not altered by propranolol [13]. It should be recalled that propranolol prevents the increase in Factor VIII activity caused by exercise or by adrenalin [13, 15, 97].

The results of a particularly long study were reported by Winther [99]. Twelve subjects were exercised for 40 minutes 3 times/week for approximately 3 months. The fibrinolytic activity was determined by a diluted blood clot lysis time method. All subjects except one, who was unable to adhere to the exercise program, showed enhanced postexercise fibrinolytic activity. A perusal of the data showed unchanged resting pre-exercise values in good agreement with our results [89]. Two of three patients with intermittent claudication became free of symptoms. Most patients with AP were reported to have a work capacity too low to produce postexercise enhancement of fibrinolysis [99a].

Groups of Subjects with Defective Fibrinolytic Response to Exercise

Iatridis and Ferguson [1] noticed that some individuals had a reduced fibrinolytic response to exercise. Altogether, 12 of their presumably normal subjects showed no evidence of exercise-enhanced fibrinolysis by their assays. However, as mentioned before, some of their negative findings could be explained by the use of insensitive methods. Other possible explanations for their results are a failure to show the usual reaction to stress or an increase in inhibitor activity. The patient with Hageman disease presented a particular problem. Despite a defective production of plasminogen activator by kaolin-activation, he produced a fibrinolytic response to exercise, suggesting that separate mechanisms may be involved. One of the subjects presented evidence of enhanced inhibition.

The existence of individuals or groups of patients not responding to exercise has created a great deal of interest and initiated several attempts to classify these nonresponders and to correlate them with certain disease patterns [80, 100]. The weak fibrinolytic response observed in some individuals [96] was investigated in more detail in a study of the effects of moderate, exhaustive, and prolonged exercise [101]. Some individuals, who were poor responders in some or all of the exercise procedures, could be separated from the remainder of the group. It was the existence of such individuals which led Cash [80] to suggest that they could represent a group of subjects exposed to a prolonged retainment of fibrin deposits and therefore particularly prone to develop thrombosis, vascular disease, and arteriosclerosis. Much of the work of Cash and associates has attempted to substantiate this concept. Of particular interest is the impaired response observed in the third trimester of pregnancy [102]. They found no correlation between baseline plasminogen activator levels and the fibrinolytic response, an observation correlating well with our observations. Thus, an impaired fibrinolytic response to exercise was observed in patients with Type IV hyperlipoproteinemia [103] in spite of the normal resting levels in these and other groups of patients with abnormal lipoprotein patterns [104]. Significantly, the diurnal rise in fibrinolytic activity was also decreased in patients with Type IV hyperlipoproteinemia [105]. Only some of the patients in these groups showed increased inhibition of fibrinolysis. The possible production of an inhibitor during prolonged exercise was mentioned previously [95].

Obviously, several problems arise in connection with the existence of groups of nonresponders to exercise [100]. The workload must be adjusted individually so that all subjects are exposed to a strenuous work effort; the possible presence of inhibitors modifying the effect must be considered; and the diurnal rise and the possibility of an emotional response must be accounted for because these might increase the baseline values. Also, the strain produced by brief periods of strenuous exercise probably differs physiologically from that produced by prolonged exposure to moderate degrees of work efforts, and the results need not be comparable. The presence of disease or of differences in physiological conditions may also influence the results. Riedler et al [106] report on a patient with march hemoglobinuria whose fibrinolytic response was enhanced after an 18-km march. The enhancement declined somewhat when the march was repeated with simultaneous heparinization, a result taken to indicate that the enhanced response was caused by a process of DIC. Cash and McGill [107] reported that young insulin-dependent diabetics had reduced fibrinolytic responses to exercise. Their resting activities were higher than in the control group, a result contrasting reports of normal or decreased resting activities [108, 109]. The diurnal variation is reported to be nearly absent in South African Bantus [110]. However, the reported data show abnormally high resting morning values in the Bantu, possibly resulting from mental strain as seen in several of our cases [90]. Berkarda et al [111] determined the fibrinolytic response to moderate exercise in young normal males, older normal males, and male patients with atherosclerosis, in order to elucidate the problem of the *poor responder*. Interestingly, all three groups developed the same degree of hypercoagulability. In contrast, the fibrinolytic response was diminished in the group of older males, and it was still lower in the atherosclerotic group. Significantly, among the 30 young men, five were *poor responders*. Also, among the subjects in our normal groups a few responded much less than the remainder [89, 100]. Berkarda et al found 12 *poor responders* among their 20 atherosclerotic patients, but only two among the 12 age-matched older normal men. The resting values in all these groups were in the normal range, in good agreement with our findings [103, 104, 105]. It is of interest that Moser and Hajjar [112] reported diminished diurnal increases in groups of older normal persons or diabetic patients. Our group of older normals could be divided into one showing the normal diurnal increase in fibrinolytic activity and another, smaller, with an impaired diurnal response. In the atherosclerotic subjects, the diurnal response was markedly decreased although they had normal resting values [105]. Chakrabarti et al [113] found 32 percent of CHD patients and 12 percent of controls to have defective fibrinolysis. Using a brief, moderate exercise, Laursen and Gormsen [114] found no significant differences in response between a group of 10 patients suffering from intermittent claudication and a control group of 11 persons. They also found no evidence of fibrinogen-fibrin degradation products which would have suggested an active coagulation process followed by fibrinolysis [114a]. This finding was recently confirmed [22a]. Chakrabarti et al [115] studied the response to various forms of stress (electroplexy, surgery, myocardial infarction) and observed a reduction in fibrinolytic activity following an immediate enhancement. This observation might be related to the decrease reported by some authors to follow prolonged periods of exercise [95], and which is believed to be caused by a release of inhibitor. Significantly, patients with hepatic cirrhosis yielded larger than normal fibrinolytic responses to electroshock [116] and exercise [117]. Finally, in regard to the possible role of the Hageman factor, Holemans and Roberts [118] reported a weak fibrinolytic response to venous occlusion in Hageman patients, corresponding well to the Iatridis and Ferguson report [1] of an impaired response to exercise. However, Nilsson and Robertson [119] were unable to correlate the fibrinolytic response following venous occlusion to the Hageman factor, and Harold and Straub [14] found the same enhancement in fibrinolytic activity following exercise in Hageman patients as in normal controls. Brief, vigorous exercise does not affect the Hageman factor cofactor which is needed for activation of blood fibrinolysis by the Hageman factor-dependent pathway [120]. Thus, the Hageman problem remains unsettled.

Exercise in Animals

Before concluding this review, it is natural to ask about the apparent absence of systematic animal studies in this field. Numerous experiments on the fibrinolytic response to vasoactive drugs have been performed on animals, by von Kaulla [51] and Holemans [121] in particular. However, the fibrinolytic system in blood from most animal species differs so much from that in human blood that few definite conclusions can be drawn from the information obtained [122, 123, 124]. Differences between species also exist in the fibrinolytic activity of the vessel wall from which the increase in blood fibrinolytic activity is believed by many to be derived. Therefore, only a few observations in animals of possible interest to our problem will be mentioned. Fantl and Simon [36], in their study of fibrinolysis following electroconvulsive therapy, produced convulsions in four calves, but no fibrinolytic activity was observed in samples of the diluted plasma or the euglobulin fractions. However, Jensen [126] found euglobulins obtained from pigs exposed to electroshock to be markedly fibrinolytic, and even more so when stunned by carbon dioxide inhalation. The euglobulin clot lysis times are also reported to be longer in unanesthetized pigs, as well as in pigs under general anaesthesia (nitrous oxide and halothane), than in man [127]. Bedrak's [82] exercise experiments on dogs might also be mentioned in this context. The dog and pig have highly reactive blood fibrinolytic systems, while those in cattle or rabbits are of very low activity [124]. Williams [128] noticed that rabbits produce little fibrinolytic activity following adrenalin injection. Interestingly, prolonged exercise in rabbits did not prevent cholesterol-induced atherogenesis [129] although it appeared to decrease the incidence of spontaneous aortic lesions [130]. The development of a micromethod made it possible to use rats instead of dogs in studies of the effects of vasoactive agents [131].

Summary

Exercise enhances blood coagulation and increases blood fibrinolytic activity. The effect on blood coagulation is mainly caused by a considerable increase (200 percent) in measured Factor VIII activity (antihemophilic factor activity). Components of the extrinsic coagulation system apparently are not affected. The effects on Hageman factor activity and platelets are debatable. The large increase in blood fibrinolytic activity is caused by an increase in concentration of a plasminogen activator. The effects of exercise on blood coagulation and fibrinolysis are independent. Administration of β-adrenergic blocking agents (propranolol) prevents the increase in Factor VIII activity, but has no influence on the increase in blood fibrinolysis. A review of the literature is presented, the reported findings examined, and their possible physiological implications and role in thrombotic disease discussed.

REFERENCES

1. Iatridis, S.G., and Ferguson, J.H. Effect of physical exercise on blood clotting and fibrinolysis. *J. Appl. Physiol.* 18:337, 1963.

2. Cannon, W.B., and Gray, H. Factors affecting the coagulation time of blood. III. The hastening or retarding of coagulation by adrenalin injections. *Am. J. Physiol.* 34:232, 1914.

3. Cannon, W.B., and Mendenhall, W.L. Factors affecting the coagulation time of blood. IV. The hastening of coagulation in pain and emotional excitement. *Am. J. Physiol.* 34:251, 1914.

4. Egeberg, O. The effect of exercise on the blood clotting system. *Scand. J. Clin. Lab. Invest.* 15:8, 1963.

5. Egeberg, O. On the nature of the blood antihemophilic A factor (AHA=F. VIII) increase associated with muscular exercise. *Scand. J. Clin. Lab. Invest.* 15:202, 1963.

6. Rizza, C.R. Effect of exercise on the level of antihaemophilic globulin in human blood. *J. Physiol.* 156:128, 1961.

7. Egeberg, O. The effect of muscular exercise on hemostasis in von Willebrand's disease. *Scand. J. Clin. Lab. Invest.* 15:273, 1963.

8. Egeberg, O. Changes in the activity of antihemophilic A factor (F. VIII) and the bleeding time associated with muscular exercise and adrenaline infusion. *Scand. J. Clin. Lab. Invest.* 15:539, 1963.

9. Overman, R.S., Newman, A.A., and Wright, I.S. Plasma prothrombin times in normal human subjects. The effects of certain factors on the prothrombin time. *Am. Heart J.* 39:56, 1950.

10. Kesseler, K., and Egli, H. Untersuchungen über die Gerinnbarkeit des Blutes während und nach körperlicher Arbeit. *Int. Z. Angew. Physiol.* 17:228, 1958.

11. Winckelmann, G., Meyer, G., and Roskamm, H. Der Einfluss körperlicher Belastung auf Blutgerinnung und Fibrinolyse bei untrainierten Personen und Hochleistungssportlern. *Klin. Wochenschr.* 46:712, 1968.

12. Keeney, C.E., and Laramie, D.W. Effect of exercise on blood coagulation. *Circulation Res.* 10:691, 1962.

13. Cohen, R.J., Epstein, S.E., Cohen, L.S., and Dennis, L.H. Alterations of fibrinolysis and blood coagulation induced by exercise, and the role of beta-adrenergic-receptor stimulation. *Lancet* II:1264, 1968.

14. Harold, R., and Straub, P.W. In vivo role of factor XII (Hageman factor) in hypercoagulability and fibrinolysis. *J. Lab. Clin. Med.* 79:397, 1972.

15. Ingram, G.I.C., and Jones, R.V. The rise in clotting factor 8 induced in man by adrenaline: effect of alpha- and beta-blockers. *J. Physiol.* 187:447, 1966.

16. Abildgaard, C.F., and Link, R.P. Blood coagulation and hemostasis in thoroughbred horses. *Proc. Soc. Exp. Biol. Med.* 119:212, 1965.

17. Sjolin, K.E. Coagulation defect in horse plasma. *Proc. Soc. Exp. Biol. Med.* 94:818, 1957.

18. Biggs, R., Macfarlane, R.G., and Pilling, J. Observations on fibrinolysis. Experimental activity produced by exercise or adrenaline. *Lancet* I:402, 1947.

19. Dawson, A.A., and Ogston, D. Exercise-induced thrombocytosis. *Acta Haemotol.* 42:241, 1969.

20. Libre, E.P., Cowan, D.C., Watkins, S.P., and Shulman, N.R. Relationships between spleen, platelets and Factor VIII levels. *Blood* 31:358, 1968.

21. Rizza, C.R., and Eipe, J. Exercise, Factor VIII and the spleen. *Brit. J. Haematol.* 20:629, 1971.

21a. Bennett, B., and Ratnoff, O.D. Changes in antihemophilic factor (AHF, Factor VIII) procoagulant activity and AHF-like antigen in normal pregnancy, and following exercise and pneumoencephalography. *J. Lab. Clin. Med.* 80:256, 1972.

22. McClure, P.D., Ingram, G.I.C., and Jones, R.V. Platelet changes after adrenaline infusions with and without adrenaline blockers. *Thromb. Diath. Haemorrh.* 13:136, 1965.

22a. Prentice, C.R.M., Hassanein, A.A., McNicol, G.P., and Douglas, H.S. Studies on blood coagulation, fibrinolysis and platelet function following exercise in normal and spleenectomized people. *Br. J. Haematol.* 23:541, 1972.

23. Wacholder, K., Parchwitz, E., Egli, H., and Kesseler, K. Der Einfluss körperlicher Arbeit auf die Zahl der Thrombocyten und auf deren Haftneigung. *Acta Haematol.* 18:59, 1957.

24. Wright, H.P. The sources of blood platelets and their adhesiveness in experimental thrombocytosis. *J. Pathol.* 56:151, 1944.

25. Yamazaki, H., Sano, T., Odakura, T., Takeuchi, K., and Shimamoto, T. Electro-cardiographic and hematological change by exercise test in coronary patients and pyridinol carbamate treatment. *Am. Heart J.* 79:640, 1970.

26. Yamazaki, H., Kobayaski, I., and Shimamoto, T. Enhancement of ADP-induced platelet aggregation by exercise test in coronary patients and its prevention by pyridinol carbamate. *Thromb. Diath. Haemorrh.* 24:438, 1970.

27. Pegrum, G.D., Harrison, K.M., Shaw, S., Haselton, A., and Wolff, S. Effect of prolonged exercise on platelet adhesiveness. *Nature* 213:301, 1967.

28. Sarajas, H.S.S., Konttinen, A., and Frick, M.H. Thrombocytosis evoked by exercise. *Nature* 192:721, 1961.

29. Ikkala, E., Myllylä, G., and Sarajas, H.S.S. Haemostatic changes associated with exercise. *Nature* 199:459, 1963.

30. Breddin, K., and Hach, W. Agglutination und Adhäsivität der Thrombozyten nach körperlicher Belastung. *Thromb. Diath. Haemorrh.* 15:109, 1966.

31. Egeberg, O. Influence of thyroid function on the blood clotting system. *Scand. J. Clin. Lab. Invest.* 15:1, 1963.

32. Macfarlane, R.G., and Pilling, J. Observations on fibrinolysis. Plasminogen, plasmin, and antiplasmin content of human blood. *Lancet* II:562, 1946.

33. Macfarlane, R.G., and Biggs, R. Observations on fibrinolysis. Spontaneous activity associated with surgical operations, trauma, etc. *Lancet* II:862, 1946.

34. Macfarlane, R.G., and Biggs, R. Fibrinolysis. Its mechanism and significance. *Blood* 3:1167, 1948.

35. Mole, R.H. Fibrinolysin and the fluidity of the blood post mortem. *J. Pathol.* 60:413, 1948.

36. Fantl, P., and Simon, S.E. Fibrinolysis following electrically induced convulsions. *Aust. J. Exp. Biol. Med. Sci.* 26:521, 1948.

37. Bidwell, E. Fibrinolysins of human plasma. A comparison of fibrinolytic plasma from normal subjects and from cadaver blood with plasmin prepared by activation with chloroform. *Biochem. J.* 55:497, 1953.

38. Müllertz, S. A plasminogen activator in spontaneously active human blood. *Proc. Soc. Exp. Biol. Med.* 82:291, 1953.

39. Astrup, T. Fibrinolysis in the organism. *Blood* 11:781, 1956.

40. Fearnly, G.R., and Tweed, J.M. Evidence of an active fibrinolytic enzyme in the plasma of normal people with observations on inhibition associated with the presence of calcium. *Clin. Sci.* 12:81, 1953.

41. Fearnly, G.R., Balmforth, G., and Fearnly, E. Evidence of a diurnal fibrinolytic rhythm; with a simple method of measuring natural fibrinolysis. *Clin. Sci.* 16:645, 1957.

42. Sherry, S., Lindemeyer, R.I., Fletcher, A.P., and Alkjaersig, N. Studies on enhanced fibrinolytic activity in man. *J. Clin. Invest.* 38:810, 1959.

43. Sawyer, W.D., Fletcher, A.P., Alkjaersig, N., and Sherry, S. Studies on the thrombolytic activity of human plasma. *J. Clin. Invest.* 39:426, 1960.

44. Truelove, S.C. Fibrinolysis and the eosinophil count. *Clin. Sci.* 10:229, 1951.

45. Truelove, S.C. Fibrinolysis in relation to ACTH and cortisone. *Clin. Sci.* 11:101, 1952.

46. Truelove, S.C. Fibrinolysis and eosinopenia after surgical operations. *Clin. Sci.* 11:107, 1952.

47. Fearnly, G.R., Revill, R., and Tweed, J.M. Observations on the inactivation of fibrinolytic activity in shed blood. *Clin. Sci.* 11:309, 1952.

48. Truelove, S.C. The lability of human fibrinolysin. *Clin. Sci.* 12:75, 1953.

49. Fearnly, G.R., and Lackner, R. The fibrinolytic activity of normal blood. *Brit. J. Haematol.* 1:189, 1955.

50. Fearnly, G.R. *Fibrinolysis.* Baltimore, Williams & Wilkins, 1965.

51. von Kaulla, K.N. *Chemistry of Thrombolysis: Human Fibrinolytic Enzymes.* Springfield, Ill., Thomas, 1963.

52. Sherry, S., Fletcher, A.P., and Alkjaersig, N. Fibrinolysis and fibrinolytic activity in man. *Physiol. Rev.* 39:343, 1959.

53. Kwaan, H.C., Lo, R., and McFadzean, A.J.S. On the production of plasma fibrinolytic activity within veins. *Clin. Sci.* 16:241, 1957.

54. Messer, D.L., Celander, D.R., and Guest, M.M. Stability of fibrin contiguous to intima of veins. *Circ. Res.* 11:832, 1962.

55. Kwaan, H.C., and McFadzean, A.J.S. On plasma fibrinolytic activity induced by ischaemia. *Clin. Sci.* 15:245, 1956.

56. Clarke, R.L., and Cliffton, E.E. Oxygen saturation and spontaneous fibrinolytic activity. *Am. J. Med. Sci.* 244:466, 1962.

57. Tighe, J.R., and Swan, H.T. Fibrinolysis and venous obstruction. *Clin. Sci.* 25:219, 1963.

58. Amery, A., Vermylen, J., Maes, H., and Verstraete, M. Enhancing the fibrinolytic activity in human blood by occlusion of blood vessels. *Thromb. Diath. Haemorrh.* 7:70, 1962.

59. Todd, A.S. The histological localisation of fibrinolysin activator. *J. Pathol.* 78:281, 1959.

60. Astrup, T., Albrechtsen, O.K., Claassen, M., and Rasmussen, J. Thromboplastic and fibrinolytic activity of the human aorta. *Circ. Res.* 7:969, 1959.

61. Coccheri, S., and Astrup, T. Thromboplastic and fibrinolytic activities in large human vessels. *Proc. Soc. Exp. Biol. Med.* 108:369, 1961.

62. Aoki, N., and von Kaulla, K.N. The extraction of vascular plasminogen activator from human cadavers and a description of some of its properties. *Am. J. Clin. Pathol.* 55:171, 1971.

63. Holemans, R. Enhancement of fibrinolysis in the dog by injection of vasoactive drugs. *Am. J. Physiol.* 208:511, 1965.

64. Menon, S. Muscles as a possible source of plasminogen activators to the circulation. *J. Assoc. Physicians India* 17:441, 1969.

65. Astrup, T. Tissue activators of plasminogen. *Fed. Proc.* 25:42, 1966.

66. Albrechtsen, O.K. The fibrinolytic agents in saline extracts of human tissues. *Scand. J. Clin. Lab. Invest.* 10:91, 1958.

67. Hamberg, U. Studies on plasminogen activators. I. Sucrose density gradient distribution of activators from normal and lytic human plasma. *Acta Chem. Scand.* 20:2539, 1966.

68. Astrup, T., Piper, J., and Rasmussen, J. The fibrinolytic system in human blood, as exemplified in a case of agammaglobulinemia and a case of macroglobulinemia. *Scand. J. Clin. Lab. Invest.* 12:336, 1960.

69. Brakman, P. *Fibrinolysis. A Standardized Fibrin Plate Method and a Fibrinolytic Assay of Plasminogen.* Amsterdam, Scheltema and Holkema, NV, 1967.

70. Brakman, P., and Astrup, T. The fibrin plate method for assay of fibrinolytic agents. *In*, Bang, N.V., Ed. *Thrombosis and Bleeding Disorders, Theory and Methods*, p. 332. New York, Academic, 1971.

71. Astrup, T., and Rasmussen, J. Estimation of fibrinolytic activity in blood. *In, Proc. VIIth International Congress of the International Society of Haematology*, p. 164. Rome, 1958.

72. Brakman, P., Albrechtsen, O.K., and Astrup, T. A comparative study of coagulation and fibrinolysis in blood from normal men and women. *Br. J. Haematol.* 12:74, 1966.

73. Rasmussen, J., Astrup, T., Geill, T., Ollendorff, P., and Lund, E. Fibrinolytic activity in blood from old age patients under influence of dietary fats. *In, Proc. 8th Congress of European Society of Haematology*, Wien, 1961. (Comm. No. 440)

74. Blix, S. Studies on the fibrinolytic system in the euglobulin fraction of human plasma. *Scand. J. Clin. Lab. Invest.* 13(Suppl. 58):1, 1961.

75. Astrup, T., Brakman, P., Ollendorff, P., and Rasmussen, J. Haemostasis in haemophilia in relation to the haemostatic balance in the organism and the effect of peanuts. *Thromb. Diath. Haemorrh.* 5:329, 1960.

76. Fearnly, G.R. Spontaneous fibrinolysis. *Am. J. Cardiol.* 6:371, 1960.

77. Chakrabarti, R., Bielawiec, M., Evans, J.F., and Fearnly, G.R. Methodological study and the recommended technique for determining the euglobulin lysis time. *J. Clin. Pathol.* 21:698, 1968.

78. Ratnoff, O.D. Studies on a proteolytic enzyme in human plasma. IV. The rate of lysis of plasma clots in normal and diseased individuals with particular reference to hepatic disease. *Bull. Johns. Hopkins. Hosp.* 83:29, 1949.

79. Ratnoff, O.D., and Donaldson, V.H. Physiologic and pathologic effects of increased fibrinolytic activity in man. With notes on the effects of exercise and certain inhibitors on fibrinolysis. *Am. J. Cardiol.* 6:378, 1960.

80. Cash, J.D. A new approach to studies of the fibrinolytic system in man. *Am. Heart J.* 75:424, 1968.

81. Menon, I.S., Burke, F., and Dewar, H.A. Effects of strenuous and graded exercise on fibrinolytic activity. *Lancet* 1:700, 1967.

82. Bedrak, E. Effect of muscular exercise in a hot environment on canine fibrinolytic activity. *J. Appl. Physiol.* 20:1307, 1965.

83. Bedrak, E., Beer, G., and Furman, K.I. Fibrinolytic activity and muscular exercise in heat. *J. Appl. Physiol.* 19:469, 1964.

84. Billimoria, J.D., Drysdale, J., James, D.C.O., and Maclagan, N.F. Determination of fibrinolytic activity of whole blood with special reference to the effect of exercise and fat feeding. *Lancet* II:471, 1959.

85. Meikle, A.W., and Graybill, J.R. Fibrinolysis and hemorrhage in a fatal case of heat stroke. *N. Engl. J. Med.* 276:911, 1967.

86. Weber, M.B., and Blakely, J.A. The haemorrhagic diathesis of heat stroke. A consumption coagulopathy successfully treated with heparin. *Lancet* I:1190, 1969.

87. Clinicopathologic Conference. A sixty-five year old woman with heat stroke. *Am. J. Med.* 43:113, 1967.

88. Bachmann, F. Evidence for hypercoagulability in heat stroke. *J. Clin. Invest.* 46:1033, 1967.

89. Moxley, R.T., Brakman, P., and Astrup, T. Resting levels of fibrinolysis in blood in inactive and exercising men. *J. Appl. Physiol.* 28:549, 1970.

90. Rosing, D.R., Brakman, P., Redwood, D.R., Goldstein, R.E., Beiser, G.D., Astrup, T., and Epstein, S.E. Blood fibrinolytic activity in man. Diurnal variation and the response to varying intensities of exercise. *Circ. Res.* 27:171, 1970.

91. Moser, K.M. The "compleat fibrinolyticist": a study in septophrenia. *Fed. Proc.* 25:94, 1966.

92. Deutsch, E., and Elsner, P. Pyrogens as thrombolytic agents. Clinical and experimental studies. *Am. J. Cardiol.* 6:420, 1960.

93. von Kaulla, K.N. Intravenous protein-free pyrogen. A powerful fibrinolytic agent in man. *Circulation* 17:187, 1958.

94. Ogston, D., and Fullerton, H.W. Changes in fibrinolytic activity produced by physical activity. *Lancet* II:730, 1961.

95. Bennett, N.B., Ogston, C.M., and Ogston, D. The effect of prolonged exercise on the components of the blood fibrinolytic enzyme system. *J. Physiol.* 198:479, 1968.

96. Cash, J.D., and Allan, A.G.E. The fibrinolytic response to moderate exercise and intravenous adrenalin in the same subjects. *Br. J. Haematol.* 13:376, 1967.

97. Cash, J.D., Woodfield, D.G., and Allan, A.G.E. Adrenergic mechanisms in the systemic plasminogen activator response to adrenaline in man. *Br. J. Haematol.* 18:487, 1970.

98. Tanser, A.R., and Smellie, H. Observations on adrenaline-induced fibrinolysis in man. *Clin. Sci.* 26:375, 1964.

99. Winther, O. Exercise and blood fibrinolysis. *Lancet* II:1195, 1966.

99a. Redwood, D.R., Rosing, D.R., and Epstein, S.E. Circulatory and symptomatic effects of physical training in patients with coronary-artery disease and angina pectoris. *N. Engl. J. Med.* 286:959, 1972.

100. Astrup, T., and Brakman, P. Responders and non-responders in exercise-induced blood fibrinolysis. *In,* Larsen, O.A., and Malmborg, R.O., Eds. *Coronary Heart Disease and Physical Fitness,* p. 130. Baltimore, University Park Press, 1971.

101. Cash, J.D., and Woodfield, D.G. Fibrinolytic response to moderate, exhaustive and prolonged exercise in normal subjects. *Nature* 215:628, 1967.

102. Woodfield, D.G., Cole, S.K., and Cash, J.D. Impaired fibrinolytic response to exercise stress in normal pregnancy. Its possible role in the development of Shwartzman-type reactions. *Am. J. Obstet. Gynecol.* 102:440, 1968.

103. Epstein, S.E., Rosing, D.R., Brakman, P., Redwood, D.R., and Astrup, T. Impaired fibrinolytic response to exercise in patients with Type IV hyperlipoproteinaemia. *Lancet* II:631, 1970.

104. Astrup, T., Brakman, P., Levy, R.I., and Fredrickson, D.S. Hyperlipoproteinemia and fibrinolysis. *Circulation* 42 (Suppl. III):49, Abstract No. 156, 1970.

105. Rosing, D.R., Redwood, D.R., Brakman, P., Astrup, T., and Epstein, S.E. Impairment of the diurnal fibrinolytic response in man: Effects of aging, Type IV hyperlipoproteinemia and coronary artery disease. (to be published in *Circ. Res.*)

106. Riedler, G., Straub, P.W., and Frick, P.G. The effects of acute intravascular hemolysis on coagulation and fibrinolysis. II. March hemoglobinemia and hemoglobiuria. *Helv. Med. Acta* 34:217, 1968.

107. Cash, J.D., and McGill, R.C. Fibrinolytic response to moderate exercise in young male diabetics and non-diabetics. *J. Clin. Pathol.* 22:32, 1969.

108. Fearnly, G.R., Chakrabarti, R., and Aois, P.R.D. Blood fibrinolytic activity in diabetes mellitus and its bearing on ischaemic heart disease and obesity. *Br. Med. J.* 1:921, 1963.

109. Tanser, A.R. Fibrinolytic response of diabetics and non-diabetics to adrenaline. *J. Clin. Pathol.* 20:231, 1967.

110. Lackner, H., and Sougin-Mibashan, R. Fibrinolysis and alimentary lipaemia in Whites and Bantus; their relationship and response to intravenous heparin. *Thromb. Diath. Haemorrh.* 11:108, 1964.

111. Berkarda, B., Akokan, G., and Derman, U. Fibrinolytic response to physical exercise in males. *Atherosclerosis* 13:85, 1971.

112. Moser, K.M., and Hajjar, G.C. Age and disease-related alterations in fibrinogen-euglobulin (fibrinolytic) behavior. *Am. J. Med. Sci.* 251:536, 1966.

113. Chakrabarti, R., Hocking, E.D., Fearnly, G.R., Mann, R.D., Atwell, T.N., and Jackson, D. Fibrinolytic activity and coronary-artery disease. *Lancet* I:987, 1968.

114. Laursen, B., and Gormsen, J. Pharmacological enhancement and short-time stimulation of blood fibrinolytic activity. *Scand. J. Haematol.* 6:402, 1969.

114a. Laursen, B., and Gormsen, J. Studies on fibrinolytic activity in normal persons and patients with atherosclerotic vascular disease after physical activity and injections of nicotinic acid. *Angiology* 21:486, 1970.

115. Chakrabarti, R., Hocking, E.D., and Fearnly, G.R. Reaction pattern to three stresses-electroplexy, surgery, and myocardial infarction–of fibrinolysis and plasma fibrinogen. *J. Clin. Pathol.* 22:659, 1969.

116. Fletcher, A.P., Biederman, O., Moore, D., Alkjaersig, N., and Sherry, S. Abnormal plasminogen-plasmin system activity (Fibrinolysis) in patients with hepatic cirrhosis: Its cause and consequences. *J. Clin. Invest.* 43:681, 1964.

117. Das, P.C., and Cash, J.D. Fibrinolysis at rest and after exercise in hepatic cirrhosis. *Br. J. Haematol.* 17:431, 1969.

118. Holemans, R., and Roberts, H.R. Hageman factor and in vivo activation of fibrinolysis. *J. Lab. Clin. Med.* 64:778, 1964.

119. Nilsson, I.M., and Robertson, B. Effect of venous occlusion on coagulation and fibrinolytic components in normal subjects. *Thromb. Diath. Haemorrh.* 20:396, 1968.

120. Ogston, D., Bennett, N.B., Ogston, C.M., and Ratnoff, O.D. The assay of a plasma component necessary for the generation of a plasminogen activator in the presence of Hageman factor (Hageman factor co-factor) *Bri. J. Haemat.* 20:209, 1971.

121. Holemans, R., and Silver, M.J. The blood fibrinolytic system. Mechanism of activation and significance. *In*, Johnson, S.A., and Guest, M.M., Eds. *Dynamics of Thrombus Formation and Dissolution*, p. 307. Philadelphia, Lippincott, 1969.

122. Astrup, T. Fibrinolytic mechanisms in man and animals. *In*, Johnson, S.A., and Guest, M.M., Eds. *Dynamics of Thrombus Formation and Dissolution*, p. 275. Philadelphia, Lippincott, 1969.

123. Cliffton, E.E., and Downie, G.R. Variations in proteolytic activity of serum of animals including man. *Proc. Soc. Exp. Biol. Med.* 73:559, 1950.

124. Olesen, E.S. Variations in non-specific activation of fibrinolytic system in sera of different species. *Acta Pharmacol. Toxicol.* 19:73, 1962.

125. Astrup, T., and Buluk, K. Thromboplastic and fibrinolytic activities in vessels of animals. *Circ. Res.* 13:253, 1963.

126. Jensen, M.M. Fibrinolytic activity in slaughter pigs stunned by electric shock or carbon dioxide inhalation. *Acta. Vet. Scand.* 7:394, 1966.

127. Blecher, T.E., and Gunstone, M.J. Fibrinolysis, coagulation and haematological findings in normal Large White/Wessex cross pigs. *Br. Vet. J.* 125:74, 1969.

128. Williams, J.R.B. The fibrinolytic activity of urine. *Br. J. Exp. Pathol.* 32:530, 1951.

129. Brainard, J.B. Effect of prolonged exercise on atherogenesis in the rabbit. *Proc. Soc. Exp. Biol. Med.* 100:244, 1959.

130. Kobernick, S.D., and Hashimoto, Y. Histochemistry of atherosclerosis. II. Spontaneous degenerative lesions of aorta of exercised and sedentary rabbits. *Lab. Invest.* 12:685, 1963.

131. Wasantapruek, S., and von Kaulla, K.N. A serial microfibrinolysis test and its use in rats with liver by-pass. *Thromb. Diath. Haemorrh.* 15:284, 1966.

12

SUBSTRATE UTILIZATION IN MUSCLE–
ADAPTATIONS TO PHYSICAL EFFORT

Hugh G. Welch, Ph.D.

Considering the importance of understanding muscle metabolism, particularly of cardiac muscle, and its implications for health and disease, it is surprising to find that knowledge in this area is quite fragmentary. The available literature on the subject indicates the source of the problem. The techniques necessary to study muscle metabolism are difficult, and can be used only under certain ideal conditions; in the case of heart muscle their use can be extremely dangerous.

Much of the early work used tissue slices or homogenates, isolated heart-lung preparation, or isolated, perfused heart. Although useful information was obtained from these studies, the results were suspect because the experiments were non-physiological. Significant progress was not made until the advent of relatively modern techniques, including cardiac catheterization.

By combining the findings of earlier studies with the results of 25 years of catheterization studies, it is now possible to construct a picture of skeletal and cardiac muscle metabolism during rest and during exercise of varying intensity. This picture, while admittedly imperfect and certainly subject to modification as more refined techniques are developed, should help in the effort to resolve questions of adaptation to physical stress and diseases of muscle.

Basic Principles

Muscle has the capacity to utilize a wide variety of substrates for the production of energy. The adaptive value of this fact should be obvious, especially for the heart. The continuous demand for energy, even during periods when the body is at rest, requires a steady supply of substrate regardless of changes in the nature of the food supply and even during periods of starvation. Therefore, it is not surprising to find that the heart can utilize an array of substrates including glucose, pyruvate, lactate, fatty acids, ketone bodies, and even amino acids. The choice of substrate is apparently determined by the arterial concentration under normal conditions [4, 5].

Fat is the most economical form for storing energy in the body. This statement is supported by the data in TABLE I. It should be clear that to store a given amount of energy, fat can provide the storage with less than half the weight required for carbohydrate (CHO). In fact, the total energy stored in the body as carbohydrate is probably less than 2000 kcal in a normal, relatively sedentary man. In contrast, a 70 kg man with a body fat content of only 8 percent (an extremely low value) would have available some 50,000 kcal from this store.

TABLE I

Caloric values for carbohydrate, fat and protein in the human body

	CHO	Fat	Protein
kcal/g	4.10	9.30	4.10
kcal/liter O$_2$ consumed	5.05	4.69	4.60

Carbohydrate is the most efficient source of energy. Although 1 gram of fat contains over twice as much energy as 1 gram of CHO, it requires almost three times as much oxygen to oxidize it to carbon dioxide and water. The result is that CHO yields more energy for a given volume of oxygen than does fat, despite its lower energy content (TABLE I). Also, if one is concerned with the biologically useful energy derived from foods, carbohydrates still have a higher yield per liter of oxygen (TABLE II). It should be noted that in this context, lactate is a more *efficient* fuel than fat when the oxygen supply is limited.

TABLE II

Energy available for biological purposes from some commonly metabolized compounds per unit volume of oxygen

(glucose	=	1.00)
glycogen		1.02
lactate		0.95
palmitate		0.89

Metabolically, cardiac muscle is similar to red skeletal muscle. The differences between cardiac muscle and skeletal muscle tissues have been overstated. It should be remembered that cardiac muscle is continually active and skeletal muscle is not. The differences between continuously contracting red skeletal muscle and cardiac muscle are small, suggesting that under appropriate conditions, data obtained from skeletal muscle may be used to enhance our understanding of cardiac muscle metabolism.

Substrate Utilization in Skeletal and Cardiac Muscle

Rest. Skeletal muscle, like cardiac muscle, utilizes a wide variety of substrates. Presumably, however, it has a preference for glucose and free fatty acids. There is evidence that, at rest, fats are the fuel of choice since glucose oxidation can account for no more than about 35 percent of the total energy requirement [6]. Resting muscle produces a small amount of lactate [13].

In the case of the heart it should be noted that, even during rest, cardiac muscle is metabolically active; indeed, its metabolic rate may be 15-20 times higher than inactive skeletal muscle [9, 10, 11, 12]. TABLE III shows the ranges of values for different substrates. The wide variability is due in part to the heart's ability to adapt to the available substrate and the availability of these substrates in the different experimental protocols.

TABLE III

Fraction of oxidative metabolism supplied by different substrates in the heart at rest

glucose	18-30%
pyruvate	0 - 1%
lactate	15-30%
free fatty acids	25-70%
amino acids	0 - 5%
ketones	0 - 5%

(Adapted from Bing [3]; Keul and Doll [8])

The utilization of lactate and the variation in the role of free fatty acids are findings of importance. There is some evidence that carbohydrates are preferred by the heart and that the use of fats is dependent upon the availability of carbohydrate [9].[1]

Exercise. During physical activity, the metabolic rates of both skeletal and cardiac muscle increase. Skeletal muscle may increase its oxygen consumption from 0.6 ml/100g/min at rest [10, 12] to as high as 20-25 ml/100g/min during high rates of contraction [14]. Cardiac muscle, which uses 8-10 ml O_2/100g/min during rest, may increase to a value several times greater with exercise [4, 11].[2]

---

[1] The preference of both the myocardium and skeletal muscle for glucose as a substrate is important in both normals and cardiacs, especially since there is a greater efficiency in terms of calories liberated per liter of oxygen consumed when carbohydrate is the substrate rather than fats. This is important particularly in patients with arteriosclerotic heart disease who have a limited blood flow and hence a reduced oxygen supply. [H.K.H. Ed.]

[2] The ratio of the myocardial oxygen intake to the total body oxygen intake remains relatively constant over a large range of oxygen intake of the body. In our study of firemen, the ratio of the myocardial oxygen intake to body oxygen intake was approximately 13 times higher in the fit, and 17 times higher in the unfit subjects. [H.K.H. Ed.]

In general, both types of muscle tend to utilize relatively more carbohydrate during exercise and the proportion of metabolism supported by carbohydrate utilization increases in proportion to the severity of the work. Skeletal muscle may derive as much as 95 percent of its energy from glucose oxidation (including glycogen) during high rates of stimulation [6]. At less intense levels, the glucose utilization is decreased and in prolonged work, the proportion of energy derived from glucose decreases over time. Data from human subjects participating in prolonged exercise also indicate that the role of carbohydrates as an energy source decreases with time, suggesting an increased use of fats [1, 2, 7]. Subjective exhaustion in these experiments was correlated with lowered levels of available carbohydrate.

During early stages of work, skeletal muscles produce large amounts of lactate, presumably as a result of insufficient oxygen in the cell. In severe exercise, arterial lactate levels may exceed 10 meq/liter. However, in prolonged work, muscles may begin to take up lactate from the blood [13]. This may indicate a decreased availability of glucose and/or glycogen and suggests the possibility that the muscle is now using lactate as an energy source.

The picture in the heart, while similar, has some interesting differences. TABLE IV shows a comparison of substrates utilized by the heart during rest, submaximal exercise, and maximal steady state exercise. While increasing levels of exercise are reflected by higher levels of carbohydrate utilization, the chief carbohydrate appears to be lactate, not glucose. There are several possible reasons. The heart does not have the endogenous glycogen stores available to it that skeletal muscle has, and, therefore, glucose metabolism must be supported largely from blood rather than from the heart muscle itself.

There are reasons to suggest that the rate of glucose penetration into cardiac muscle cells is slower than that of lactate. TABLE II shows that the energy yield from lactate approximates that of glucose; if the rate of entry is faster, conceivably it could be a more useful fuel for heart muscle than glucose. Since cardiac muscle metabolism is influenced by arterial concentration of a substrate, the high arterial levels of lactate during exercise probably enhance its utilization by the myocardium. In fact, the idea of the utilization of lactate by the

TABLE IV

Fraction of oxidative metabolism supplied by different
substrates in the heart during exercise (in percent)

Substrate	rest	600 kgm/min	1200 kgm/min
glucose	31	17	16
lactate	28	50	61
pyruvate	2	1	–
free fatty acids	34	30	21
ketones	5	2	2

(Adapted from Keul and Doll [8])

myocardium, at a time when that source is normally available, suggests an attractive adaptive mechanism.

Summary

Muscle has the capacity to utilize a wide variety of substrates for the production of energy. Fat is the most economical form for storing energy in the body. Carbohydrate is the most *efficient* source of energy. Metabolically, cardiac muscle is similar to red skeletal muscle. Both skeletal muscle and cardiac muscle utilize a wide variety of substrates; at rest, fats are the fuel of choice. During severe exercise, carbohydrate utilization from endogenous glycogen increases in the skeletal muscle, and in the heart muscle utilization is predominately from glucose and lactate.

REFERENCES

1. Bergstrom, J., Hermansen, L., Hultman, E., and Saltin, B. Diet, muscle glycogen and physical performance. *Acta Physiol. Scand.* 71:129-139, 1967.

2. Bergstrom, J., and Hultman, E. A study of glycogen metabolism during exercise in man. *Scand. J. Clin. Lab. Invest.* 19:218-228, 1967.

3. Bing, R.J. Myocardial metabolism. *Circulation* 12:635-647, 1955.

4. Bing, R.J. Cardiac metabolism. *Physiol. Rev.* 45:171-213, 1965.

5. Bing, R.J. Coronary circulation and cardiac metabolism. *In*, Fishman, A.P., and Richards, D.W., Eds., *Circulation of the Blood*, pp. 199-264. New York, Oxford Univ. Press, 1964.

6. Chapler, C.K., and Stainsby, W.N. Carbohydrate metabolism in contracting dog skeletal muscle *in situ*. *Am. J. Physiol.* 215:995-1004, 1968

7. Costill, D.L., Bowers, R., Branam, G., and Sparks, K. Muscle glycogen utilization during prolonged exercise on successive days. *J. Appl. Physiol.* 31:834-841, 1971.

8. Keul, J., and Doll, E. The influence of exercise and hypoxia on the substrate uptake of human heart and human skeletal muscles. *In*, Poortmans, J.R., Ed., *Biochemistry of Exercise*, pp. 41-46. Baltimore, University Park Press, 1968.

9. Olson, R.E. Physiology of cardiac muscle. *In*, Hamilton, W.F., Ed., *Handbook of Physiology.* Sect. 2 *Circulation*. Vol. 1, pp. 199-235. Washington, American Physiological Society, 1962.

10. Piiper, J., DiPrampero, P.E., and Cerritelli, P. Oxygen debt and high-energy phosphates in gastrocnemius muscle of the dog. *Am. J. Physiol.* 215:523-531, 1968.

11. Scott, J.C. Physical activity and the coronary circulation. *Can. Med. Assoc. J.* 96:853-859, 1967.

12. Stainsby, W.N., and Otis, A.B. Blood flow, blood oxygen tension, oxygen uptake and oxygen transport in skeletal muscle. *Am. J. Physiol.* 206:858-866, 1964.

13. Stainsby, W.N., and Welch, H.G. Lactate metabolism of contracting dog skeletal muscle *in situ*. *Am. J. Physiol.* 211:177-183, 1966.

14. Welch, H.G., and Stainsby, W.N. Oxygen debt in contracting dog skeletal muscle *in situ*. *Respir. Physiol.* 3:229-242, 1967.

13

BIOCHEMICAL ADAPTATION IN THE HEART
SECONDARY TO PHYSICAL EFFORT

Menard M. Gertler, M.D. and *Hillar E. Leetma*, M.D.

The ability to perform exercise depends on the capacity of the myocardium to extract and utilize oxygen from the coronary arteries. This process is dependent on the physiologic and/or pathologic status of the coronary arteries, as well as upon the myocardium. Myocardial oxygen consumption in ml/min (MVO_2) may be estimated from the relationship of the product heart rate (HR) and systolic blood pressure (SBP) (mm Hg) [1]. This assumption is based on the high degree of correlation between the equation of HR $\times$ SBP and actual MVO_2 measurements. Because the theoretical implications of the basic physiological reasons responsible for O_2 consumption of the heart are so important to exercise stress testing and prescription, certain basic biochemical facts will be reviewed [2].

Basic Biochemical Facts

The minute cardiac oxygen consumption (MVO_2) is determined by a combination of mechanisms:
1. Intramyocardial tension (pressure $\times$ stress).
   The evidence for this is well-documented and has firm foundation in La Place's phenomenon.
2. Contractile state of the heart.
   It has been observed that inotropic stimulation of the heart with norepinephrine, paired electric stimulation, or calcium produces a significant increase in MVO_2 while substances known to have a negative inotropic influence (procainamide or propranolol) reduce MVO_2. The influence of myocardial contractility is proportionately greater than intramyocardial tension on MVO_2 if the percentage increase of each required to increase an equal MVO_2 is measured.

Study supported by grants from the Social and Rehabilitation Service, HEW, Grant No. RD-1715-M-67-C2, and the Cardiac Welfare Fund.

3. Heart rate.

The influence of the heart rate on MVO_2 is not as easy to dissect as the tension or contractility phenomena. The heart rate will influence the aforementioned factors. The total MVO_2 will depend upon the interaction of the previously mentioned influences which usually result in an increase of MVO_2 as the heart rate increases.

4. Other influences on MVO_2.

External work, e.g., aortic stenosis and hypertension usually result in an increase in MVO_2. There is some evidence that depolarization of the heart will contribute to MVO_2. Finally, MVO_2 is influenced by the conditions of the resting or basal state as well. This is probably related to activation energy and cellular processes since the heart only *rests* during the absolute refractory state.

The challenge of a supervised exercise program is to restore coronary circulation and cardiac muscle metabolism to the appropriate physiologic state and reserve necessary for the individual's activities of daily living. Thus, an exercise program must achieve at least two goals:

Increase coronary circulation by increasing blood flow and increasing coronary collaterals.

Increasing myocardial energy production, utilization, and transference in readiness for increased myocardial demand. These may be accomplished by:

- increasing the substrate flow
- increasing the efficiency of oxidative phosphorylation
- maintaining the cardiac muscle proteins and ions in readiness to accept and be stimulated by high-energy compounds to affect adequate contractility.

An exercise program may be challenged in these quests by at least two obstacles:

a. Coronary artery disease so advanced that any attempt to increase coronary blood flow is impeded by the obstacles of an irreversibly narrow lumen.
b. Myocardial fibrosis secondary to multiple myocardial infarctions (MI) so advanced that there is an inadequate amount of myocardial tissue available to convert biochemical energy to mechanical energy adequate to meet the body's requirements.

Myocardial Energy

The myocardium derives its energy chiefly from aerobic sources (Fig. 1). This is the most effective and efficient manner of metabolism. Each gram molecule of glucose yields 690,000 calories. This energy output may be divided into the anaerobic (Embden-Meyerhoff) phase which yields 58,000 calories and the aerobic (citric acid or Kreb's cycle) phase which yields 450,000 calories. Nearly

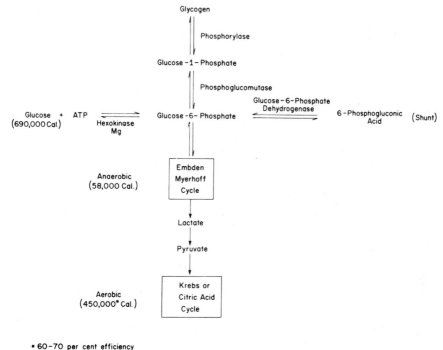

Fig. 1.   Schematic of glucose oxidation.

all other energy-yielding compounds, e.g., amino acids or free fatty acids, are degraded and processed so they enter the citric acid or aerobic cycle at various places yielding their maximal energy (glutamate into α ketoglutarate; proprionic acid into succinate; tyrosine into fumarate).

Therefore, in order to achieve the same amount of work under anaerobic conditions, approximately 10 times more oxygen is required than if the work is accomplished under aerobic conditions. Under anaerobic conditions, more glucose (6-8 times) is oxidized than under aerobic conditions. If there is interference with the aerobic cycle, the heart must either utilize more oxygen to compensate via the anaerobic cycle or utilize more substrate at a very low efficiency. Neither of these mechanisms has any teleological heritage.

The coronary blood flow has been measured to be 0.7-0.9 ml/g left ventricle/ min. This approximates 105-135 ml/min for a 150-lb man assuming that the heart weighs 300 g and the left ventricle 150 g. The coronary blood flow may be increased two- to threefold during exercise and as much as six- to sevenfold during anoxia secondary to oxygen deprivation or to histotoxic anoxia secondary to uncouplers of oxidative phosphorylation such as 2,4-dinitrophenol, CO, or azide (Fig. 2).

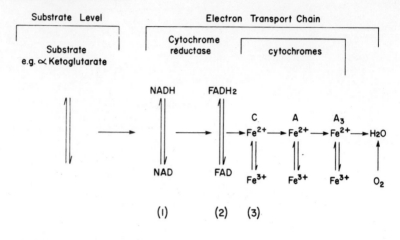

Blockers at I. barbiturates
Blockers at 2. dicumarol
Blockers at 3. CO azide cyanide

Fig. 2.   Schematic of oxidative phosphorylation.

The A-V extraction of oxygen by the coronary circulation is the most efficient in the body. Seventy percent of the available O_2 is extracted, and this equals 0.12 ml/ml of coronary flow. Accordingly, myocardial oxygen consumption is 0.8-1.0 ml/min/g which equals 30 ml/O_2/min. The myocardium utilizes about 7-10 percent of the total O_2 body consumption. The oxygen demand varies according to the functional state of the heart, i.e., normal function, congestive heart failure, or exercise. The O_2 consumption is a satisfactory general index of the functional state of the heart and is also related to systolic blood pressure and heart rate, but does not reflect the basic biochemical changes in cardiac muscle at the cellular level.

The myocardial cell, through the mitochondria, will harness the energy available from oxygen through the process of oxidative phosphorylation (Fig. 2). This is the means by which the oxidative energy, i.e., energy available from oxygen, is transferred and kept available for future cellular function in the form of high-energy phosphates [from ATP (adenosine triphosphate) and to a lesser degree from CP (creatine phosphate)]. The latter reaction is a far more sensitive measure of cardiac anoxia than is oxygen intake by the myocardium and/or total body oxygen consumption [3].

The myocardium obtains its contractile energy from this process. The heart cannot continue to function for any length of time if there is oxygen deprivation or any biochemical process which is an uncoupler of oxidative phosphorylation. Carbon monoxide, azide, cyanide, and to a lesser degree, sodium amytal will produce a cessation of cardiac energy production in the face of adequate oxygenation. The degree and severity of influence on the electron transport chain

depends on the site of stimulation or inhibition. The most effective and ir-
reversible uncoupling takes place at the cytochrome oxidase level, e.g., cyanide,
CO, and azide. The uncouplers at the NADH level or FADH level, barbiturates
and Dicumarol (Fig. 2), can be reversed more easily.

Myocardial metabolism. The myocardium metabolizes various substances including glucose, free fatty acids, citric acid intermediates, and amino acids. All
of these intermediate metabolites must pass through the Krebs (citric acid or
aerobic) cycle to be utilized in cardiac metabolism. There are elegant descrip-
tions of changes in the serum and urinary contents of such substances as lactic
acid, free fatty acids, and catecholamines which point to profound biologic
readjustments to physical stress. The central theme in these observations is that
the urinary excretion of norepinephrine and epinephrine increases from five- to
fifteenfold during exercise. This increase may be more meaningful when considered in the light of cyclic AMP, the second hormone messenger.

Cyclic AMP is derived from the action of adenyl cyclase on ATP. The co-
factors involved in this reaction are epinephrine, norepinephrine, glucagon, and
dopamine. It may be reasoned that, during exercise, when there is a great
demand for high-energy phosphates, as well as for substrate intermediates, the
presence of epinephrine may enhance the production of cyclic AMP. The conversion of phosphorylase b to phosphorylase a is enhanced by cyclic AMP to
stimulate increased glycogenolysis (TABLE I).

TABLE I

Effect of long-term training in humans

	Before	After	P
Muscle glycogen mg/g wet weight	12.4	17.7	<0.001
Muscle triglycerides μM/g dry weight	27.6	50.5	<0.001
Urinary secretion of norepinephrine ng/liter	25.0	390.0	<0.001

Theoretically, the cardiac demand for glucose and free fatty acids during high
oxygen utilization is supported by experimental observations. Several investigators have reported that during epinephrine release, there is a rise in the serum
glucose and free fatty acids. An ancillary and supporting observation is the
accumulation of glycogen in all muscles during training. It has also been reported
that free fatty acids inhibit the anaerobic metabolism of glucose at the level of
glucose-6-phosphate. This action appears to accomplish several important metabolic phenomena which, if left unchecked, may produce histotoxic anoxia of
cardiac muscle. That these observations go beyond theoretical concepts are supported by Oliver and Opie, who observed that the degree and frequency of
cardiac arrhythmias are correlated with the rise in free fatty acid levels [4, 5].
Thus, during exercise, the trained individual will utilize glucose as a substrate
and receive his energy from aerobic sources (glycogenolysis). The untrained

individual, whose glycogen stores may be low, will resort to utilization of free fatty acids as a source of energy and during the process, will inhibit the aerobic pathways producing histotoxic anoxia with its dire consequences.

Responses to Acute and Chronic Exercise

The concept of exercise by untrained and trained individuals requires definition and standardization. For example, a weight lifter may have well-trained arm and skeletal muscles, but be unable to cope with the stress of a 1-mile run. Thus, the weight lifter is untrained from the viewpoint of leg muscles and perhaps the cardiovascular response to running. On the other hand, a runner may be unable to press 100 pounds efficiently because of his underdeveloped arm muscles. Exercise, as discussed here, implies a cardiovascular response to running, walking, or mountain climbing.

Two types of response to exercise are: acute, and chronic. The data, referred to herein, were from both animal and man and are supportive of certain conclusions because of the observations made following acute and prolonged training periods.

The general observations are: acute exercise in men over age 40 results in an increase in serum glutamic oxaloacetate transaminase (SGOT); serum glutamic-pyruvic transaminase (SGPT); creatine phosphokinase (CPK); lactic dehydrogenase (LDH); and lactic dehydrogenase isoenzymes (except LDH-2). The enzyme changes are more difficult to assess with chronic or long-term training. There is general agreement that the oxidative enzymes increase with training. The evidence for this statement is derived from muscle examinations of orthopedic patients with prolonged rest periods compared with early ambulation and activity periods; excised muscles from animals such as rats or rabbits during prolonged training procedures; and prolonged military training.

Available information reveals a rise in the enzymes involved in oxidative phosphorylation and the citric acid cycle, e.g., cytochrome oxidase, succinic oxidase, NADH dehydrogenase, and NADH-cytochrome reductase. Malic dehydrogenase and isocitric dehydrogenase increased in blood serum during prolonged military training. There is no evidence to indicate whether these rises in enzyme levels are due to enzyme induction or to enlargement of muscle mass. The latter theory gains support from Holloszy's studies demonstrating a rise in mitochondrial protein (nitrogen) from 2.97 ± 0.2 to 4.67 ± 0.3 mg/g muscle after training [6].

Serum Lipids

The effect of long-term rigorous exercise on serum lipids has been studied in several groups of individuals including Marine Corps recruits. One study involved 101 Marine Corps trainees whose average age was 20.5 (range 17 to 25 years). The basic training was accomplished over a 22-week period; 12 weeks at the

Marine Corps Recruit Depot, Parris Island, S.C., and the remaining 10 weeks at Camp Lejeune, N.C. Their diet consisted of milk ad lib (average 3.3 pints/man daily). Other dairy products, butter, ice cream (average of 4 ounces or 113.3 grams) daily, cheese, and eggs (2 to 3 eggs five times/week) were also plentiful. The intake of animal fats was not rationed. The average caloric intake was 4,500 of which fat contributed 225 grams or 2,025 calories, carbohydrates 506 grams or 2,025 calories, and proteins 112 grams or 450 calories. For 12 weeks at Parris Island, the recruits averaged 16 hrs/day of rigorous drill and disciplinary activity which included a daily 5-mile forced march. The activity at Camp Lejeune was almost as rigorous.

The study was, in reality, a direct challenge to exercise as a catabolic agent or caloric utilizer and a compensator for a diet high in saturated fat and caloric intake. The vigorous exercise program met the challenge and the data are summarized in TABLE II. It should be noted that, in spite of the large caloric intake, there was virtually no weight gain. The mean serum cholesterol level did not change appreciably. The mean lipid phosphorus and triglyceride levels rose to a statistically significant degree ($p < 0.001$). There were no significant changes in either the systolic or diastolic blood pressure.

TABLE II

Evaluation of clinical and biochemical variables in Marine Corps
subjects before and after 22 weeks of basic training

Age Range 17-25

Variable	Mean	S.D.	Mean	S.D.	t	p
Weight lbs.	162.	±21.	166.	±16.	1.52	NS
Systolic blood pressure mmHg	118.	±13.	118.	± 8.	0.00	NS
Cholesterol mg %	176.	±35.	183.	±36.	1.40	NS
Lipid phosphorus mg %	8.2	± 1.3	9.4	± 1.8	5.43	<.001
Triglycerides mg %	42.	±22.	91.	±23.	15.47	<.001
Uric acid mg %	4.8	± 1.1	5.0	± 1.4	1.12	NS
Lactic dehydrogenase (LDH)	244.	±54.	231.	±49.	1.79	NS
Malic dehydrogenase (MDH)	72.	±18.	91.	±25.	6.19	<.001
Isocitric dehydrogenase (ICDH)	6.6	± 2.7	3.4	± 1.4	10.58	<.001

The serum enzyme levels did not reveal any change in lactic dehydrogenase. However, there was a significant decline in isocitric dehydrogenase and a significant rise in malic dehydrogenase. It would be folly to speculate on the effect that exercise could have on the serum lipid levels if the caloric intake had consisted of more protein and carbohydrate. It is interesting, however, that the variations were miniscule except for the significantly elevated triglyceride and lipid phosphorus levels. Both of these substances are derived from L-alpha-glycerol nucleus with added fatty acids in positions 1, 2, and 3 in the former, and fatty acids in positions 1 and 2, phosphorus and an amino acid in position 3 in the latter.

Stress Testing in Sedentary vs Active Subjects

The coagulation and metabolic variables have been evaluated before and immediately after step-wise submaximal treadmill stress testing in sedentary and physically active healthy men whose physical fitness and work tolerance were determined prior to enrollment in an exercise training program. All participants in the study were volunteers employed by a large insurance company in New York City.

The age range of the sedentary men was 30 to 56 and the mean age 46.3 ± 8.1. The mean height and weight for this group was 69.3 ± 3.7 inches and 180 ± 21.2 pounds, respectively. The age range of the physically active men was 35 to 57 and the mean age 45.2 ± 7.4. The mean height was 69.8 ± 2.1 inches and the mean weight 180 ± 18.9 pounds. All subjects were active in sports or already enrolled in a training program prior to exercise stress testing.

In the sedentary men the kaolin activated PTT and euglobulin lysis time were significantly shortened ($p < 0.05$) during exercise stress testing, indicating that there is a change in homeostasis and a tendency toward coagulation which is simultaneously counteracted by a significant increase in fibrinolytic activity (TABLE III). A significantly shortened euglobulin lysis time ($p < 0.05$) was also observed in individuals who were physically active prior to exercise stress testing. However, there was no significant change in kaolin-activated PTT, which was 3.41 seconds longer at rest than in sedentary men (TABLE IV). Therefore, it is reasonable to assume that peak performances and uncontrolled exercise, particularly in the poorly conditioned individuals, carry a certain amount of risk of increasing thrombotic activity, which could lead to an acute thrombotic event. This could explain the occurrence of sudden deaths during unaccustomed physical activity, such as shoveling snow.

Following exercise stress testing, the lactate, cholesterol, and uric acid levels were significantly elevated in both groups; lipid phosphorus only in the sedentary; and triglycerides only in the physically active men (TABLES III and IV). There were no significant changes in glucose, immunoreactive insulin, and free fatty acid levels in either group.

The effect of a well-controlled and individually prescribed training program of 6 months' duration on physical, coagulation, and biochemical variables was also evaluated. The training consisted of jogging 4 times/week on an indoor track under the supervision of a physician and physical educator. The jogging and calisthenic exercises were interrupted by rest periods when the subject's age-determined target heart rate was reached.

At the completion of the 6-month training program, it was noted that the work tolerance of the subjects, who were physically active prior to enrollment, had increased significantly ($p < 0.001$). This was accompanied by significant weight reduction ($p < 0.05$).

TABLE III

Coagulation and metabolic variables before and after submaximal treadmill stress testing in sedentary healthy male subjects

Variable	N	B.E.[1]	A.E.[2]	Mean[3]	S.D.	S.E.	t	p
Prothrombin TAME units	11	51.72	53.04	-1.32	3.78	1.14	-1.16	NS
Kaolin PTT seconds	12	38.71	37.49	1.22	1.67	.48	2.53	$< .05$
Fibrinogen mg %	11	386.8	400.2	-13.36	43.14	13.01	-1.03	NS
Euglobulin lysis minutes	12	292.1	278.3	13.75	21.55	6.22	2.21	$< .05$
Plasminogen (caseinolytic units)	12	1.266	1.218	-.047	.199	.0576	-.825	NS
Platelet count ($\times 100$)	7	2,771.	2,795.	-24.0	99.5	37.6	-.6	NS
Adhesiveness %	7	53.91	51.49	2.43	3.83	1.45	1.68	NS
Glucose mg %	12	98.8	98.5	.25	6.25	1.81	.14	NS
Insulin (IRI) μ units/ml	12	18.9	17.6	1.25	5.33	1.54	.81	NS
FFA μ Eq/L	8	549.9	503.4	46.5	160.97	56.9	.82	NS
Lactate μ moles/ml	4	1.168	1.856	-.69	.36	.18	-3.79	$< .05$
Cholesterol mg %	12	267.5	252.7	-14.8	8.91	2.57	-5.77	$< .001$
Lipid phosphorus mg %	12	10.18	10.93	-.75	.69	.20	-3.75	$< .01$
Triglycerides mg %	12	124.0	143.9	-19.9	38.9	11.2	-1.77	NS
Uric acid mg %	12	6.35	6.49	-.14	.138	.040	-3.56	$< .01$

[1] Mean before exercise stress testing.

[2] Mean after exercise stress testing.

[3] Mean differences i.e. $\frac{1}{n} \Sigma$ (X before $-$ X after exercise stress testing).

TABLE IV

Coagulation and metabolic variables before and after submaximal treadmill stress testing in physically active healthy male subjects

Variable	N	B.E.[1]	A.E.[2]	Mean[3]	S.D.	S.E.	t	P
Prothrombin TAME units	12	45.58	46.06	-.48	4.00	1.16	-.42	NS
Kaolin PTT seconds	12	42.16	41.03	1.13	2.02	.58	1.94	NS
Fibrinogen mg %	12	334.7	343.1	-8.42	16.13	4.66	-1.81	NS
Euglobulin lysis minutes	12	268.3	244.6	23.75	38.3	11.1	2.15	<.05
Plasminogen (caseinolytic units)	11	1.24	1.30	-.0636	.108	.033	-1.95	NS
Platelet count (× 100)	8	2,734.	3,099.	-365.	346.1	122.	-2.98	<.05
Adhesiveness %	8	56.48	57.00	-.525	5.87	2.07	-.25	NS
Glucose mg %	12	97.25	99.75	-2.50	5.96	1.72	-1.45	NS
Insulin (IRI) μ units/ml	12	13.70	13.13	.58	3.34	.96	.60	NS
FFA μ Eq/L	10	662.4	563.0	99.4	270.4	85.5	1.16	NS
Lactate μ moles/ml	8	1.10	3.44	-2.34	.99	.35	-6.65	<.001
Cholesterol mg %	12	225.3	234.3	-9.00	8.89	2.57	-3.51	<.01
Lipid phosphorus mg %	12	10.40	10.66	-.25	.715	.207	-1.21	NS
Triglycerides mg %	10	132.1	123.7	8.4	12.28	13.88	2.17	<.05
Uric acid mg %	12	6.26	6.45	-.19	.27	.077	-2.48	<.05

[1] Mean before exercise stress testing.
[2] Mean after exercise stress testing.
[3] Mean differences, i.e., $1/n \Sigma$ (X before − X after exercise stress testing).

REFERENCES

1. Blackburn, H., Winkler, G., Vilandre, J., Hodgson, J., and Taylor, H.L. Exercise tests. Comparison of the energy cost and heart rate response to five commonly-used single-stage, non-steady-state, submaximal work procedures. *In*, Brunner, D., and Jokl, E., Eds. *Physical Activity and Aging*. Baltimore, University Park Press, 1970. *Medicine and Sport* 4:28-36, 1970.

2. Sonnenblick, E.H., and Skelton, C.L. Oxygen consumption of the heart: Physiological principles and clinical implications. *Mod. Concepts Cardiovasc. Dis.* XL, No. 3:9-16, 1971.

3. Gertler, M.M. Differences in efficiency of energy transfer in mitochondrial systems derived from normal and failing hearts. *Proc. Soc. Exp. Biol. Med.* 106:109-112, 1961.

4. Oliver, M.F. Metabolic response during impending myocardial infarction. Clinical implications. *Circulation* XLV: 491-500, 1972.

5. Opie, L.H. Metabolic response during impending myocardial infarction. 1. Relevance of studies of glucose and fatty acid metabolism in animals. *Circulation* XLV: 483-490, 1972.

6. Holloszy, J.O. Morphological and enzymatic adaptations to training: A review. *In*, Larson, O.A., and Malmborg, R.O., Eds. *Coronary Heart Disease and Physical Fitness*, pp.147-151. Baltimore, University Park Press, 1970.

14

LONG-TERM METABOLIC ADAPTATIONS IN MUSCLE TO ENDURANCE EXERCISE

John O. Holloszy, M.D.

Introduction

A marked change has occurred in the living habits of the populations of the wealthy industrialized nations over the past century. As a result of extensive mechanization and automation, it has, for the first time in man's history, become possible for large population groups to go through life with a minimum of physical activity.

Vigorous exercise was a consistent component of man's everyday life, necessary for survival, throughout the course of his evolution. It is a natural consequence of adaptation by natural selection that a species is best adapted to the environment of its remote ancestors, perhaps a hundred or more generations back. It seems likely, therefore, that the currently prevalent lack of exercise represents an environmental situation to which man is poorly adapted in genetic terms. However, with the advent of the machine age, both the medical profession and the lay public began not only to question the need for exercise but also to feel that vigorous exercise might be detrimental to health.

This development was probably a direct result of the close contact that people living in industrialized nations have with machines. Their familiarity with the manner in which machines function makes it natural for them to think of the human body in the same terms. Since the rate at which a machine wears out is related to how long and hard it is run, it might seem reasonable that one's body would also wear out faster, if it was repeatedly subjected to hard physical work. A more sophisticated variation of this concept, in the form of a stress and strain hypothesis, was promulgated among biological scientists and physicians by a school of physiologists whose intellectual leader was Hans Selye. This hypothesis is best summarized in Selye's own words, " . . . later, after these original findings, we showed that stress is the rate of wear and tear in the human machinery which accompanies any vital activity. In a sense it parallels and is a reasonably accurate indicator of the intensity of one's life. The rate is increased during nervous tension, physical injury, infections, muscular work, or any other strenuous activity . . . " [1].

That a biologist could, in all seriousness, equate the effects of muscular work with those of infections or nervous tension seems quite bizarre in the context of present-day knowledge. Yet, these ideas were taken seriously by many until quite recently.

Needless to say, living organisms are not machines. In contrast to machines, which wear out and deteriorate faster the more they are used, biological systems generally develop an adaptive increase in functional capacity in response to increased workloads, and undergo a decrease in functional capacity or *disuse atrophy* when subjected to inactivity. In general, within genetically determined limits, the capacity of an individual to perform a function depends on the demands placed on him in the preceding period. The same applies to a specific organ or organ system. For example, the capacity of the kidney to conserve salt increases as salt intake decreases; the capacity of the liver to cat..bolize protein varies with protein intake; and the strength of a muscle group decreases with inactivity, and increases as the habitual workload is increased.

Not only the state of the skeletal muscles, but also the state of the cardio-vascular system, some components of the autonomic nervous system, and of bones, ligaments, and tendons, depend on the habitual level of physical activity. All these systems deteriorate with lack of exercise. This phenomenon is not dependent on the present of disease, but also occurs in normal, healthy individuals if they are immobilized.

Types of exercise

The nature of the increase in functional capacity that occurs in response to physical activity depends on the type of exercise stimulus. The term exercise includes three different types of stimulus, each with its own specific pattern of response.

One type is heavy resistance or strength exercise, which involves very forceful muscle contractions and is exemplified by activities such as weight lifting and isometric exercises. It results in muscle hypertrophy with an increase in strength.

A second type of exercise involves the learning of movement patterns and results in the development of skill, with an increase in coordination and agility. This type of exercise is exemplified by such activities as fencing, the various ball games, driving a car, or playing a musical instrument. The primary adaptive changes in response to this type of exercise take place in the central nervous system, and must involve a programming process initiated by repeated performance of a movement pattern until it becomes a conditioned reflex.

The third type is endurance exercise which is exemplified by activities such as long-distance running, swimming, or bicycling. It results in an increase in the capacity for prolonged aerobic exercise, made possible by adaptations in the cardiovascular system, the skeletal muscles, and the autonomic nervous system. The changes seen in the skeletal muscles are quite different from those seen with strength exercise. There is no muscle hypertrophy or increase in strength. In stead, there is an increase in the capacity for aerobic metabolism with an increase in endurance.

The Potential Role of Exercise in
Preventive and Therapeutic Medicine

The realization that the functional capacity of a number of tissues and organ systems increases in response to regularly performed exercise, and decreases with inactivity, has recently resulted in a rise in interest in the possible roles of exercise in preventive and therapeutic medicine. Contributing to this interest is the suspicion that the increase in the incidence of coronary heart disease (CHD), obesity, and adult onset of diabetes mellitus that appears to have occurred in the past 100 years or so in the wealthy industrialized nations may, in part, represent long-term metabolic repercussions from the very low levels of habitual physical activity currently prevalent in these areas.

Carefully controlled clinical studies are needed to test the possibility that exercise may have important health benefits. In addition, if exercise is to become a scientifically acceptable therapeutic modality, a better understanding is needed of the biochemical and physiological adaptations that occur at the cellular level in response to exercise.

Some progress has been made in the latter direction in the past few years. This report will describe recent advances in the understanding of the adaptive response to the type of exercise which probably has the greatest potential as a tool in preventive medicine: endurance exercise.

Adaptive Responses to Endurance Exercise

It has long been known that endurance exercise training can result in an increase in an individual's maximum capacity to utilize oxygen ($\dot{V}_{O_2}$max), as well as in his maximum work capacity. Major effects of training can also be demonstrated at submaximal work levels. If a previously sedentary individual is retested at the same submaximal work level following an intensive program of endurance exercise training, he is found to have lower concentrations of lactate in his muscles [2] and blood [2, 3, 4]; his muscle glycogen level decreases at a slower rate [2]; he has a lower respiratory quotient, indicating that he is oxidizing more fat and less carbohydrate [2, 5]; and his endurance is greatly increased.

For many years it was believed that lactate production by working muscles reflects muscle hypoxia even during relatively mild exercise. In this context, it was believed that the lower lactate levels and greater endurance seen in trained individuals during submaximal exercise were due to improved delivery of oxygen to the working muscles made possible by the well-documented cardiovascular adaptations brought about by exercise. This interpretation no longer seems reasonable in light of the information that has accumulated.

It has been clearly established that well-oxygenated muscles can produce large amounts of lactate during work [6] . This happens when glycogenolysis is turned on to a greater extent than respiration in a working muscle, or when the rate of glycogenolysis exceeds the capacity of the muscle mitochondria to oxidize pyruvate and DPNH.

Secondly, if untrained muscles were hypoxic during submaximal exercise, and if trained muscles produced less lactate because of a better oxygen supply, then one would expect the trained individual to have a higher oxygen consumption than the untrained at the same submaximal work level. In other words, if a tissue were hypoxic, one would expect its oxygen consumption to increase if its oxygen supply was increased. However, no increase in oxygen consumption occurs at the same absolute, submaximal work level with training. It is well-documented that oxygen consumption is the same in the trained and untrained states at the same submaximal work load [2, 7, 8, 9, 10] .

Lastly, blood flow to the working muscles is actually lower in trained, than in sedentary individuals at the same absolute, submaximal work level [9, 11, 12] . The working muscles compensate for the lower blood flow in the trained state by extracting more O_2, as reflected in a greater arteriovenous O_2 difference during submaximal exercise [7, 10, 13, 14] .

Since neither oxygen delivery to, nor oxygen utilization by skeletal muscle during submaximal exercise are increased by exercise training, it seemed likely that other adaptations, probably within the muscles themselves, must be primarily responsible for the lower lactate levels, the slower glycogen depletion, the lower respiratory quotient, the increased extraction of O_2, and the greater endurance, observed in trained individuals. One line of evidence that stimulated an investigation of this possibility came from comparative studies which reported that a good correlation exists between the ability of a muscle to perform prolonged exercise and its content of respiratory enzymes. For example, the breast muscles of the domestic chicken, which does not fly, have a low oxidative capacity, while the breast muscles of mallards and pigeons, which spend long periods in flight, are rich in mitochondria, and have approximately ten times as great a capacity for oxidative metabolism as chicken breast muscle [15] . Similarly, the levels of cytochrome oxidase and succinate dehydrogenase activity in psoas muscles of sedentary laboratory rabbits are only one-third as high as those of the active wild rabbit [16] . Although these differences may be largely on a genetic basis, it seemed possible that an adaptive response might also be playing a role. This turned out to be the case.

Biochemical Adaptations to Endurance Exercise in
Rat Skeletal Muscle

In our studies, young male rats are trained to run on a treadmill. The speed and duration of the run are progressively increased over a period of 3 months until the animals run continuously at 31 m/min, up an 8° incline, for 2 hours, 5 days/week. This program results in a great increase in endurance capacity, but does not result in hypertrophy of the leg muscles [17, 18].

On visual examination, the leg muscles and homogenates of the muscles of the exercised animals have a deeper red color. The myoglobin concentration is increased approximately 80 percent in the leg muscles of the runners [17]. Only the muscles directly involved in the exercise have an increased myoglobin content. It has been observed in in vitro studies that myoglobin can increase O_2 transport across a fluid layer [19 20, 21]. It seems likely that myoglobin may also facilitate oxygen utilization in tissues by enhancing oxygen transport through the cytoplasm.

An approximately twofold increase also occurs in the levels of activity of the mitochondrial respiratory chain enzymes involved in the oxidation of DPNH and succinate, in the leg muscles of the exercised animals [18, 22]. Mitochondrial coupling factor 1, which is closely associated with the respiratory chain in the mitochondrial cristae and catalyzes the oxidative phosphorylation of ADP to ATP coupled to electron transport, increases in parallel with the components of the respiratory chain [23].

The levels of activity of the mitochondrial citric acid cycle enzymes also increase significantly in the leg muscles of the runners [24].

As might be expected from these increases in enzyme levels, the running program results in an increase in the capacity of the leg muscles to oxidize pyruvate. This increase is approximately twofold, both for the mitochondrial fraction from leg muscles and for whole homogenates [18, 22, 25].

Measurements of respiratory quotient and of the rate of conversion of ^{14}C-labeled fatty acids to [14]CO_2 have shown that physically trained individuals oxidize more fat and less carbohydrate than untrained ones during submaximal exercise [2, 5, 26]. These findings led us to examine the adaptive response to exercise of the pathway of fatty acid oxidation in skeletal muscle [27, 28]. The levels of ATP-dependent palmityl CoA synthetase, carnitine palmityltransferase, and palmityl CoA dehydrogenase, which are involved in the activation, transport, and catabolism of long chain fatty acids, all increased approximately twofold in hind limb muscles of the runners [28]. The capacity of the mitochondrial fraction and of whole homogenates to oxidize palmitate, oleate, and linoleate also doubled [27, 28]. This difference in the capacity to oxidize fatty acids was demonstrated over a wide physiological range of fatty acid concentrations [28].

In addition to increasing the capacity of muscle to oxidize fatty acids, endurance exercise training appears to produce adaptations which result in a greater rate of release of fatty acids from adipose tissue and higher levels of free fatty acids in blood in trained, than in untrained subjects during exercise [29, 30]. The increase in the capacity of muscle to oxidize fat and the greater mobilization of fatty acids probably act synergistically to account for the physically trained individuals' greater utilization of fat as an energy source during exercise.

The mitochondria obtained from the exercised animals exhibit a high level of respiratory control and tightly coupled oxidative phosphorylation with either pyruvate or fatty acids as substrate [1, 28]. This finding demonstrates that the increase in oxidative capacity is accompanied by a parallel rise in the capacity to regenerate ATP via oxidative phosphorylation.

The increases in enzymatic activity and oxidative capacity are apparently related to an increase in enzyme protein. This is evidenced by a doubling of the concentration of cytochrome c and an approximately 60 percent increase in the protein content of the mitochondrial fraction of skeletal muscle [18, 22, 23, 24, 25, 28, 31]. The finding that mitochondrial protein increases only by about 60 percent can probably be explained by the fact that, although some mitochondrial enzymes increase twofold, others increase only by 35 to 50 percent. Others do not increase at all.

Among the enzymes that do not increase are mitochondrial α-glycerophosphate dehydrogenase [31], creatine phosphokinase, and adenylate kinase [23]. The activities of these enzymes are unchanged when expressed per gram of muscle; however, as a result of the increase in mitochondrial protein, the specific activities of these enzymes are significantly decreased when expressed per milligram of mitochondrial protein [23, 31]. The finding that mitochondrial adenylate kinase, creatine phosphokinase, and α-glycerophosphate dehydrogenase do not increase in muscle in response to exercise seems consistent with what is known regarding the adaptation to endurance exercise. As previously described, *the major feature of the adaptation in skeletal muscle is an increase in the capacity of the involved muscles for aerobic metabolism.* In contrast, glycolytic capacity does not increase [32] and may even decrease [33].

It is well-documented that the capacity of a muscle to oxidize α-glycerophosphate parallels its glycolytic capacity and is inversely related to its capacity for aerobic metabolism [34]. White muscle, which has a high capacity for glycolysis and a low capacity for aerobic metabolism, has high levels of α-glycerophosphate dehydrogenase, adenylate kinase, and creatine phosphokinase, relative to cardiac muscle which has a very high capacity for oxidative metabolism and a relatively low glycolytic capacity [34, 35, 36, 37].

It appears that when skeletal muscle adapts to endurance exercise, it becomes more like cardiac muscle in that its content of mitochondria and its capacity to generate ATP from oxidation of pyruvate and fatty acids increases. Skeletal muscle mitochondria also become more like heart mitochondria in their enzyme pattern as a result of the decrease in the specific activities of creatine phosphokinase, adenylate kinase, and α-glycerophosphate dehydrogenase expressed per milligram of mitochondrial protein [23, 31].

Mixed muscles, such as the gastrocnemius and quadriceps, on which these studies were carried out, are a mixture of three different fiber types in rodents, and a variety of other species. The white fibers have a low capacity for oxidative metabolism, a high glycogenolytic capacity, a high myosin ATPase activity, and are fast twitch. The intermediate fibers have a moderately high capacity for oxidative metabolism, a very low capacity for glycogenolysis, low myosin ATPase activity, and are slow twitch. The red fibers have a high oxidative capacity, a high glycolytic capacity, a high myosin ATPase activity, and are fast twitch [38, 39, 40]. The capacity of all three muscle fiber types for aerobic metabolism increases approximately twofold in rats subjected to the running program used in this laboratory [25]. This was demonstrated by measurements of (1) the capacity to oxidize pyruvate and fatty acids; (2) levels of activity of cytochrome oxidase, citrate synthase, and carnitine palmityltransferase; and (3) concentration of cytochrome c. All of these factors increased approximately twofold in all three muscle types [25]. Thus, the differences in oxidative capacity between the fiber types are maintained, and, although the respiratory capacity of the white fibers increases, they are not converted to red fibers.

These biochemical findings have stimulated a number of investigators to study the effect of endurance exercise training on the electron microscopic appearance of skeletal muscle. Gollnick and King [41] have reported an increase in both the size and number of muscle mitochondria in rats. Morgan et al [42] and Kiessling et al [43] have reported similar changes in muscle biopsies from men subjected to programs of endurance exercise. Varnauskas et al [12] and Morgan and coworkers [42] also reported significant increases in the levels of activity of a number of mitochondrial enzymes in muscle biopsies from humans, demonstrating that human and rat skeletal muscle undergo similar adaptations in response to endurance exercise.

To summarize, regularly performed endurance exercise, such as prolonged running, results in an adaptive increase in skeletal muscle mitochondria, with an increase in capacity to generate ATP via oxidation of pyruvate and fatty acids, which involves all three muscle fiber types and makes their enzyme pattern more like that of heart muscle.

Mechanisms by Which the Biochemical Adaptations in Skeletal Muscle Contribute to the Increase in Endurance Seen with Training

The rate of oxygen consumption by muscle cells during exercise is determined primarily by work rate. When muscles are stimulated to contract in situ, under conditions in which oxygen supply is not limiting, the steady state, submaximal level of oxygen intake attained is a function of the stimulation rate (i.e., the number of contractions per minute) [44, 45]. In studies of this type, supramaximal shocks are used so that all the fibers in the muscle are stimulated to contract.

As a result of the tight coupling of oxidative phosphorylation to electron transport in intact mitochondria, the rate of oxygen consumption is largely determined by the intramitochondrial concentrations of ADP and Pi; the rate of respiration appears to be an inverse function of the ratio ATP/(ADP + Pi) [46, 47, 48, 49]. Studies on frog and toad sartorius muscles, using the decrease in respiratory chain DPNH fluorescence to estimate ADP concentration, have shown that the increase in intramitochondrial ADP concentration, produced by a series of contractions, follows a saturation curve. The plateau or steady state level of ADP and, therefore, of O_2 consumption, is attained after about 30 twitches [50, 51]. The magnitude of the steady state concentration of ADP, and, therefore, of the rate of oxygen consumption attained, is a function of the stimulation frequency [51].

At work rates resulting in a submaximal rate of oxygen intake, once the steady state level of oxygen consumption is attained in a muscle cell, the rate of ATP formation via oxidative phosphorylation, during and between muscle contractions, must balance the ATP breakdown associated with the muscle contractions. During the interval between the onset of work and the attainment of the steady state, when ATP hydrolysis is not balanced by oxidative phosphorylation, the concentrations of creatine phosphate (CP) and ATP drop, resulting in the so-called muscle oxygen deficit [51]. Simultaneously, the concentrations of Pi, ADP, AMP, and probably also of NH_3, rise to the steady state levels determined by the work rate. In other words, Pi and ADP concentrations rise until they turn on electron transport, O_2 intake, and oxidative phosphorylation sufficiently to balance ATP breakdown.

Since skeletal muscle that has adapted to strenuous endurance exercise contains up to twice as many mitochondrial cristae per gram as untrained muscle, the concentrations of ADP and Pi must increase less and attain lower steady state levels at a given submaximal rate of work and oxygen consumption, in muscles of trained as compared to sedentary individuals. Expressed as O_2 consumption per muscle cell, the greater the number of mitochondria in a cell, the lower must be the O_2 intake per mitochondrion at a given submaximal rate of O_2 consumption. Thus, to attain a given steady state, submaximal level of O_2 con- sumption, a smaller increase in ADP and Pi concentrations must occur in the trained individuals' muscles, since, with more mitochondria, each mitochondrion has to be *turned on* to a lesser extent to balance a given rate of ATP hydrolysis by the myofibrils. A smaller initial drop in CP and ATP concentrations should result in lower steady state concentrations of AMP, also of NH_3.

The rate of glycogenolysis in muscle is, to a large extent, controlled by the intracellular concentrations of ATP, CP, Pi, ADP, AMP, and NH_3 [53, 54, 55, 56, 57]. Phosphofructokinase is inhibited by ATP and CP, and this inhibition is counteracted by Pi, ADP, AMP, and NH_3 [53, 54, 55, 56, 57]. Therefore, because of lower steady state levels of ADP, AMP, and Pi, and higher concentrations of ATP and CP in the trained state, glycogenolysis should occur at a slower rate at a given absolute, submaximal level of O_2 consumption and work. This should result in a slower rate of muscle glycogen depletion and lower lactate concentrations at the same absolute, submaximal work level in the trained, as compared to the untrained state.

Empirical evidence supporting this line of reasoning comes from muscle biopsy studies on humans. Saltin and Karlsson [2] reported that at the same absolute, submaximal work level, the fall in CP and ATP concentrations, the rate of glycogen depletion, and the concentration of lactate in quadriceps muscle are lower, in the same individual, in the trained than in the untrained state.

Another factor which probably plays an important role in accounting for the decreased rate of glycogen depletion and lactate production is the shift in the source of carbon for the citric acid cycle with, as discussed earlier, the physically trained individual deriving a greater percent of his energy from oxidation of fatty acids. An increase in the oxidation of fat decreases carbohydrate utilization (58, 59, 60).

Cardiovascular Effects of Endurance Exercise Training

Certain adaptations brought about by endurance exercise training interact to result in a reduction in the amount of work performed and the quantity of oxygen required by the heart when an individual performs a standard submaximal exercise. For example, when CHD patients or normal subjects are retested at the same submaximal workload following a program of exercise, they have a slower heart rate, a lower blood pressure, a reduced tension time index, decreased blood flow to the working muscles, and, frequently, a lower cardiac output [4, 7, 9, 10, 11, 12, 13, 14, 61, 62, 63, 64, 65], while O_2 consumption remains unchanged. The muscles maintain their O_2 consumption despite the reduction in blood flow by extracting more oxygen, as reflected in an increased arteriovenous O_2 difference [4, 7, 14].

Both the decrease in blood flow to, and the increased extraction of O_2 by the working muscles are very likely secondary to the adaptations induced in skeletal muscle by training. Even the slower heart rate seen during submaximal exercise following training may, in part, be mediated by the adaptive changes in skeletal muscle. This is evidenced by the findings of Clausen, Trap-Jensen, and Lassen that training of the arm muscles reduced the heart rate only during arm work, while training of the leg muscles only reduced the heart rate during leg work [66]. Thus the reduction in heart rate obtained by training one group of muscles was not transferred to work performed with untrained muscle groups. These investigators interpreted their results to indicate that the reduction in heart rate is not dependent on cardiac factors, but probably on changes in the trained muscles [66]. The mechanism by which this effect is mediated is, at present, purely speculative. In any case, it does appear that the adaptations in skeletal muscle may make an important contribution to the improved (more efficient) cardiac function, during submaximal exercise, of CHD patients following endurance exercise training.

In contrast to skeletal muscle, heart muscle does not undergo an adaptive increase in respiratory capacity in response to endurance exercise [67, 68]. Expressed per gram of heart, the levels of activity of a variety of mitochondrial marker enzymes, and the concentrations of cytochrome c and mitochondrial protein are unchanged in trained animals [67, 68]. Also in contrast to skeletal muscle, the heart hypertrophies in response to strenuous endurance exercise, so that trained individuals have heavier hearts than sedentary controls of the same body weight. This increase in the size of the heart relative to the body could play an important role, in normal individuals, in the increase in work capacity brought about by training. In the absence of cardiovascular pathology, there appears to be a good correlation between heart size and maximum cardiac output [69]. An increase in the ratio of heart weight to body weight should, therefore, result in an increase in the maximum capacity to deliver blood to the working muscles. As a consequence, the hypertrophied *trained* heart should be able to supply oxygen to a larger mass of muscle during exercise.

REFERENCES

1. Selye, H. On just being sick. *Nutr. Today*, 5:2, 1970.
2. Saltin, B., and Karlsson, J. *In*, Pernow, B., and Saltin, B., Eds. *Muscle Metabolism During Exercise*, pp. 289 and 395. New York, Plenum, 1971.
3. Robinson, S., and Harmon, P.M. Lactic acid mechanism and certain properties of blood in relation to training. *Am. J. Physiol.* 132:757, 1941.
4. Ekblom, B., Astrand, P.-O., Saltin, B., Stenberg, J., and Wallström, B. Effect of training on circulatory response to exercise. *J. Appl. Physiol.* 24:518, 1968.
5. Christensen, E.H., and Hansen, O. Arbeitsfähigkeit and Ernährung. *Skand. Arch. Physiol.* 81:160, 1939.
6. Jobsis, F.F., and Stainsby, W.N. Oxidation of NADH during contractions of circulated mammalian skeletal muscle. *Respir. Physiol.* 4:292, 1968.
7. Varnauskas, E., Bergman, H., Houk, P., and Björntorp, P. Haemodynamic effects of physical training in coronary patients. *Lancet* 2:8, 1966.
8. Frick, M.H., and Katila, M. Hemodynamic consequences of physical training after myocardial infarct. *Circulation* 37:192, 1968.
9. Clausen, J.P., Larsen, O.A., and Trap-Jensen, J. Physical training in the management of coronary artery disease. *Circulation* 40:143, 1969.
10. Saltin, B., Blomqvist, G., Mitchell, J.H., Johnson, R.L., Wildenthal, K., and Chapman, C.B. Response to exercise after bed rest and after training. *Circulation* 38 (Suppl. 7):1, 1968.
11. Grimby, G., Häggendal, E., and Saltin, B. Local xenon-133 clearance from the quadriceps muscle during exercise in man. *J. Appl. Physiol.* 22:305, 1967.
12. Varnauskas, E., Björntorp, P., Fahlen, M., Prerovsky, I., and Stenberg, J. Effects of physical training on exercise blood flow and enzymatic activity in skeletal muscle. *Cardiovasc. Res.* 4:418, 1970.
13. Ekblom, B., Astrand, P.-O., Saltin, B., Stenberg, J., and Wallström, B. Effect of training on circulatory response to exercise. *J. Appl. Physiol.* 24:518, 1968.
14. Detry, J.-M.R., Rousseau, M., Vandenbroucke, G., Kusumi, F., Brasseur, L.A., and Bruce, R.A. Increased arteriovenous oxygen difference after physical training in coronary heart disease. *Circulation* 44:109, 1971.
15. Paul, M.H., and Sperling, E. Cyclophorase system; correlation of cyclophorase activity and mitochondrial density in striated muscle. *Proc. Soc. Exp. Biol. Med.* 79:352, 1952.
16. Lawrie, R.A. The activity of the cytochrome system in muscle and its relation to myoglobin. *Biochem. J.* 55:298, 1953.
17. Pattengale, P.K., and Holloszy, J.O. Augmentation of skeletal muscle myoglobin by a program of treadmill running. *Am. J. Physiol.* 213:783, 1967.
18. Holloszy, J.O. Biochemical adaptations in muscle. Effects of exercise on mitochondrial oxygen uptake and respiratory enzyme activity in skeletal muscle. *J. Biol. Chem.* 242:2278, 1967.
19. Hemmingsen, E.A. Enhancement of oxygen transport by myoglobin. *Comp. Biochem. Physiol.* 10:239, 1963.
20. Scholander, P.F. Oxygen transport through hemoglobin solutions. *Science* 131:585, 1960.
21. Wittenberg, J.B. The molecular mechanism of hemoglobin-facilitated oxygen diffusion. *J. Biol. Chem.* 241:104, 1966.
22. Fuge, K.W., Crews, E.L., Pattengale, P.K., Holloszy, J.O., and Shank, R.E. Effects of protein deficiency on certain adaptive responses to exercise. *Am. J. Physiol.* 215:660, 1968.

23. Oscai, L.B., and Holloszy, J.O. Biochemical adaptations in muscle. II. Response of mitochondrial adenosine triphosphatase, creatine phosphokinase, and adenylate kinase activities in skeletal muscle to exercise. *J. Biol. Chem.* 246:6968, 1971.

24. Holloszy, J.O., Oscai, L.B., Don, I.J., and Molé, P.A. Mitochondrial citric acid cycle and related enzymes: adaptive responses to exercise. *Biochem. Biophys. Res. Commun.* 40:1368, 1970.

25. Baldwin, K.M., Klinkerfuss, G.H., Terjung, R.L., Molé, P.A., and Holloszy, J.O. Respiratory capacity of white, red, and intermediate muscle: adaptative response to exercise. *Am. J. Physiol.* 222:373, 1972.

26. Issekutz, B., Jr., Miller, H.I., and Rodahl, K. Lipid and carbohydrate metabolism during exercise. *Fed. Proc.* 25:1415, 1966.

27. Molé, P.A., and Holloszy, J.O. Exercise-induced increase in the capacity of skeletal muscle to oxidize palmitate. *Proc. Soc. Exp. Biol. Med.* 134:789, 1970.

28. Molé, P.A., Oscai, L.B., and Holloszy, J.O. Adaptation of muscle to exercise. Increase in levels of palmityl CoA synthetase, carnitine palmityltransferase, and palmityl CoA dehydrogenase, and in the capacity to oxidize fatty acids. *J. Clin. Invest.* 50:2323, 1971.

29. Havel, R.J., Carlson, L.A., Ekelund, L.-G., and Holmgren, A. Turnover rate and oxidation of different free fatty acids in man during exercise. *J. Appl. Physiol.* 19:613, 1964.

30. Issekutz, B., Jr., Miller, H.I., Paul, P., and Rodahl, K. Aerobic work capacity and plasma FFA turnover. *J. Appl. Physiol.* 20:293, 1965.

31. Holloszy, J.O., and Oscai, L.B., Effect of exercise on alpha-glycerophosphate dehydrogenase activity in skeletal muscle. *Arch. Biochem. Biophys.* 130:653, 1969.

32. Holloszy, J.O., Oscai, L.B., Molé, P.A., and Don, I.J. *In*, Pernow, B., and Saltin, B., Eds. *Muscle Metabolism During Exercise*, p.51. New York, Plenum, 1971.

33. Baldwin, K.M., Terjung, R.L., Winder, W.W., and Holloszy, J.O. Glycolytic enzymes in different types of skeletal muscle: adaptation to exercise. *Am. J. Physiol.* In Press.

34. Pette, D. *In*, Tager, J.M., Papa, S., Quagliariello, E., and Slater, E.C., Eds. *Regulation of Metabolic Processes in Mitochondria*, p.28. Amsterdam, Elsevier, 1966.

35. Sacktor, B., and Cochran, D.C. The respiratory metabolism of insect flight muscle. I. Manometric studies of oxidation and concomitant phosphorylation with sarcosomes. *Arch. Biochem. Biophys.* 74:266, 1958.

36. Shonk, C.E., and Boxer, G.E. Enzyme patterns in human tissues. I. Methods for the determination of glycolytic enzymes. *Cancer Res.* 24:709, 1964.

37. Dart, C.H., and Holloszy, J.O. Hypertrophied non-failing rat heart: partial biochemical characterization. *Circulation Res.* 25:245, 1969.

38. Edgerton, V.R., and Simpson, D.R. The intermediate muscle fiber of rats and guinea pigs. *J. Histochem. Cytochem.* 17:828, 1969.

39. Gauthier, G.F. *In*, Briskey, E.J., Cassens, R.G., and Marsh, B.B., Eds. *The Physiology and Biochemistry of Muscle as a Food*, 2nd ed., p. 103. Madison, Univ. Wis. Press, 1970.

40. Barnard, R.J., Edgerton, V.R., Furukawa, T., and Peter, J.B. Histochemical, biochemical, and contractile properties of red, white, and intermediate fibers. *Am. J. Physiol.* 220:410, 1971.

41. Gollnick, P.D., and King, D.W. Effect of exercise and training on mitochondria of rat skeletal muscle. *Am. J. Physiol.* 216:1502, 1969.

42. Morgan, T.E., Cobb, L.A., Short, F.A., Ross, R., and Gunn, D.R. *In*, Pernow, B., and Saltin, B., Eds. *Muscle Metabolism During Exercise*, p. 87. New York, Plenum, 1971.

43. Kiessling, K.H., Piehl, K., and Lundqvist, C.-G. *In*, Pernow, B., and Saltin, B., Eds. *Muscle Metabolism During Exercise*, p. 97. New York, Plenum, 1971.

44. Folkow, B., and Halicka, H.D. A comparison between "red" and "white" muscle with respect to blood supply, capillary surface area and oxygen uptake during rest and exercise. *Microvasc. Res.* 1:1, 1968.

45. Chapler, C.K., and Stainsby, W.N. Carbohydrate metabolism in contracting dog skeletal muscle *in situ. Am. J. Physiol.* 215:995, 1968.

46. Chance, B. The response of mitochondria to muscular contraction. *Ann. N.Y. Acad. Sci.* 81:477, 1959.

47. Lardy, H.A., and Wellman, H. The catalytic effect of 2, 4-dinitrophenol on adenosine triphosphate hydrolysis by cell particles and soluble enzymes. *J. Biol. Chem.* 201:357, 1953.

48. Chance, B., and Williams, G.R. The respiratory chain and oxidative phosphorylation. *Adv. Enzymol.* 17:65, 1956.

49. Klingenberg, M., and Von Hafen, H. Hydrogen pathway in mitochondria. I. Hydrogen transfer from succininate to acetoacetate. *Biochem. Z.* 337:120, 1963.

50. Jöbsis, F.F. Spectrophotometric studies on intact muscle. II. Recovery from contractile activity. *J. Gen. Physiol.* 46:929, 1963.

51. Jöbsis, F.F., and Duffield, J.C. Oxidative and glycolytic recovery metabolism in muscle: flurometric observations on their relative contributions. *J. Gen. Physiol.* 50:1009. 1967.

52. Piiper, J., DiPrampero, P.E., and Cerretelli, P. Oxygen debt and high-energy phosphates in the gastrocnemius muscle of the dog. *Am. J. Physiol.* 215:523, 1968.

53. Wu, R., and Racker, E. Regulatory mechanisms in carbohydrate metabolism. III. Limiting factors in glycolysis of ascites tumor cells. *J. Biol. Chem.* 234:1029, 1959.

54. Passonneau, J.V., and Lowry, O.H. P- fructokinase and control of the citric acid cycle. *Biochem. Biophys. Res. Commun.* 13:372, 1963.

55. Uyeda, K., and Racker, E. Regulatory mechanisms in carbohydrate metabolism. VII. Hexokinase and phosphofructokinase. *J. Biol. Chem.* 240:4682, 1965.

56. Williamson, J.R. Glycolytic control mechanisms. II. Kinetics of intermediate changes during the aerobic-anoxic transition in perfused rat heart. *J. Biol. Chem.* 241:5026, 1966.

57. Krzanowski, J., and Matschinsky, F.M. Regulation of phosphofructokinase by phosphocreatine and phosphorylated glycolytic intermediates. *Biochem. Biophys. Res. Commun.* 34:816, 1969.

58. Paul, P., Issekutz, B. and Miller, H.I. Interrelationship of free fatty acids and glucose metabolism in the dog. *Am. J. Physiol.* 211:1313, 1966.

59. Newsholme, E.A., and Randle, P.J. Regulation of glucose uptake by muscle. 7. Effects of fatty acids, ketone bodies and pyruvate, and of alloxan-diabetes, starvation, hypophysectomy and adrenalectomy on the concentrations of hexose phosphates, nucleotides and inorganic phosphate in perfused rat heart. *Biochem. J.* 93:641, 1964.

60. Parmeggiani, A., and Bowman, R.H. Regulation of phosphofructokinase activity by citrate in normal and diabetic muscle. *Biochem. Biophys. Res. Commun.* 12:268, 1963.

61. Naughton, J., Shanbour, K., Armstrong, R., McCoy, J., and Lategola, M.T. Cardiovascular responses to exercise following myocardial infarction. *Arch. Int. Med.* 117:541, 1966.

62. Whitsett, T., and Naughton, J. Systolic time intervals following exercise in patients with ASHD. *Clin. Res.* 16:438, 1968.

63. Hellerstein, H.K., and Hornsten, T.R. Assessing and preparing the patient for return to a meaningful and productive life. *J. Rehabil.* 32:48, 1966.

64. Hellerstein, H.K., Hornsten, T.R., Goldbarg, A., Burlando, A.G., Friedman, E.H., Hirsch, E.Z., and Marik, S. The influence of active conditioning upon subjects with coronary artery disease: cardio-respiratory changes during training in 67 patients. *Can. Med. Assoc. J.* 96:758, 1967.

65. Hanson, J.S., Tabakin, B.S., Levy, A.M., and Nedde, W. Long-term physical training and cardiovascular dynamics in middle-aged men. *Circulation* 38:783, 1968.

66. Clausen, J.P., Trap-Jensen, J., and Lassen, N.A. The effects of training on the heart rate during arm and leg exercise. *Scand. J. Clin. Lab. Invest.* 26:295, 1970.

67. Oscai, L.B., Molé, P.A., Brei, B., and Holloszy, J.O. Cardiac growth and respiratory enzyme levels in male rats subjected to a running program. *Am. J. Physiol.* 220:1238, 1971.

68. Oscai, L.B., Molé, P.A., and Holloszy, J.O. Effects of exercise on cardiac weight and mitochondria in male and female rats. *Am. J. Physiol.* 220:1944, 1971.

69. Grande, F., and Taylor, H.L. *In*, Hamilton, W.F., Ed. *Handbook of Physiology.* Section 2, *Circulation*, Vol. III, p. 2615. (Washington, D.C., Am. Physiol. Soc.) Baltimore, Williams & Wilkins, 1965.

PART II

Psychology, Psychiatry, and Sociology

15

INFLUENCE OF PSYCHOSOCIAL FACTORS
ON CORONARY RISK AND ADAPTATION TO A
PHYSICAL FITNESS EVALUATION PROGRAM

Ernest H. Friedman, M.D., and *Herman K. Hellerstein,* M.D.

In a study of 3,954 Cleveland attorneys, the prevalence of coronary heart disease (CHD) in subjects aged 24 to 59 correlated to economic background and status as determined by the quality of law school attended [1]. The coronary prevalence rate of the highest status group was significantly less than the middle but not significantly less than the lowest status group. Hinkle replicated this finding in a broader sample of 270,000 Bell System employees, followed 3 years for coronary incidence. The major difference was a lower incidence in executives compared with foremen, the workmen being slightly less than the foremen [2, 3].

The purpose of the present study is to relate position in the socioeconomic hierarchy in a group of middle-aged men to: the coronary risk factors of blood pressure and body weight; psychosocial factors (Behavior Pattern A, a measure of self-esteem and The Hollingshead Two-Factor Index of Social Position); adherence to a prescribed physical fitness regimen; and modification of blood pressure and body weight as determined at the time of 6-month followup examination.

Materials and Methods

The study population consisted of 173 middle-aged predominantly Jewish upper middle class business and professional male volunteer participants in the Case Western Reserve University-Jewish Community Center (CWRU-JCC) physical fitness program. These men were classified as highly coronary-prone on the

From the Coronary Prevention Program of The Jewish Community Center and The School of Medicine, Case Western Reserve University. This study was supported in part by grants from the U.S. Public Health Service to the Clinical Heart Center (HE 06304) and to the Division of Biometry (GM 12302) of Case Western Reserve University; and from The American Heart Association, Northeast Ohio Chapter, Inc., to The Jewish Community Center of Cleveland.

basis of possessing three or more of the characteristics which indicate an increased susceptibility to the premature development of coronary heart disease [4]. The methodology employed in this study has been described previously [5].

Psychosocial evaluation. On the day of the first physical fitness test, psychosocial evaluation was performed. The methods included the Rosenman-Friedman structured tape-recorded interview, designed to elicit Behavior Pattern A (Pattern A), the booklet form of the Minnesota Multiphasic Personality Inventory (MMPI) [6] which was hand-scored, and a rating of each subject and his father on The Hollingshead Two-Factor Index of Social Position based on education and occupation [7].

*Quantitative Analysis of
Rosenman-Friedman Behavior Patterns Technique*

The tape-recorded interview designed to elicit Pattern A was administered by a trained technician. A Roberts 1630 Stereophonic tape recorder was used with two Phillips close-talking microphones. Our quantitative rating method consisted of a scoring sheet composed of the 62 questions in the interview which permitted the technician to rate the response to each question by content and style, according to the criteria of Rosenman and Friedman (Appendix A). A total of 45 of the 62 questions could be rated by content and all 62 questions were rated by style.

For the questions dealing with content, the possible ratings ranged from 1 as the extreme type A to 5 as the extreme type B. An example: How much exercise do you schedule a day intentionally?

    1 — amount only
    2 — amount plus other words
    3 — varies
    4 — can't recall
    5 — indefinite

In other words, a score of 1 meant the subject gave the briefest possible response by only giving the amount of exercise without elaboration. A score of 2 indicated an answer of amount plus additional words or statements. A score of 3 meant that the amount of exercise varied.

Style ratings based on the degree of abrupt, terse, emphatic, hurried, or staccato responses ranged from 1 to 4, with 1 being the extreme Pattern A and 4 the extreme Pattern B. If a subject failed to answer the question or if the answer was not intelligible, the question was omitted from the rating. The scores of the content and style responses were summed separately and divided by the respective number of questions involved (Content = 45; Style = 62), thus providing an average content rating (content rating) and an average style rating (style rating) for each subject.

Validation of quantitative method. To validate this method, a separate subsample of 25 subjects drawn from a larger group of 327 CWRU-JCC subjects originally rated by this method [8], were independently rated by one of us (EHF), and his content and style ratings were correlated with those of the technician. The mean content and style ratings of EHF and the technician did not differ: EHF, content rating = 2.06 standard error of the mean (SE) 0.07 and style rating = 2.08 SE 0.11; technician, content rating = 2.09 SE 0.08 and style rating = 2.07 SE 0.09. As a measure of the representativeness of the 173 subjects under study, the mean content and style ratings of the 25 subjects and the 173 subjects in the main study sample (TABLE I) were compared and found similar. Content and style ratings by EHF and the technician of the 25 subjects matched by subjects correlated significantly, both $p < 0.01$, content rating $r = 0.85$, and style rating $r = 0.50$. These data support an earlier finding of a high degree of replicability of the behavior pattern rating method as determined by Rosenman's 84.1 percent categorical agreement with EHF [9].

Comparison of Categorical and Quantitative
Content and Style Ratings

A second way of validating the quantitative method was by comparing the quantitative analysis with the categorical A and B ratings of 60 consecutive interviews drawn from the original sample of 327 subjects. These were rated according to the original Rosenman-Friedman method: A1, A2, B3, B4. The mean content and style ratings were calculated for categorical A (A1 and A2) and B (B3 and B4) patterns.

Categorical A and B ratings of 60 subjects yielded 44 subjects of the A type (73.3 percent) and 16 subjects of the B type (26.7 percent). These findings were similar to those previously reported by Friedman and Rosenman [10] and by our group demonstrating 72 percent of patients with clinical coronary heart disease and with valvular rheumatic heart disease exhibiting Pattern A [11]. This finding suggests consistency with the random sample of Rosenman and Friedman despite the fact that the present population sample is volunteer, not randomly selected, and is narrow in terms of being a highly selected middle-aged, urban, upper middle class Jewish group of males.

The technician's quantitative content and style ratings of these 60 subjects yields a mean content rating of 2.13 and a mean style rating of 1.96 for the A subjects, and a mean content rating of 2.45 and a mean style rating of 2.48 for the B subjects which differ at the 0.01 and 0.001 levels of significance, respectively. The significantly different content and style mean ratings for the two groups divided by the categorical ratings demonstrates the utility of this quantitative content and style rating system.

Average Heineman Rating Scale of the
Minnesota Multiphasic Personality Inventory (MMPI)

An indirect measure of the subject's tendency to present himself in a favorable or unfavorable light was developed by adapting Dr. Charles E. Heineman's

TABLE I

Summary of findings of 173 noncoronary men, classified by annual income on entering a physical fitness program and 6-month adherence rating (see text)

Income Group		Age (Years)	Body Height (Inches)	Index of Social Position[f] and Class — Subject	Father	Behavior Pattern Interview — Content Rating	Style Rating	Average Heineman Rating – MMPI[g]	Adherence Rating[e]
I	Mean	45.9	68.9	20.2 II	41.2 III	2.12	1.85	2.55	2.31
	SE[h]	1.05	0.35	1.49	2.05	0.05	0.07	0.03	.20
	N	32	31	32	32	30	30	30	26
II	Mean	45.6	68.9	21.0 II	40.8 III	2.09	2.08[c]	2.65[c]	1.78[d]
	SE	0.85	0.43	1.20	2.06	0.04	0.05	0.02	.16
	N	48	48	47	47	46	46	46	41
III	Mean	45.5	67.9	27.5[a] II	49.7[a] IV	2.19[b]	2.01	2.60	1.64[c]
	SE	1.60	0.81	1.15	1.29	0.03	0.04	0.02	.10
	N	93	92	91	91	88	88	88	84

[a]Compared with Group I or II, p <0.001

[b]Compared with Group II, p <0.05

[c]Compared with Group I, p <0.01

[d]Compared with Group I, p <0.05

[e]Lower Value Denotes Greater Adherence

[f]Lower value denotes higher social position

[g]Lower value denotes more favorable presentation of self

[h]Standard error of the mean

Social Class	
I	11-17
II	18-31
III	32-47
IV	48-63
V	64-77

rating scale [6]. He asked 108 students in an introductory psychology class at the State University of Iowa to indicate the degree to which an answer of *True* to each MMPI item would give a favorable or an unfavorable impression about the respondent: 1, very favorable; 2, somewhat favorable; 3, neutral; 4, somewhat unfavorable; 5, very unfavorable. The class average of each of the 566 MMPI items was expressed as a 3 digit number to the second decimal. In the present investigation, each of the 566 true or false MMPI responses for every subject was keypunched into standard IBM computer cards. The computer was programmed to average the Heineman ratings corresponding to the MMPI items answered *True* by the subject. Thus, each subject received an Average Heineman Rating with the higher value denoting presentation of self in a less favorable light.

Validation of the Average Heineman Rating as a measure of unfavorable presentation of self was demonstrated by its high positive correlation to the F minus K scale (low self-esteem) of the MMPI, $r = 0.87$, $p < 0.005$, strongly suggesting that they measured a similar personality factor [8].

The Hollingshead Two Factor Index of Social Position based on education and occupation was calculated for each subject and his father, thus providing an estimate of current status and intergenerational mobility.

Physiological Parameters

On entry into the program (Test 1) and 6 months later (Test 2), resting systolic and diastolic blood pressures were determined by the standard cuff technique with the subject seated on a bicycle ergometer in the *get ready* position just prior to physical fitness testing. Physical fitness, determined by multi-level bicycle ergometer testing, was expressed as the highest workload and maximal oxygen intake [5]. During the 6-month period between physical fitness tests, the subject's adherence to the physical fitness regimen was determined from attendance records as described previously [5]; exercise sessions were scheduled three times per week. The adherence rating was: 1 = good; 2 = fair; 3 = poor; and 4 = none.

Income groups. Subjects were classified by annual income in dollars in three groups: Group I, $35,000 or more; Group II, $20,000-$35,000; and Group III, less than $20,000. These income groups were compared by the t-test of difference between means of all variables described above.

Results

Data in TABLE I demonstrate that on entry into the physical fitness program, the three income groups were alike in age and body height. The social class in all three groups was higher than in their fathers'. Groups I and II were similar in terms of their own and their fathers' index of social position, whereas income Group III was significantly lower on both ratings. Hollingshead's Social Class categorization demonstrated that the intergenerational mobility of Group III was greater, being mobile from Class IV to Class II, whereas income Groups I and II were mobile from Social Class III to Class II.

Behavior Pattern A (Pattern A) content and style ratings of the income groups exhibited dissimilar patterns. Pattern A content of Group II was significantly greater than of Group III but insignificantly greater than Group I. Group I's Pattern A style was significantly greater than Group II but not greater than Group III. F minus K scores were similar in Groups I, II, and III, averaging minus 12.

The average Heineman Rating demonstrated the unfavorable self-presentation of Group I to be significantly less than Group II (p < 0.01) but not less than Group III.

Data in TABLE II demonstrate significant differences between income groups in blood pressure and body weight on entry into the fitness program, which were no longer present after 6 months' participation in the program. On entry, systolic blood pressure and body weight correlated negatively to annual income. Diastolic blood pressure was significantly greater in Group II than in Group I, p < 0.01, and significantly less greater in Group III than in Group I, p < 0.02. There were no significant differences in the highest workload or the maximal oxygen intake in the three income groups on entry into the program.

The adherence rating correlated inversely to annual income (TABLE I).

Insignificant differences in body weight and blood pressure after 6 months' physical fitness training was achieved by decreases in Groups II and III toward the levels of Group I and accompanied by very significant increases in highest workload and maximal oxygen intake in Groups II and III. Improvement of fitness was not as striking in Group I.

Discussion

Although this population sample is upper middle class, Jewish, volunteer, and not randomly selected, it is comparable in terms of height, weight, and aerobic capacity to a French-Canadian white male population sample [12]. Nevertheless, caution should be exercised in generalizing to other populations.

The findings of this study support the hypothesis relating socioeconomic status to coronary risk, and suggest that economic position of the individual and the social position of the father are more selective than social position of the individual in discriminating high- and low-risk groups. Similarly, a previous report of sexual activity in another subsample of the CWRU-JCC population showed that the frequency of orgasms per week correlated positively to income but not to social position [5].

The pattern of coronary prevalence in the socioeconomic hierarchy in attorneys is replicated in this investigation on several scales. In the present report, Group I with the highest income and hypothesized to be at lowest coronary risk compared with Group II, the *highest risk* category (Group III, intermediate) exhibited on entry into the program, lower resting diastolic blood pressure, more

TABLE II

Summary of findings of noncoronary men on entry (*Test 1*) and after 6 months' participation (*Test 2*) in a physical fitness program (classified by annual income)

Income Group		Blood Pressure (mm Hg) Systolic	Diastolic	Body Weight (pounds)	Highest Work-load (kilopond-meters/min)	Maximal O_2 Intake (ml O_2/kg body wt/min)
TEST 1						
I	Mean	117.6	81.3	175.6	679.7	25.3
	SE[1]	1.97	1.46	3.54	23.30	0.86
	N	32	32	32	32	31
II	Mean	124.3^c	87.5$^{a'}$	180.3	663.8	25.2
	SE	2.24	1.54	4.17	16.90	0.71
	N	47	47	48	47	46
III	Mean	126.1^a	85.9^b	183.6^c	657.1	24.5
	SE	2.05	1.25	2.97	17.01	0.50
	N	92	92	92	92	88
TEST 2						
I	Mean	117.3	81.5	176.9	738.9^f	27.2
	SE	2.45	2.25	2.39	27.64	1.08
	N	26	26	27	27	28
II	Mean	119.6	81.8	175.6	760.9^d	28.4^e
	SE	2.30	1.78	4.80	20.56	0.82
	N	41	41	40	41	40
III	Mean	119.3	81.2	176.6	753.4^d	28.3^d
	SE	1.92	1.22	2.89	19.09	0.61
	N	86	86	87	88	83

Compared with Group I in TEST 1:

a, $p < 0.01$

b, $p < 0.02$

c, $p < 0.05$

Change from Test 1:

d, $p < 0.001$

e, $p < 0.01$

f, $p < 0.10$

[1] Standard Error of the Mean

Pattern A style, and more favorable presentation of self, suggesting greater self-esteem.

This consistent pattern of physiological and psychological parameters assumes greater significance in the light of recent research, demonstrating the influence of excess sympathetic activity on essential hypertension. Resting diastolic blood pressure correlated closely to basal norepinephrine concentrations, $p < 0.001$. After ganglionic blockade there was a highly significant correlation between change in resting blood pressure and change in plasma norepinephrine, $p < 0.001$ [13]. It is tempting to speculate about the interrelationships among modifications of physical fitness, physiologic and psychologic parameters. It appears plausible that, physically activating and enhancing the physiologic function of previously phlegmatic individuals with compromised self-images, could have a beneficial effect in these areas by mechanisms not elucidated by the present investigation. Unfortunately, repeat measures of Pattern A and the Average Heineman Rating at 6 months were not evaluated. This remains a subject for future investigation.

Social position data. Although the data regarding social position show no difference in background or intergenerational mobility of Group I compared with Group II, the relative contribution of intragenerational mobility is unclear. The latter is supported as a factor by the discrepancy in incomes between Groups I and II despite ostensibly similar backgrounds. Kaplan et al demonstrated a lower coronary risk in upwardly mobile subjects originating from Social Classes I through III [14].

Pattern A style may reflect drive which could explain the difference in income between Groups I and II despite their similar backgrounds. Outwardly directed activity as a defense against passive dependency, less influence of the latter on sexual activity, higher income, and more children characterized normal coronary-prone compared with postcoronary subjects. These psychological differences were hypothesized to be longstanding antedating the onset of clinical coronary heart disease [5].

Greater self-esteem or favorable self-presentation might also lead to more success, other factors being constant. However, drive, responsiveness, self-esteem, and mode of presentation may be results as well as causes of change in economic position in society. This study, while unable to resolve the question, does suggest that the phlegmatic individual whose behavior reflects low self-esteem is at higher coronary risk.

The significance of a lack of emotional responsiveness to coronary risk has been discussed by Minc as *action without emotion.* He reasoned that recurrent, unemotive, civilized stress adversely affects the cardiovascular system, particularly in persons whose feelings are suppressed by rationality [15].

Pattern A content. Group II was highest in Pattern A content, lowest in Pattern A style, and least in physiologic rest. These findings are discrepant with the Rosenman-Friedman hypothesis since content and style are poorly correlated with each other, tending toward a negative relationship. Furthermore, style correlated very significantly to coronary risk but in the *reverse* direction as would be predicted by Rosenman and Friedman. Pattern A content was highest in Group II, the *highest risk* category, but only intermediate in the *lowest risk* category, Group I.

These data suggest that separate content and style ratings can discriminate between groups of patients in ways not previously demonstrated by the global rating method of Rosenman and Friedman. The limitations of their methodology are evidenced by the results of their prospective study. There was a higher coronary incidence only in incompletely developed Pattern A whereas the incidence in exaggerated Pattern A was no greater than in Pattern B [16, 17]. It is noteworthy that in the Bell System study, there was little difference between the higher coronary risk workmen and the lower coronary risk managers, or between the lower risk *college* and higher risk *no college* men in the amount of their goal-directed purposeful activity—in the perceived pressures and tensions of their daily lives, or in the personality traits and behavior patterns that could be detected by psychological tests. In this study, Hinkle and collaborators could find among 75 men with definite coronary heart disease only eight men with personality traits like those of Rosenman and Friedman's "Type A" and four men who appeared to be repressing such personality traits [3].

Heineman rating. The Average Heineman Rating is a new scale we developed and, although not standardized in other population samples, does (as mentioned earlier) correlate very significantly to the self-esteem scale of the MMPI (F minus K) and is more selective in identifying socioeconomic classes. This Heineman rating scale, while not easily scored by hand, lends itself readily to computerized scoring of the MMPI by a modest addition to an existing program.

Socioeconomic status correlated negatively with body weight, systolic blood pressure on entry, and adherence to the program. In the attorney study, background and status were related negatively to pounds overweight, $p < 0.0005$ [1]. No separate statistical analysis was made in the present investigation to identify interrelationships among weight, blood pressure, and adherence. The negative correlation of adherence to socioeconomic status is unexplained.

Group III, with parents from the lowest social class, exhibited the heaviest weight, highest systolic blood pressure, and the least Pattern A content on entry, and the closest adherence to the fitness regimen accompanied by the greatest improvement in maximal oxygen intake. The enhancement of fitness in Group II as well as in Group III with attendant improvements in weight and blood pressure demonstrates that the lower socioeconomic groups originally at higher coronary risk, secured the greatest benefit from the physical fitness regimen.

The findings of this study indicate that active participation in a physical fitness program is accompanied by reduction in risk factors in coronary-prone subjects. The methodology developed in this investigation can be utilized in future studies of interrelationships among psychosocial factors, physical fitness, and the development and course of coronary artery disease.

Summary

A total of 173 normal coronary-prone men entering a physical fitness program were stratified by annual income into three groups: I, $35,000 or more; II, $20,000 to $35,000; and III, less than $20,000. These groups were compared by mean age, body height and weight, scale scores of the Minnesota Multiphasic Personality Inventory, content and style ratings of subject responses to the Rosenman-Friedman structured interview designed to elicit Behavior Pattern A, blood pressure, and physical fitness on the bicycle ergometer. Six months later, subjects were rated by degree of adherence to the fitness regimen and repeat physical measurements were secured. Group III subjects, derived from lowest social class fathers, had the lowest income, the best adherence to the training program, greatest improvement in physical fitness, maximal oxygen intake, weight loss, and reduction of systolic blood pressure. Group II subjects, initially at least physiologic rest in terms of systolic and diastolic blood pressure, demonstrated the *least* Pattern A style, the most unfavorable presentation of self and similar reductions of weight and blood pressure with enhanced physical fitness. The findings are discrepant with the Pattern A hypothesis; suggest that the phlegmatic individual with low self-esteem is a high coronary risk; and relate economic position to coronary risk and its reduction by an intervention program.

ACKNOWLEDGMENTS

We wish to express gratitude to Misses Nancy Galambush and Nancy Symons, and to Mrs. Marjorie Stonebrook and Mrs. Norine Wild for excellent technical assistance.

REFERENCES

1. Friedman, E.H., and Hellerstein, H.K. Occupational stress, law school hierarchy and coronary artery disease in Cleveland attorneys. *J. Psychosom. Med.* 30:72-86, 1968.

2. Hinkle, L.E., Whitney, L.H., Lehman, E.W., Dunn, J., Benjamin, B., King, R., Plakun, A., and Flehinger, B. Occupation, education and coronary heart disease. *Science* 161:238-246, 1968.

3. Hinkle, L.E., Jr. An estimate of the effects of "stress" on the incidence and prevalence of coronary heart disease in a large industrial population in the United States. *Thromb. Diath. Haemorrh.* Suppl. 51:15-65, 1972.

4. Epstein, F.H. The epidemiology of coronary heart disease: a review. *J. Chron. Dis.* 18:735-774, 1965.

5. Hellerstein, H.K., and Friedman, E.H. Sexual activity and the postcoronary patient. *Arch. Intern. Med.* 125:987-999, 1970.

6. Dahlstrom, W.G., and Welsh, G.S. *An MMPI Handbook.* Minneapolis, Univ. Minn. Press, 1960.

7. Hollingshead, A.B. *Two Factor Index of Social Position.* New Haven, Conn., privately printed, 1957.

8. Friedman, E.H., Hellerstein, H.K., and Hsi, B.P. Validation of Behavior Pattern A. *Circulation* Suppl. 2 to 43 and 44:166, 1971.

9. Friedman, E.H., Hellerstein, H.K., Eastwood, G.L., and Jones, S.E. Behavior patterns and serum cholesterol in two groups of normal males. *Am. J. Med. Sci.* 255:237-244 and 269-271, 1968.

10. Rosenman, R.H., Friedman, M., Straus, R., Wurm, M., Jenkins, C.D., and Messinger, H.B. Coronary heart disease in the western collaborative group study: a follow-up experience of two years. *J.A.M.A.* 195:86-92, 1966.

11. Hellerstein, H.K., Friedman, E.H., Brdar, P.J., Weiss, M., Dupertuis, C.W., Turell, D.J., and Rumbaugh, D. A comparison of the personality of adult subjects with rheumatic heart disease and with arteriosclerotic heart disease. In, *Rehabilitation of Non-Coronary Heart Disease*, pp.220-282. Symposium. Höhenried, Bayern, International Society of Cardiology, June, 1969.

12. Allard, C., Goulet, C., Choquette, G., and David, P. Submaximal work capacity of a French-Canadian male population. *In*, Raab, W., Ed. *Prevention of Ischemic Heart Disease*, pp. 226-235. Springfield, Ill., Thomas, 1966.

13. Louis, W.J., Doyle, A.E., and Onavekas, S. Plasma norepinephrine levels in essential hypertension. *N. Engl. J. Med.* 228:599-601, 1973.

14. Kaplan, B.H., Cassel, J.C., Tyroler, H.A., Cornoni, J.C., Kleinbaum, D.G., and Hames, C.G. Occupational mobility and coronary heart disease. *Arch. Intern. Med.* 128:938-942, 1971.

15. Minc, S. Psychological factors in coronary artery disease. *Geriatrics* 20:747-755, 1965.

16. Rosenman, R.H., Friedman, M., Straus, R., Jenkins, C.D., Zyzanski, S.J., and Wurm, M. Coronary heart disease in The Western Collaborative Group Study. A follow-up experience of 4½ years. *J. Chron. Dis.* 23:173-190. 1970.

17. Friedman, E.H. Personality types and coronary artery disease. (Letter to Editor) *J.A.M.A.* 219:385, 1972.

APPENDIX A

BEHAVIOR PATTERN INTERVIEW TRANSCRIPTION SHEET

Content

1 — yes
2 — qualified "yes"
3 — qualified "no"
4 — no
5 — indefinite
6 — both
7 — neither
8 — question not answered
9 — question not asked

Style

1 — very abrupt, terse, emphatic, hurried or staccato response
2 — moderately abrupt, terse, emphatic, hurried or staccato response
3 — moderately relaxed, unhurried, essentially opposite of 2
4 — very relaxed, unhurried, essentially opposite of 1
7 — can't evaluate
8 — not answered
9 — not asked

Column Number

1, 2, 3	☐ ☐ ☐	Study Number
4, 5	☐ ☐	
6, 7, 8	☐ ☐ ☐	Identification number of subject
9	☐	May I ask your age, Mr. _____?
10	☐	Style (1, 2, 3, 4, 7, 8, 9)
11	☐	How much exercise do you schedule a day intentionally?
12	☐	Style (1, 2, 3, 4, 7, 8, 9)
13	☐	Do you actually accomplish what you planned?

Do you actually accomplish what you planned?

1 – yes   5 – indefinite
2 – qualified yes   8 – not answered
3 – qualified no   9 – not asked
4 – no

14	☐	Style (1, 2, 3, 4, 7, 8, 9)

(APPENDIX A continued)

STYLE CODE
1. very abrupt, tense, emphatic, hurried or staccato response
2. moderately abrupt, tense, emphatic, hurried or staccato response
3. moderately relaxed, unhurried, essentially opposite of no. 2
4. very relaxed, unhurried, essentially opposite of no. 1
7. can't evaluate   8. not answered   9. not asked

---

15 ☐   What is your present position?
                   1 – stated in one sentence
                   2 – stated in more than one sentence
                   5 – indefinite
                   8 – not answered
                   9 – not asked

16 ☐   Style (1, 2, 3, 4, 7, 8, 9)

17 ☐   How long have you held this position?
                   1 – precise period of time (in years, months)
                   2 – precise (years)
                   3 – imprecise (years)
                   4 – imprecise (decades)
                   5 – indefinite
                   8 – not answered
                   9 – not asked

18 ☐   Style (1, 2, 3, 4, 7, 8, 9)

19 ☐   Would you say your job has heavy responsibilities?
                   1 – yes   5 – indefinite
                   2 – qualified yes   8 – not answered
                   3 – qualified no   9 – not asked
                   4 – no

20 ☐   Style (1, 2, 3, 4, 7, 8, 9)

21 ☐   Do you participate in any community activities?
                   1 – yes   5 – indefinite
                   2 – qualified yes   8 – not answered
                   3 – qualified no   9 – not asked
                   4 – no

22 ☐   Style (1, 2, 3, 4, 7, 8, 9)

23 ☐   When you were in high school or college, were you on
                   any athletic teams?
                   –1 – yes   5 – indefinite
                   2 – qualified yes   8 – not answered
                   3 – qualified no   9 – not asked
                   4 – no

(APPENDIX A continued)

STYLE CODE
1. very abrupt, tense, emphatic, hurried or staccato response
2. moderately abrupt, tense, emphatic, hurried or staccato response
3. moderately relaxed, unhurried, essentially opposite of no. 2
4. very relaxed, unhurried, essentially opposite of no. 1
7. can't evaluate   8. not answered   9. not asked

---

24 ☐   Style (1, 2, 3, 4, 7, 8, 9)

25 ☐   If yes, were you captain of any?
                  1 — yes   5 — indefinite
                  2 — qualified yes   8 — not answered
                  3 — qualified no   9 — not asked
                  4 — no

26 ☐   After you began making a living, did you attend night
               school or take any extension courses to further your
               career?
                  1 — yes   5 — indefinite
                  2 — qualified yes   8 — not answered
                  3 — qualified no   9 — not asked
                  4 — no

28 ☐   Style (1, 2, 3, 4, 7, 8, 9)

29 ☐   Were you in any branch of the armed forces during
               the war? (Or between?)
                  1 — yes   5 — indefinite
                  2 — qualified yes   8 — not answered
                  3 — qualified no   9 — not asked
                  4 — no

30 ☐   Style (1, 2, 3, 4, 7, 8, 9)

31 ☐   If "yes," what rank did you enter the service with?
                  1 — officer   5 — indefinite
                  2 — n.c.o.   8 — not answered
                  3 — enlisted man   9 — not asked

32 ☐   Style (1, 2, 3, 4, 7, 8, 9)

33 ☐   What was your rank on discharge?
                  1 — officer   5 — indefinite
                  2 — n.c.o.   8 — not answered
                  3 — enlisted man   9 — not asked

34 ☐   Style (1, 2, 3, 4, 7, 8, 9)

(APPENDIX A continued)

STYLE CODE
 1. very abrupt, tense, emphatic, hurried or staccato response
 2. moderately abrupt, tense, emphatic, hurried or staccato response
 3. moderately relaxed, unhurried, essentially opposite of no. 2
 4. very relaxed, unhurried, essentially opposite of no. 1
 7. can't evaluate   8. not answered   9. not asked

---

35 ☐   Advancement in service — leave blank if not asked
                1 — enlisted man to officer
                2 — enlisted man advancing two or more ranks to
                    enlisted status
                3 — officer advancing two or more ranks
                4 — enlisted man advancing one rank to enlisted status
                5 — officer advancing one rank
                6 — enlisted man not advancing
                7 — officer not advancing
                8 — enlisted man demoted
                9 — officer demoted

36 ☐   How long were you in the service?
                1 — precise answers (years, months)
                2 — precise answer (years)
                3 — imprecise (years)
                4 — can't recall
                5 — indefinite
                8 — not answered
                9 — not asked

37 ☐   Style (1, 2, 3, 4, 7, 8, 9)

38 ☐   If not in the service, why?
                1 — disability
                2 — deferment because of essential job
                3 — family hardship
                4 — conscientious objector
                5 — indefinite
                6 — not called
                8 — not answered
                9 — not asked

39 ☐   Style (1, 2, 3, 4, 7, 8, 9)

40 ☐   Are you content with your present job level or are you
                striving for further advancement?
                1 — no & striving   5 — indefinite
                2 — no & not striving   8 — not answered
                3 — yes & striving   9 — not asked
                4 — yes & not striving (content)

(APPENDIX A continued)

STYLE CODE
1. very abrupt, tense, emphatic, hurried or staccato response
2. moderately abrupt, tense, emphatic, hurried or staccato response
3. moderately relaxed, unhurried, essentially opposite of no. 2
4. very relaxed, unhurried, essentially opposite of no. 1
7. can't evaluate   8. not answered   9. not asked

---

41 ☐   Style (1, 2, 3, 4, 7, 8, 9)

42 ☐   When you were younger, were you aware that you were
                consciously striving for advancement?
                  1 — yes   5 — indefinite
                  2 — qualified yes   8 — not answered
                  3 — qualified no   9 — not asked
                  4 — no

43 ☐   Style (1, 2, 3, 4, 7, 8, 9)

44 ☐   Do you still think you strive to advance?
                  1 — yes   5 — indefinite
                  2 — qualified yes   8 — not answered
                  3 — qualified no   9 — not asked
                  4 — no

45 ☐   Style (1, 2, 3, 4, 7, 8, 9)

46 ☐   Would you describe yourself as a hard-driving and
                aggressive individual, or relaxed and easy going?
                  1 — hard-driving and aggressive
                  2 — qualified hard-driving and aggressive
                  3 — qualified easy going
                  4 — easy going
                  5 — indefinite
                  6 — both
                  7 — neither
                  8 — not answered
                  9 — not asked

47 ☐   Style (1, 2, 3, 4, 7, 8, 9)

48 ☐   Are you married?
                  1 — yes   5 — indefinite
                  2 — widowed   8 — not answered
                  3 — divorced &   9 — not asked
                      separated

49 ☐   Style (1, 2, 3, 4, 7, 8, 9)

(APPENDIX A continued)

STYLE CODE
1. very abrupt, tense, emphatic, hurried or staccato response
2. moderately abrupt, tense, emphatic, hurried or staccato response
3. moderately relaxed, unhurried, essentially opposite of no. 2
4. very relaxed, unhurried, essentially opposite of no. 1
7. can't evaluate   8. not answered   9. not asked

---

50 ☐   Does your wife think of you as aggressive and hard-driving?
           1 — yes   6 — both
           2 — qualified yes   7 — neither
           3 — qualified no   8 — not answered
           4 — no   9 — not asked
           5 — indefinite

51 ☐   Style (1, 2, 3, 4, 7, 8, 9)

52 ☐   Concordance of subject's and wife's estimate (46 and 50)
           1 — concordant   4 — information not available
           2 — discordant   5 — indefinite

53 ☐   Does she say slow down?
           1 — yes   5 — indefinite
           2 — qualified yes   8 — not answered
           3 — qualified no   9 — not asked
           4 — no

54 ☐   Style (1, 2, 3, 4, 7, 8, 9)

55 ☐   Does she say get on with it?
           1 — yes   5 — indefinite
           2 — qualified yes   8 — not answered
           3 — qualified no   9 — not asked
           4 — no

56 ☐   Style (1, 2, 3, 4, 7, 8, 9)

57 ☐   Would you rather have **admiration** and **respect** from
           friends and work associates, or would you rather have
           their **affection**?
           1 — admiration and respect
           2 — qualified admiration and respect
           3 — qualified affection
           4 — affection
           5 — indefinite
           6 — both (admiration, respect, & affection)
           7 — neither
           8 — not answered
           9 — not asked

(APPENDIX A continued)

STYLE CODE
1. very abrupt, tense, emphatic, hurried or staccato response
2. moderately abrupt, tense, emphatic, hurried or staccato response
3. moderately relaxed, unhurried, essentially opposite of no. 2
4. very relaxed, unhurried, essentially opposite of no. 1
7. can't evaluate   8. not answered   9. not asked

---

58 ☐   Style (1, 2, 3, 4, 7, 8, 9)

59 ☐   Do you have children?
       1 – yes   5 – indefinite
       2 – qualified yes   8 – not answered
       3 – qualified no   9 – not asked
       4 – no

60 ☐   Style (1, 2, 3, 4, 7, 8, 9)

61 ☐   Do you (did you) find time to play games with them?
       1 – yes   5 – indefinite
       2 – qualified yes   8 – not answered
       3 – qualified no   9 – not asked
       4 – no

62 ☐   Style (1, 2, 3, 4, 7, 8, 9)

63 ☐   I'm curious to know if you always purposely let them win?
       1 – yes   5 – indefinite
       2 – qualified yes   8 – not answered
       3 – qualified no   9 – not asked
       4 – no

64 ☐   Style (1, 2, 3, 4, 7. 8, 9.

65 ☐   Did you ever let them win?
       1 – yes   5 – indefinite
       2 – qualified yes   8 – not answered
       3 – qualified no   9 – not asked
       4 – no

66 ☐   Style (1, 2, 3, 4, 7, 8, 9)

67 ☐   Do you engage in any competitive activities with your
       contemporaries such as cards or sports?
       1 – yes   5 – indefinite
       2 – qualified yes   8 – not answered
       3 – qualified no   9 – not asked
       4 – no

68 ☐   Style (1, 2, 3, 4, 7, 8, 9)

(APPENDIX A continued)

STYLE CODE
1. very abrupt, tense, emphatic, hurried or staccato response
2. moderately abrupt, tense, emphatic, hurried or staccato response
3. moderately relaxed, unhurried, essentially opposite of no. 2
4. very relaxed, unhurried, essentially opposite of no. 1
7. can't evaluate   8. not answered   9. not asked

---

69   ☐   If yes, do you play for all you're worth, fighting all the
                 way, or do you play for the **fun** of it?
                 1 – fighting   6 – both
                 2 – qualified fighting 7 – neither
                 3 – qualified fun   8 – not answered
                 4 – fun   9 – not asked
                 5 – indefinite

70   ☐   Style (1, 2, 3, 4, 7, 8, 9)

71   ☐   Do you have much competition in your work?
                 1 – yes   5 – indefinite
                 2 – qualified yes   8 – not answered
                 3 – qualified no   9 – not asked
                 4 – no

72   ☐   Style (1, 2, 3, 4, 7, 8, 9)

73   ☐   Do you enjoy it?
                 1 – yes   5 – indefinite
                 2 – qualified yes   8 – not answered
                 3 – qualified no   9 – not asked
                 4 – no

74   ☐   Style (1, 2, 3, 4, 7, 8, 9)

75   ☐   Do you have many deadlines in your work?
                 1 – yes   5 – indefinite
                 2 – qualified yes   8 – not answered
                 3 – qualified no   9 – not asked
                 4 – no

76   ☐   Style (1, 2, 3, 4, 7, 8, 9)

77   9   Blank

78   1   Test Number

79, 80 6 8   Card Number

(APPENDIX A continued)

STYLE CODE
1. very abrupt, tense, emphatic, hurried or staccato response
2. moderately abrupt, tense, emphatic, hurried or staccato response
3. moderately relaxed, unhurried, essentially opposite of no. 2
4. very relaxed, unhurried, essentially opposite of no. 1
7. can't evaluate   8. not answered   9. not asked

1, 2, 3   ☐ ☐ ☐   Study number

4, 5   ☐ ☐

6, 7, 8   ☐ ☐ ☐   Identification number of subject

9   ☐   Did you find them exciting and enjoyable?
     1 – yes   5 – indefinite
     2 – qualified yes   8 – not answered
     3 – qualified no   9 – not asked
     4 – no

10   ☐   Style (1, 2, 3, 4, 7, 8, 9)

11   ☐   Most persons prefer to awaken before 9 A.M. What time do you like to –uh–uh–uh– get up?
     1 – subject interrupted before question completed
     2 – word "get" was said before subject replied
     3 – words "get up" were said before subject replied
     8 – not answered
     9 – not asked

12   ☐   Style (1, 2, 3, 4, 7, 8, 9)

13   ☐   Do you retire early or do you **prefer** to stay up and work late to get more things done each day?
     1 – stays up and works late
     2 – stays up late, doesn't work
     3 – retires early
     5 – indefinite
     8 – not answered
     9 – not asked

14   ☐   Style (1, 2, 3, 4, 7, 8, 9)

15, 16
17, 18   ☐ ☐ ☐ ☐   What time do you usually retire? (actual time 24-hour clock)
     55 – indefinite
     88 – not answered
     99 – not asked

(APPENDIX A continued)

STYLE CODE
1. very abrupt, tense, emphatic, hurried or staccato response
2. moderately abrupt, tense, emphatic, hurried or staccato response
3. moderately relaxed, unhurried, essentially opposite of no. 2
4. very relaxed, unhurried, essentially opposite of no. 1
7. can't evaluate   8. not answered   9. not asked

---

19 ☐   Some people write with pen, some with pencil. Which do you prefer —uh—uh—uh— to use?
       1 – subject interrupted before question completed
       2 – word "to" was said before subject replied
       3 – words "to use" were said before subject replied
       8 – not answered
       9 – not asked

20 ☐   Style (1, 2, 3, 4, 7, 8, 9)

21 ☐   If you tell your wife or friend that you'll meet them somewhere at a definite time, will you be there?
       1 – yes   5 – indefinite
       2 – qualified yes   8 – not answered
       3 – qualified no   9 – not asked
       4 – no

22 ☐   Style (1, 2, 3, 4, 7, 8, 9)

23 ☐   Do you work up to the last moment before leaving to keep an appointment?
       1 – yes   5 – indefinite
       2 – qualified yes   8 – not answered
       3 – qualified no   9 – not asked
       4 – no

24 ☐   Style (1, 2, 3, 4, 7, 8, 9)

25 ☐   Does it bother you to be kept waiting?
       1 – yes   5 – indefinite
       2 – qualified yes   8 – not answered
       3 – qualified no   9 – not asked
       4 – no

26 ☐   Style (1, 2, 3, 4, 7, 8, 9)

27 ☐   Do you make any remarks about it?
       1 – yes   5 – indefinite
       2 – qualified yes   8 – not answered
       3 – qualified no   9 – not asked
       4 – no

(APPENDIX A continued)

STYLE CODE
1. very abrupt, tense, emphatic, hurried or staccato response
2. moderately abrupt, tense, emphatic, hurried or staccato response
3. moderately relaxed, unhurried, essentially opposite of no. 2
4. very relaxed, unhurried, essentially opposite of no. 1
7. can't evaluate   8. not answered   9. not asked

---

28 ☐   Style (1, 2, 3, 4, 7, 8, 9)

29 ☐   Are you apt to get impatient when you see something
                being done more slowly than you think it should be done?
                    1 — yes   5 — indefinite
                    2 — qualified yes   8 — not answered
                    3 — qualified no   9 — not asked
                    4 — no

30 ☐   Style (1, 2, 3, 4, 7, 8, 9)

* 31 ☐   When you have this feeling, are you apt to take the job
                away from people simply because you think you could
                do it better or faster?
                    1 — yes   5 — indefinite
                    2 — qualified yes   8 — not answered
                    3 — qualified no   9 — not asked
                    4 — no

32 ☐   Style (1, 2, 3, 4, 7, 8, 9)

* 33 ☐   Do you often try to get something else done, like calcu-
                lating or reading trade material, while going to the
                bathroom or while shaving?
                    1 — yes   5 — indefinite
                    2 — qualified yes   8 — not answered
                    3 — qualified no   9 — not asked
                    4 — no

34 ☐   Style (1, 2, 3, 4, 7, 8, 9)

* 35 ☐   Are you a fast walker?
                    1 — yes   5 — indefinite
                    2 — qualified yes   8 — not answered
                    3 — qualified no   9 — not asked
                    4 — no

36 ☐   Style (1, 2, 3, 4, 7, 8, 9)

(APPENDIX A continued)

STYLE CODE
1. very abrupt, tense, emphatic, hurried or staccato response
2. moderately abrupt, tense, emphatic, hurried or staccato response
3. moderately relaxed, unhurried, essentially opposite of no. 2
4. very relaxed, unhurried, essentially opposite of no. 1
7. can't evaluate   8. not answered   9. not asked

---

* 37   ☐   Do you like to dawdle around the dining room table
                   after dinner or do you prefer to eat fast and then get on
                   to more important things?
                   1 – eat fast
                   2 – qualified "eat fast"
                   3 – qualified "dawdle"
                   4 – dawdle
                   5 – indefinite
                   6 – both
                   8 – not answered
                   9 – not asked

   38   ☐   Style (1, 2, 3, 4, 7, 8, 9)

* 39   ☐   Does it irritate you to go to a restaurant and have to
                   wait in line for a table?
                   1 – yes   5 – indefinite
                   2 – qualified yes   8 – not answered
                   3 – qualified no   9 – not asked
                   4 – no

   40   ☐   Style (1, 2, 3, 4, 7, 8, 9)

* 41   ☐   Have you ever left a restaurant because you saw a lot of
                   people waiting?
                   1 – yes   5 – indefinite
                   2 – qualified yes   8 – not answered
                   3 – qualified no   9 – not asked
                   4 – no

   42   ☐   Style (1, 2, 3, 4, 7, 8, 9)

* 43   ☐   Is this habitual?
                   1 – yes   5 – indefinite
                   2 – qualified yes   8 – not answered
                   3 – qualified no   9 – not asked
                   4 – no

   44   ☐   Style (1, 2, 3, 4, 7, 8, 9)

(APPENDIX A continued)

STYLE CODE
1. very abrupt, tense, emphatic, hurried or staccato response
2. moderately abrupt, tense, emphatic, hurried or staccato response
3. moderately relaxed, unhurried, essentially opposite of no. 2
4. very relaxed, unhurried, essentially opposite of no. 1
7. can't evaluate   8. not answered   9. not asked

---

*   45   ☐   Do you often find yourself listening to someone talking but all the while thinking of something other than what he is talking about?
     1 – yes   5 – indefinite
     2 – qualified yes   8 – not answered
     3 – qualified no   9 – not asked
     4 – no

    46   ☐   Style (1, 2, 3, 4, 7, 8, 9)

*   47   ☐   If this person takes too long to come to the point, do you feel like hurrying him along to make him get to the point more quickly?
     1 – yes   5 – indefinite
     2 – qualified yes   8 – not answered
     3 – qualified no   9 – not asked
     4 – no

    48   ☐   Style (1, 2, 3, 4, 7, 8, 9)

*   49   ☐   Do you actually put words in his mouth?
     1 – yes   5 – indefinite
     2 – qualified yes   8 – not answered
     3 – qualified no   9 – not asked
     4 – no

    50   ☐   Style (1, 2, 3, 4, 7, 8, 9

*   51   ☐   Do you often have the feeling that time is passing too quickly each day to get everything done that you want to do?
     1 – yes   5 – indefinite
     2 – qualified yes   8 – not answered
     3 – qualified no   9 – not asked
     4 – no

    52   ☐   Style (1, 2, 3, 4, 7, 8, 9)

*   53   ☐   Do you get this feeling on the job or at home?
     1 – both   5 – indefinite
     2 – on the job   8 – not answered
     3 – at home   9 – not asked

(APPENDIX A continued)

STYLE CODE
1. very abrupt, tense, emphatic, hurried or staccato response
2. moderately abrupt, tense, emphatic, hurried or staccato response
3. moderately relaxed, unhurried, essentially opposite of no. 2
4. very relaxed, unhurried, essentially opposite of no. 1
7. can't evaluate   8. not answered   9. not asked

---

54   ☐   Style (1, 2, 3, 4, 7, 8, 9)

* 55   ☐   Does this sense of time urgency make you feel that you
                 have to do everything in a hurry?
                 1 — yes   5 — indefinite
                 2 — qualified yes   8 — not answered
                 3 — qualified no   9 — not asked
                 4 — no

56   ☐   Style (1, 2, 3, 4, 7, 8, 9)

* 57   ☐   Are you a fast car driver?
                 1 — yes   5 — indefinite
                 2 — qualified yes   8 — not answered
                 3 — qualified no   9 — not asked
                 4 — no

58   ☐   Style (1, 2, 3, 4, 7, 8, 9)

* 59   ☐   Does it usually irritate you to be held up by a car in
                 front of you?
                 1 — yes   5 — indefinite
                 2 — qualified yes   8 — not answered
                 3 — qualified no   9 — not asked
                 4 — no

60   ☐   Style (1, 2, 3, 4, 7, 8, 9)

* 61   ☐   Do you blow your horn to get him to **move** out of
                 your way?
                 1 — yes   5 — indefinite
                 2 — qualified yes   8 — not answered
                 3 — qualified no   9 — not asked
                 4 — no

62   ☐   Style (1, 2, 3, 4, 7, 8, 9)

(APPENDIX A continued)

STYLE CODE
1. very abrupt, tense, emphatic, hurried or staccato response
2. moderately abrupt, tense, emphatic, hurried or staccato response
3. moderately relaxed, unhurried, essentially opposite of no. 2
4. very relaxed, unhurried, essentially opposite of no. 1
7. can't evaluate   8. not answered   9. not asked

---

* 63 ☐   Do you feel you get upset and angry very often?
     1 — yes   5 — indefinite
     2 — qualified yes   8 — not answered
     3 — qualified no   9 — not asked
     4 — no

64 ☐   Style (1, 2, 3, 4, 7, 8, 9)

65 ☐   Do you keep it in or let it out?
     1 — keep it in
     2 — qualified "keep it in"
     3 — qualified "let it out"
     4 — let it out
     5 — indefinite
     6 — varies
     8 — not answered
     9 — not asked

66 ☐   Style (1, 2, 3, 4, 7, 8, 9)

67 ☐   Have you ever noticed that you grind your teeth when you're feeling tense?
     1 — yes   5 — indefinite
     2 — qualified yes   8 — not answered
     3 — qualified no   9 — not asked
     4 — no

68 ☐   Style (1, 2, 3, 4, 7, 8, 9)

69 ☐   Has your wife or dentist ever remarked about your teeth grinding?
     1 — yes   5 — indefinite
     2 — qualified yes   8 — not answered
     3 — qualified no   9 — not asked
     4 — no

70 ☐   Style (1, 2, 3, 4, 7, 8, 9)

(APPENDIX A continued)

STYLE CODE
1. very abrupt, tense, emphatic, hurried or staccato response
2. moderately abrupt, tense, emphatic, hurried or staccato response
3. moderately relaxed, unhurried, essentially opposite of no. 2
4. very relaxed, unhurried, essentially opposite of no. 1
7. can't evaluate   8. not answered   9. not asked

---

* 71   ☐   Do you feel rested when you awaken in the morning?
                     1 – yes   5 – indefinite
                     2 – qualified yes   8 – not answered
                     3 – qualified no   9 – not asked
                     4 – no

72   ☐   Average Content – Observer Impression (1, 2, 3, 4)

73   ☐   Average Style – Observer Impression (1, 2, 3, 4)

74   ☐   Total Content and Style – Observer Impression (1, 2, 3, 4)

75, 76, 77   ☐ ☐ ☐   Meter Reading

78   ☐1   Test Number

79, 80   ☐6 ☐9   Card Number

16

PSYCHOLOGICAL ADAPTATION TO
CONVALESCENCE IN MYOCARDIAL INFARCTION PATIENTS

Thomas P. Hackett, M.D., and *Ned H. Cassem,* M.D.

The emotional response of patients to myocardial infarction (MI) is shaped largely by two sources of psychological stress. The first, which occurs during the acute phase of MI, is the immediate threat to life. The second, generally experienced by the third hospital day, is the threat that coronary heart disease (CHD) will irreparably alter the patient's life-style and livelihood. Most patients, expectedly, respond to the threat of death by developing anxiety, just as they react to anticipated restrictions and limitations by becoming depressed. These unpleasant affects are, in turn, modified by a variety of coping mechanisms, each fashioned by the individual's personality. The authors feel that the defense of denial in one form or another is the principal such mechanism used, and central to nearly all the coping tactics dealing with the anxiety and depression experienced by patients with CHD.

Denial

Denial is defined as "the conscious or unconscious repudiation of all or part of the total available meaning of an event to allay anxiety or other unpleasant affects" [1]. A common example taken from the prehospital phase of MI is that of the patient who develops sudden, crushing precordial pain, similar to the distress he felt during a previous MI, but who holds to the conviction that it is indigestion. By doing this, he denies the most threatening aspects of chest pain, that it signals the presence of heart trouble, by identifying a less ominous condition as the cause. Since this rationalization in the service of denial results in delay in seeking help, it is maladaptive. On the other hand, there is a type of denial that might (and probably does) work in the patient's best interest.

A 56-year-old architect with a recent anterior MI impressed the examiner as being unusually complacent and unperturbed in the face of his illness. He explained his peace of mind by stating that he was "indestructible." A Texan by birth and inclination, he identified with former President Lyndon B. Johnson, who had also sustained an MI and survived. Furthermore, both his father and a paternal uncle had done well following heart attacks, and the patient firmly believed he shared their immunity to harm. There was no evidence to doubt that his confidence and composure were anything but genuine. Without denying the heart attack itself, this man denied all of its threatening aspects and accentuated the potential for survival in his family background.

Fig. 1 depicts a distribution of consultation requests from a Coronary Care Unit (CCU) to the psychiatrist according to the CCU day on which the request was made [2]. There are three categories of problems, only two of which concern us. It is evident that anxiety begins early and peaks by the second day, whereas depression comes to the fore by the third day. If hypothetical curves are superimposed on this histogram (in Fig. 2) and denial is added, it can be seen that the latter acts to stem anxiety, yet bears little or no obvious relationship to depression. Fortunately, anxiety is the easiest symptom with which to contend in treating CHD patients. Denial alone can often reduce anxiety. Realistic reassurance offered by physicians and nurses is of great help in calming patients. The very atmosphere of the CCU with its monitoring devices, alarm systems, and the constant attention to vital signs fosters a sense of protection that powerfully assuages apprehension. Finally, a variety of safe and effective tranquilizers can be employed.

Depression

Depression, unfortunately, is not as readily managed as anxiety. It is not easily denied and there are no drugs available at present to use safely as antidepressants. In our opinion, *depression remains the most formidable problem in cardiac convalescence and rehabilitation*. The psychological adaptation referred to in the title applies, by and large, to the ways in which CHD patients cope with depression.

The depression in the wake of MI is reactive and exogenous in type. Like grief following the loss of a loved one, it occurs in response to an incident that all would agree is appropriate for its development. In other words, it is not abnormal or neurotic to get depressed after MI. This classification separates it from endogenous depressive reactions which are apt to be cyclical and unpredictable in origin, and require different management. The principal danger in either type is suicide. Although no studies cite the incidence of suicide in post-MI depressions, our opinion is that deliberate self-destructive acts are unusual in this population. Rather, the course of the depression, if plotted on a graph, would resemble a plateau with few ups and downs but with a gradual slope returning to baseline in a year or two.

Although the depression generally begins on the third CCU day, it may not be obvious to the casual examiner at that time. In a study of 100 CHD patients recently completed [3], the incidence of depression in the CCU was examined. We divided depression into four categories: severe, moderate, mild, and none.

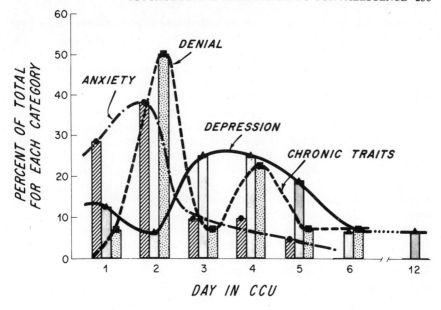

Fig. 1. Distribution of requests for psychiatric consultations in a Coronary Care Unit.

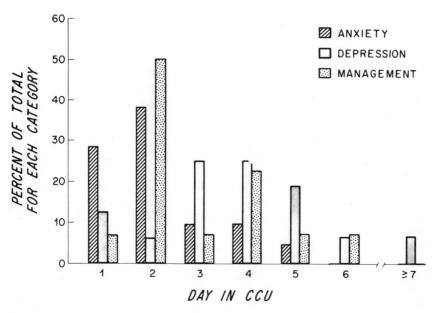

Fig. 2. Hypothetical curves of emotional responses of patients in a Coronary Care Unit. (Discussed in text)

The rating was severe when the patient complained of great discouragement and viewed his future without hope. His manner was agitated, retarded, or withdrawn. Vegetative signs and tears were often present. Moderate depression was rated when the patient either openly acknowledged despondency or admitted to it when asked. Hope, however, had not been abandoned. His appearance was depressed and his manner was withdrawn, retarded, or agitated, but to a lesser degree than in the severely depressed patient. Mild depression was rated when the patient intermittently, but not consistently, acknowledged despondency, or while denying it, appeared sad when discussing his illness and exhibited signs of retardation in behavior and speech. A judgement of none was made when the patient denied being depressed and gave no evidence to the contrary.

Of 100 patients, six were rated severely depressed, 36 moderately depressed, 33 mildly depressed, and 25 not depressed. Whereas 75 of these patients were depressed, it was obvious in only 42. Furthermore, of the 25 patients listed as not depressed, in our opinion if a measure sensitive enough were available, the majority of these would demonstrate depression. We believe that depression is almost universal following MI and the patient should be considered depressed even though it may not be clinically obvious. We therefore believe that all post-MI patients should be treated for depression. Treatment consists of inaugurating a program of physical conditioning appropriate to the patient's physical status by the time he has reached the third CCU day.

Basis for Depression

Our theory, supported by considerable fact, is that the basis for this depression is the threat of invalidism and the loss of autonomy and independence. Much of this centers about being unable to get around and perform what were normal activities before the MI. The sooner a patient's sense of self-esteem is restored, the more rapidly the depression will resolve. There is no better approach to this task than to make the patient active again.

It usually happens, in the absence of a conditioning program, that by the third CCU day the patient's physical condition has stabilized and he generally feels quite fit. Typically, such a patient begins to wonder whether his heart is damaged as seriously as the doctors claim. When the customary regimen of bed rest is enforced and no activity is allowed, this spurt of good feeling is ignored and the stage is set for the development of what we call *the homecoming depression.*

In order to explain this term, we must acquaint you with an investigation we conducted 3 years ago [4]. In followups on 50 patients we had interviewed and seen regularly during hospitalization for MI, we visited 24 patients in their homes. All visits were made from 6 to 12 months after the patient had been discharged. The most common complaint expressed by the group was weakness. Twenty patients found it distressing and two considered it a harbinger of cardiac decline. The feeling itself was described as one of exhaustion or physical weakness with minimal effort.

A typical example is that of a 39-year-old teacher who did very well following his MI until he returned home. In his words, "I felt great in the hospital. No matter what anyone told me, I pictured myself breaking records getting back to work. The first week home I could hardly walk the length of the house without feeling exhausted. I felt like a cooked goose, like I was done for. It took me another two weeks until I started to feel better." This is a prototypical statement, one that would apply to the majority of MI patients in early convalescence at home. This sense of weakness is often the trigger that springs an underlying depression into the open.

The symptom of weakness must stem from a variety of sources. Deranged cardiovascular physiology, as a result of the MI, must play a part, as must the inactivity and resulting inanition typical of CHD convalescence. Since weakness is a cardinal symptom of depression, it is likely that the latter adds to this sense of exhaustion.

Initially we wondered why the complaint of weakness was not voiced until the patient had returned home. The main reason that homecoming is necessary to elicit the symptom has to do with the minimal amount of physical activity that is possible in the hospital setting. For the most part, patients are discouraged from wandering out of range of the nurses' desk, and little provision is made for exercise at the bedside. As a consequence, the hospitalized convalescent rarely has the opportunity to test his capacity for activity unless he is willing to break a regulation or has the good fortune of being treated by an enlightened physician. It is only after his return home that he can move about enough to experience fatigue and weakness.

Vagueness of Symptom

The majority of the patients we have interviewed would not have been apt to complain spontaneously of this weakness to their physician. The symptom is too vague and nonspecific, about which they would not want to bother their doctor. By the time they are seen for the first followup visit 3 months later, the weakness has gone and the doctor is none the wiser. Their reticence to complain should not, however, be taken as evidence that weakness was regarded lightly. It was the most distressing symptom of early convalescence for these 20 patients. The reason for its importance is not difficult to establish. The feeling of weakness and easy fatigue accentuated the patient's underlying fear that he might soon become a cardiac cripple.

The threat of a substantial reduction in the amount of physical activity in which one can engage may pose no special concern to the laggard, the dawdler, or the leisure-seeker. However, we know of no study that depicts indolence, listlessness, and laxity as being characteristic of the CHD patient. On the contrary, the majority of research, especially the work of Friedman and Rosenman [5], points out that the very opposite traits are more common in coronary-prone people. They are *work addicts* with a keen awareness of time and deadlines who are seldom able to relax, even on vacation. As a consequence, a restriction in activity, either physical or mental, imposes an enormous tax on their emotional economy. The burden of enforced passivity accentuated by the feeling of weakness results in the appearance of an overt depression, the *homecoming depression*, in contrast to the more covert depression of the CCU.

Let us consider this depressive response. Depression is characterized by the look of sadness and the sense of loss, possibly accompanied by the feeling of hopelessness. There are vegetative disturbances, loss of appetite, and sleep derangements. There is undoubtedly a specific biochemistry of depression, but its composition has not as yet been elucidated. The importance of depression is that it often sets the stage for a recurrence of illness. The depressed patient population, in general, probably has a higher morbidity and greater mortality. Many current studies point in that direction [7, 8, 9, 10]. It is wrong, in our opinion, to think of depression solely as a state of protective withdrawal from a noxious situation, a notion popularly espoused by many psychiatrists. That it represents a withdrawal no one would contest; but to regard it as protective rides in the face of considerable evidence. Furthermore, the state of depression is seldom unalloyed. Anxiety, frustration, anger, and resentment accompany it in varying degrees and these unpleasant affects possess little utility in any man's language. Twenty-one out of 24 patients in our study rated themselves as being anxious as well as depressed.

At this point, a tally of the various stresses the convalescent MI operates under are:

1. The threat of sudden death. Although, as mentioned earlier, this is more extreme (and realistic) in the first few days in the CCU, it can and frequently does persist for years after the attack.

2. Depression due to inactivity and job uncertainty.

3. Depression due to deprivations: give up cigarettes, reduce eating, avoid excitement.

Deprivation

A word about deprivations. In our home-visit study of 24 people, nine out of 14 who resolved to stop smoking failed. Seven out of nine who determined to lose weight failed to do so, and five out of six who vowed to stop drinking failed. These individuals were blue-collar patients. In subsequent work we found that individuals from a higher socioeconomic class and with more education are more successful in controlling harmful habits; however, these restrictions and deprivations are very taxing and physicians have provided next to nothing in the way of help. A psychiatrist, particularly one who does a good deal of hypnosis, would never attempt to stop an individual from smoking, over-eating, and drinking simultaneously because the venture would be doomed to fail. It is asking too much. And yet that is what the post-MI patient is expected to do. We have no suggestions to offer. We can only point out the magnitude of the task. The small management aid we can offer is to point out that occasionally the irritation which inevitably occurs in the wake of dieting and stopping smoking is sometimes helped by the use of tranquilizers such as the benzodiazepines.

Some practical suggestions can be given for help in management in medication, physical conditioning, education, anticipation, and telephone followup.

Medication

The majority of patients discharged for home CHD convalescence are given neither a tranquilizer to help with daily stress nor a hypnotic for bedtime use. Since sleep disturbances are very common in the first 3 months at home and sound sleep is important, we feel that a hypnotic should be given and the patient should be encouraged to use it if needed. The same is true with tranquilizers. The benzodiazepines are non-addicting if used judiciously and do a good job in relieving emotional stress and irritability. Patients should be encouraged to use them, and their tendency to equate regular use with being unmanly should be undercut. These drugs should be accorded the same importance in the therapeutic armamentarium as diuretics, digitalis, and other more strictly medical drugs. Caution should be exercised in the use of phenothiazines (Thorazine, Stelazine, Mellaril, etc.) to control anxiety. These are antipsychotic preparations and are not designed to relieve anxiety. Furthermore, they possess hypotensive properties and increase cardiac irritability.

Within the past 10 years, psychopharmacologists have developed a powerful, potent array of antidepressants, namely the tricyclic group of drugs such as amitriptyline (Elavil), imipramine (Tofranil), and doxepin (Sinequan). Unfortunately, good data support the fact that use is associated with arrhythmias and sudden deaths. Consequently, they are not a safe group of drugs to use in the convalescent MI patient who is depressed. It has been said that doxepin (Sinequan) is devoid of these cardiac effects, but there has, as yet, been no large, double-blind, controlled study to demonstrate its freedom from untoward cardiac side effects. As a consequence, the physician must employ other means to cope with depression in these patients. It has been said that certain preparations like diazepam (Valium) and chlordiazepoxide (Librium) have antidepressant qualities as well as being effective tranquilizers. This undoubtedly is true in some cases but it would be foolhardy to depend upon them to do the full job.

Physical Conditioning

We have already mentioned physical conditioning as a way of preventing the covert depression of the CCU and of reducing or eliminating the more serious *homecoming depression*. Physical conditioning is perhaps the most important aspect of convalescence in terms of its ability to control depression by raising self-esteem and the sense of independence. The program of physical conditioning must be carried through into convalescence until it becomes a way of life with the patient.

Many patients, if not the majority, complain of having no structure to their days of convalescence. The doctor tells them to increase their activity slowly but does not specify where or how. Conditioning programs provide this guidance. Some patients, especially those with compulsive traits, must have a schedule of hourly activities set out for them, by a skilled nurse or physical therapist. It is surprising how much direction the post-MI patient needs, especially those in the blue collar category.

Physical conditioning has one strong advantage in structuring a post-MI course. It is something to do. In a long list of don'ts—don't smoke, don't eat ice cream, don't rush—physical conditioning stands out as an affirmation of life.

Dr. Fox has justified exercise on the grounds of prudent reasoning [11]: (1) as a stimulus to more prudent activity in general; (2) to increase one's sense of well-being; and (3) to increase the quality of living and encourage men to improve their diet and sleep. Dr. Friedman [12] has suggested that activity helps maintain defenses against dependency. These are true and excellent reasons for including exercise in a program for post-MI care. Another reason, however, is that activity (exercise) is the primary bulwark against depression. When deprived of it, self-esteem falters and living becomes hollow for the majority of men. Living, after all, is activity, and depression, as someone said, is death's waiting room.

Education

Each patient, upon discharge, should be informed about the nature of the infarction and the process of repair. Misconceptions must be sought and corrected. The most commonly harbored myths are:

1. Even mild exertion kills.
2. Sexual intercourse should never again be attempted.
3. Repeat infarctions tend to occur at orgasm.
4. Recurrences are apt to take place on the anniversary of the first infarction.
5. The patient is apt to die at the same age a parent did when that parent succumbed to heart disease.
6. Repeat infarctions are apt to take place in sleep.

Finally, in any educational campaign, the patient's close relatives, especially the spouse and children, should be included.

Anticipation

Telling a patient what to expect almost always reduces the anxiety of an event. If the patient is told to expect to feel weak when he returns home from the hospital and that it is a normal response, anguish can be spared. Similarly, anxiety at attempting new types of activity or extending the range of activity can be anticipated. The tendency of the family to be overprotective, and the patient to become irritable and rebellious, can also be predicted. All of these maneuvers have proved helpful to us.

Telephone Followup

For the first 2 months following discharge, having a nurse telephone the patient and his family to ask if anything occurred about which advice is needed was found to be greatly appreciated by our patient population [13]. Numerous issues arise over which the patient would not ordinarily feel justified in bothering his doctor. Nonetheless, he is faced with a problem which needs an answer. This is especially true in conditioning programs where activity is stressed and the patient is often unsure about how far he should go. Fears concerning sexual activity comprise a considerable portion of telephone queries.

SUMMARY

Although exercise may be irrelevant in terms of altering morbidity and mortality (although we do not think so), it is still the most potent antidote and prophylaxis against depression that we know. There is little doubt that depression heightens mortality.

Exercise, therefore, is right on!

REFERENCES

1. Weisman, A.D., and Hackett, T.P. Predilection to death: Death and dying as a psychiatric problem. *Psychosom. Med.* 23:232-257, 1961.
2. Cassem, N.H., and Hackett, T.P. Psychiatric consultation in a coronary care unit. *Ann. Intern. Med.* 75:9-14, 1971.
3. Hackett, T.P., and Cassem, N.H. White- versus blue-collar responses to having a heart attack. *Annual Meeting of American Psychosomatic Association*, April 16, 1972. (Abstract to be published in *Psychosom. Med.*).
4. Wishnie, H.A., Hackett, T.P., and Cassem, N.H. Psychological hazards of convalescence following myocardial infarction. *J.A.M.A.* 215: 1292-1296, 1971.
5. Rosenman, R.M., Friedman, M., Straus, R., et al. A predictive study of coronary heart disease. WCGS. *J.A.M.A.* 189:15-22, 1964.
6. Kits van Heijningen, H., and Treurniet, N. Psychodynamic factors in acute myocardial infarction. *Int. J. Psychoanal.* 47:370-374, 1966.
7. Bruhn, J.G., Wolf, S., and Philips, B.V. Depression and death in myocardial infarction: A psychosocial study of screening male coronary patients over nine years. *J. Psychosom. Res.* 15:305-313, 1971.
8. Greene, W.A. Psychological factors and reticuloendothelial disease. *Psychosom. Med.* 16:220, 1954.
9. Schmale, A.H., and Engel, G.L. The giving up-given up complex. *Arch. Gen. Psychiat.* 17:135, 1967.

10. Schmale, A.H. Relationship of separation and depression to disease. *Psychosom. Med.* 20:259, 1958.

11. Fox, S.M., III. Relationship of activity habits to coronary heart disease. *In,* Naughton, J., and Hellerstein, H.K., Eds. *Exercise Testing and Exercise Training in Heart Disease.* New York Academic, 1973.

12. Friedman, E.H., and Hellerstein, H.K. Influence of psychosocial factors on coronary risk and adaptation to a physical fitness program. *In,* Naughton, J., and Hellerstein, H.K., Eds. *Exercise Testing and Exercise Training in Coronary Heart Disease.* New York, Academic, 1973.

13. Bilodeau, C.J., and Hackett, T.P. Issues raised in a group setting by patients recovering from initial myocardial infarction. *Am. J. Psychiat.* 128:7378, 1971.

17

OBTAINING AND INTERPRETING PSYCHOSOCIAL DATA IN STUDIES OF CORONARY HEART DISEASE

John G. Bruhn, Ph.D.

Methodological difficulties in studying psychological and sociological factors in coronary heart disease (CHD) are well documented [1, 2, 3, 4]. These difficulties are due largely to the complex interrelationships between psychosocial factors and changes in the nature and degree of their interaction over time. In CHD these interactions are further modified by the disease process. The development of precise, objective, and replicable methods for studying psychosocial factors is, therefore, difficult. The nature of the variables involved and their changes do not lend themselves to the research approach used in a controlled laboratory setting. Indeed, to study behavioral factors in CHD in controlled settings would eliminate many environmental and situational factors that are important in understanding the disease process.

Despite the limitations of psychosocial methodology, similar findings from studies of CHD have been reported by several social scientists, using a variety of research techniques [5]. Certain basic methodological considerations, however, should be reexamined on the basis of experience in past studies. Too often we have repeated techniques because they are well-known or widely accepted, and have not adequately refined existing methods and developed new ones.

Uses of Psychosocial Data

Psychosocial data are collected too frequently without having a clear purpose for their later use, or data collected for one purpose are inappropriately used later for another purpose. Psychosocial data can be collected for many purposes, including description, assessment, prediction, or evaluation. Expectations of the data should be geared to the purpose for which they are gathered. For example, it should not be expected that purely descriptive data will yield precise indices of prediction. Too often we look to statistical techniques to provide rigor and sophistication to psychosocial data after the fact, when the fault rests with a choice of techniques which are inappropriate for the purpose for which the data are to be used. Certainly, combinations of techniques and approaches are desirable to provide a more complete picture of the patient, as well as to check the reliability of information obtained using several different techniques. An examination of the methodological difficulties and pitfalls in the uses of psychosocial data will help to clarify these points.

Description

The case study approach, as an example of the descriptive use of psychosocial data, is a qualitative method which does not lend itself to rigorous statistical analysis or to generalizations. However, it is useful in exploring directions for future research, establishing hypotheses, and in assembling a patient profile. The case study approach permits probing many facets of a patient's life, and gathering data about a patient's overt behavior and his responses to life events; it allows flexibility in adjusting the interview approach to the situation of each patient. The case study approach also allows the patient to be viewed in the context of a set of social relationships through time.

Numerous case studies have been performed with CHD patients, particularly in describing emotional stress preceding myocardial infarction (MI), the production of arrhythmia by emotion, and the role of emotion in patients' adjustments to their infarctions. Some case studies have been used to illustrate relationships between psychosocial and clinical phenomena, others have attempted to uncover common traits among a series of CHD patients, and still others have compared a series of CHD patients and controls with the aim of elucidating differences between them. These data usually have been obtained through psychiatric or medical interviews, which are impossible to replicate; such data have been broad in scope, often interpreted on the basis of impressions, and could not be submitted to statistical analysis. These factors underlie criticisms of the use of the case study approach in investigating the role of psychosocial factors in CHD. The danger in the case study method, however, does not lie so much with the method or technique as with the false sense of certainty the researcher feels about his conclusions.

Assessment

Psychosocial data can be used to assess the clinical progress of a patient. Psychosocial factors and clinical changes are interrelated. Changes in one sphere may produce changes in the other. Depression provides an example of these interrelationships. The high incidence of moderate and severe depression within the first 3 years following MI is particularly interesting in view of the fact that mortality is also highest during this time. Both depression and mortality decrease with increasing time following first infarction [6, 7].

Patients hospitalized more than once every 15 months experience significantly more episodes of moderate and severe depression than patients hospitalized less frequently. Depression accompanies frequent hospitalization irrespective of the severity of the disease [7]. Hospitalization, immobilization, and the life-threatening implications of an MI may alter the concept of self and result in depression. As soon as a patient perceives himself disabled, he is likely to continue functioning at a low level. Depressive feelings, in turn, may inhibit his activity and any psychological or physical distress provides further proof to him of his disability.

Miller reported that, while CHD patients as a group were more emotionally disturbed than controls, those patients over age 55 were less disturbed and more optimistic than patients under age 55 [8]. In a prospective study of these same patients, we found that those patients under age 50 maintained a higher level of anxiety than patients over age 50 for as long as 5 years following infarction [9]. With regard to depression, we found that patients who died from first or recurrent MIs were more depressed prior to death than those who survived [10, 11]. Of interest, however, was the finding that surviving patients with angina pectoris (AP) had personality profiles more similar to those of the deceased patients, indicating that surviving patients with angina were more psychologically disturbed than surviving patients without angina. As a group, surviving patients also showed greater variability in mood, serum cholesterol, uric acid, triglyceride, and fibrinogen levels during their bimonthly clinic visits over a period of 53 months than the controls. This points to the necessity for assessing mood and physiological change concomitantly among CHD patients over an extended period.

A study was also made with the same subjects on how physicians and patients evaluate depression and anxiety, and the degree of agreement in their evaluations. Physicians were asked to evaluate depression and anxiety in patients they had seen regularly over a 5-year period, and to base their evaluations on observations of patients. overt behavior and responses to questions. They rated each patient along a 3-point scale, separately for depression and anxiety. The patients, on the other hand, responded *true* or *false* to a list of symptoms and behavior indicative of depression and anxiety. The lists were scored for depression and anxiety. Both physicians and patients performed this procedure at each clinic visit over a period of 18 months.

TABLE I shows that the ratings of the majority of controls and their physicians agreed that depression was absent or minimal. Physicians, however, rated the patients as more depressed (moderate or high) than the patients rated themselves. With respect to anxiety, TABLE II shows that physicians rated both patients and controls as more anxious (moderate or high) than the patients and controls rated themselves. The more comprehensive assessment by the physicians, based on knowing the individual and his observations of the individual's behavior, appears more helpful in providing insights into understanding mood than relying solely on the patient's objective reporting of mood, which undoubtedly is influenced by denial or the concealment of symptomatology.

Prediction

Increasing interest has been shown in the use of psychosocial data in predicting first or recurrent MI. One of the more useful and highly replicable techniques

TABLE I

Agreement between the self-ratings of coronary patients and
controls on depression and physicians' ratings of their depression

Subjects' Self-Ratings of Depression[1]

Physicians' Ratings of Depression[2]	None or Minimal		Moderate		High	
	Patients N=	Controls N=	Patients N=	Controls N=	Patients N=	Controls N=
None or Minimal	6	17	1	1	–	1
Moderate	7	8	1	3	2	1
High	1	–	7	–	5	–
TOTALS	14	25	9	4	7	2

[1] Subjects were asked to complete the Welsh Depression subscale of the MMPI at each clinic visit over a period of 18 months. Categories represent a mean of these ratings.
[2] Each patient's physician was asked to rate the depressive state of his patient at each clinic visit using a scale: 0 = none or minimal, 1 = moderate, 2 = high.

TABLE II

Agreement between the self-ratings of coronary patients and
controls on anxiety and physicians' ratings of their anxiety

Subjects' Self-Ratings of Anxiety[1]

Physicians' Ratings of Anxiety	None or Minimal		Moderate		High	
	Patients N=	Controls N=	Patients N=	Controls N=	Patients N=	Controls N=
None or Minimal	4	7	–	1	1	–
Moderate	2	10	5	4	2	1
High	6	2	3	2	7	3
TOTALS	12	19	8	7	10	4

[1] Subjects were asked to complete the Bendig Anxiety subscale of the MMPI at each clinic visit over a period of 18 months. Categories represent a mean of these ratings.

is the A-B behavioral pattern typology developed by the Western Collaborative Group [12, 13]. This approach elicits clusters of factors based on the assessment of overt behavior and verbal analysis. The technique is reasonably short and easy to use with appropriate training. The elements of high achievement drive with time urgency and behavioral restlessness, which are difficult to elicit in traditional psychological tests, or which may be overlooked in favor of verbal content in interviews, emerge as highly predictive. While the behavioral factors included in the A-B typology have been described in case studies by many investigators, none had previously worked toward developing a simplified, replicable scheme for testing them.

Another related technique (not yet widely used in studies of CHD) is the Holmes Social Readjustment Rating Scale (SRRS) [14], which is reported to predict the onset of all types of illness. The scale is composed of 43 life events derived from clinical experience. Subjects are asked to indicate the number of times each event occurred in their lives during the previous 3 years. They determine the weighting of each life event according to the amount of adjustment it would require. The number of reported events are multiplied by their respective weights to form a total Life Change Unit (LCU) score, which indicates whether the subject is in a low, moderate, or high-risk group with respect to life change. The scale reliably predicts that individuals with high LCU scores become sick more often than individuals with low LCU scores. In applying the SRRS retrospectively to CHD patients, Theorell and Rahe reported that patients with no previous history of CHD showed a significant increase in their LCU scores during the 2 years prior to infarction. The severity of the infarction did not affect patients' reporting of life change [15]. The combined use of the A-B typology and the SRRS could help in assessing behavioral and life situational changes in prospective studies of CHD.

Psychosocial data have been used in predicting patients' adjustments to MI and their likelihood of survival. Evidence suggests that patients who exhibit behavioral disturbance and poor adaptation during the acute phase of hospitalization have a higher mortality rate than those who adapt successfully [16]. Indeed, there is further evidence that after 9 years of survival, the Minnesota Multiphasic Personality Inventory (MMPI) profiles of CHD patients do not differ from those of controls [17].

While some researchers report age differences in the psychological reactions to MI, these differences diminish or disappear with increasing time following the attack. These findings point to the need for repeated psychosocial measurements for several years following infarction in order to monitor patients' adjustment. This is especially true for blue-collar patients, who often have the greatest difficulty in returning to their former jobs and who are least able to afford the layoff imposed by MI. Because of lower educational levels, work skills, and often unstable work histories, job opportunities for them are limited [18, 19]. The need to feel useful and productive is important in reestablishing a positive self-image among CHD patients, which does not come about as a function of time alone.

Evaluation

Psychosocial factors have been studied in evaluating the influence of intervention and rehabilitation programs on CHD patients. McPherson and colleagues studied the impact of a 24-week physical activity program on the personalities and moods of post-infarct and healthy adult men [20]. Prior to the exercise program, CHD men were more tense, aloof, emotional, hurried, and aggressive than the healthy men. After 24 weeks, the CHD men increased their levels of physical fitness, demonstrated an improved sense of well-being, and a decrease in anxiety and depression. The experienced exercisers in the program showed fewer personality changes than the CHD patients who exercised.

In other studies of CHD patients who became regular participants in supervised programs of physical activity, it is reported that there are attitudinal, mood, and/or life-style changes [21, 22]. In our studies of physical rehabilitation and personality change, we compared the MMPI profiles of three groups of men: (1) those who reduced their physical activity; (2) those who did not change their activity patterns, but were adjusting adequately to their infarct; and (3) those who increased their physical activity. The three groups were relatively homogeneous with regard to social characteristics (TABLE III). We found that those patients who increased their physical activity had significantly lower scores ($p<0.05$) on the Hypochondriasis (Hy) and Depression (D) scales and significantly higher scores on the Ego Strength (ES) scale of the MMPI (Fig. 1). Similarly, Hellerstein reported that patients actively engaged in physical reconditioning programs showed decreases in Depression (D) and Psychasthenia (Pt) scores on the MMPI. These changes corresponded with positive physical changes, including diminution of AP [23].

Numerous psychological and sociological factors influence whether a CHD patient will elect a rehabilitative effort if it is recommended. It has been reported, for example, that wives are often protective of their husbands in regard to physical activity following an infarction [24]. The attitude of the patient's

TABLE III

Characteristics of coronary patient and control groups

Group[1]	N	Mean Age	I.Q. (WAIS)	Mean yrs. education	Mean SES[2]	Times in mos. since coronary
Total controls	31	56.2	115.7	13.5	2.7	—
Total patients	31	56.7	113.2	11.9	3.2	78.8
Patient Subgroups[3]						
Reduced activity	14	55.5	110.3	10.6	3.4	66.9
Adequate adjustment	11	57.7	116.3	13.5	3.1	66.5
Increased activity	6	57.6	114.5	12.3	2.8	103.0
F		.12	.80	1.93	.70	1.01
p		NS	NS	NS	NS	NS

[1] All subjects were males
[2] Hollingshead's Index of Social Position used.
[3] Categories are the result of an activity questionnaire completed by the patients.

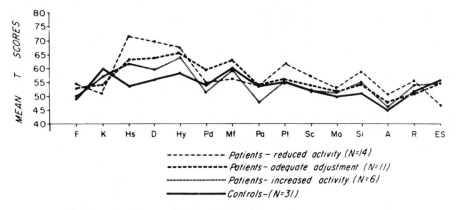

Fig. 1.   M.M.P.I. mean T scores and levels of postcoronary adjustment.

spouse and degree of family support for engaging in a physical activity program are often crucial to the patient's decision to enter a program and continue. In addition, the way the patient defines his own functioning capacity, especially in terms of his daily activities, will determine what he does, regardless of any objective criteria which the rehabilitative staff may have as indicators of progress [25]. Evaluative studies of intervention and rehabilitation programs should elicit data from the patient's family and his employer to ascertain their attitudes and degree of support for the patient's efforts. The motivation of CHD patients alone is most likely insufficient to sustain continued participation. A brief structured interview designed to tap life-style and habit changes, and short, selected psychological tests to elicit mood changes are important aids in monitoring patients' progress in rehabilitation programs. Personality tests are unlikely to reveal significant changes on a short-term basis.

The Interpretation of Psychosocial Data

Interviews

Interview data may be biased toward what the patient wants to tell, or toward the interviewer through his techniques of eliciting information. The personality of the interviewer, his style of interviewing, and/or the setting in which the interview is conducted may affect what, and how much, the patient tells. Often, the presence of the patient's spouse or other family members may cause him to deny or minimize important events. Patients are often good historians regarding their illness, but often spouses are better in relating life circumstances and events which may be relevant to the illness. The sex of the interviewer may also influence a patient's willingness to discuss certain topics [26]. Background characteristics of patients are often less important in predicting their level of responsiveness or cooperation than learning their motivation for cooperating. The needs of the patient vis-a-vis the interviewer, who may also be seen as a helper, might also influence the amount and type of information related [27]. The patient may regard the interviewer as an agent to help influence a job transfer, a source of emotional support, or an intervener in a domestic problem. A good interview, therefore, is not necessarily determined by the quantity of data obtained.

Since interviews are often obtained after an individual has developed the disease being studied, a patient's recall may be affected by the disease process and, in turn, his assessment of its impact on his life, especially if the disease has life-threatening consequences or an uncertain prognosis. A patient's denial or repression of past experiences or events may prohibit the interviewer from exploring crucial areas in the patient's life, especially if only a single interview is conducted [28, 29]. The type of interview chosen, therefore, should be determined by the purposes for which the information is being obtained [30].

All interviews need not be composed solely of unstructured questions. Certain data about the patient, such as job history, patterns of physical activity, and characteristics of his family, may be elicited through structured questions. Most information-getting interviews can be structured, while interviews designed to elicit feelings, attitudes, or opinions should be unstructured to permit flexibility for the interviewee and the interviewer in pursuing certain topics. Interviews which combine both structured and unstructured questions have the advantage of eliciting both objective and subjective information. Rapport is perhaps most difficult to establish when a totally structured interview is used, since the flow of information is uneven and the interviewer often gives the impression that only the information asked for is pertinent. Certain techniques for coding interview data can help to minimize the biases of the researcher. Independent judges can categorize subjective responses, and the degree of inter-rater reliability obtained provides an indication of the effectiveness of the interview instrument.

Psychological Tests

In the wide variety of psychological tests administered to CHD patients, the two most commonly used are the MMPI and the Cattell 16 P-F test. While personality tests have an important role in characterizing CHD patients, the results of testing alone, or testing at one point in time, have often caused researchers to refute or accept the importance of psychological factors. A single administration of a personality test will not elicit subtle mood and personality changes. Short versions of tests, particularly those designed to elicit mood, seem more pertinent in the long-term followup of CHD patients. Personality tests would be more appropriately administered to establish baseline information; tests administered subsequently at 2- to 3-year intervals would allow assessment of changes in personality traits.

There are methodological problems involved in the frequent repetition of instruments. Both interviews and psychological tests have educational value. Just as a patient may learn an interviewer's technique and adapt to his responses, he may learn test items, adopt a test-taking attitude in accordance with what he thinks the test measures, how it might be used, or reflect his antagonism toward the test in his responses. Patients' responses, therefore, might more accurately reflect their attitudes or feelings toward the test and tester than measure what the test seeks to measure. The attitude of the tester, the explanation given for administering the test and its subsequent use, and the nature of the test items can influence patients' responses. The issue of feedback is of particular importance. Often CHD patients ask how they performed on a psychological test. The researcher encounters the dilemma of explaining the results to him and possibly biasing patient's responses in future administrations of the same test, discussing the meaning of the patient's performance, or evading feedback. How the researcher copes with requested feedback will be tied to the purposes for obtaining the data.

Other Factors

Numerous other factors can influence the interpretation of psychosocial data. The patient's age, education, duration and severity of illness, denial, and degree of communicativeness influence the interpretation of both interviews and tests. The timing of when psychosocial information is obtained is important. Interviews or tests given during hospitalization might elicit, for example, apathy or pessimism. Indeed, while interviews and tests can have therapeutic value, they can also precipitate depression or angina, depending on the nature of the test or questions asked. The hospital or clinic is not an ideal setting for obtaining psychosocial data, especially if privacy cannot be assured. In addition, there is often an *institutional set* that can influence responses. We have found that patients welcome home visits for interviews. This setting provides the additional opportunity for another interviewer to visit with the patient's spouse separately and observe the family environment. Separate interviews with the patient and his spouse are essential. Wives of CHD patients are often protective, anxious regarding the uncertain future, and may have guilt feelings about how they might have contributed to their husbands' attacks [31]. Therefore, denial can be reinforced when partners are interviewed together.

Obviously, no psychosocial technique or researcher is free of bias. It is important that potential sources of bias be recognized and efforts made to minimize their effects. Careful attention should be given to the selection of psychosocial techniques with respect to the short- or long-term nature of the study and whether the techniques chosen will elicit descriptive characteristics, behavior patterns, or subtle changes in mood, attitude, or life-style. The selection of techniques solely on the basis of common usage, easy administration, or the time required, should be avoided. These guidelines can help to enhance the methodology of future psychosocial studies of CHD.

REFERENCES

1. Syme, S.L., and Reeder, L.G., Eds. Social stress and cardiovascular disease. *Milbank Mem. Fund. Q.* Vol. 45, Part 2, April, 1967.

2. Wardwell, W.I., and Bahnson, C.B. Problems encountered in behavioral science research in epidemiological studies. *Am. J. Public Health* 54:972-981, 1964.

3. Lehav, E. Methodological problems in behavioral research on disease. *J. Chron. Dis.* 20:333-340, 1967.

4. Croog, S.H., Levine, S., and Lurie, Z. The heart patient and the recovery process: A review of the directions of research on social and psychological factors. *Soc. Sci. Med.* 2:111-164, 1968.

5. Jenkins, C.D. Psychologic and social precursors of coronary disease. *N. Engl. J. Med.* 284:244-255; 307-317, Feb. 4 and 11, 1971.

6. Dovenmuehle, R.H., and Verwoerdt, A. Physical illness and depressive symptomatology. II. Factors of length and severity of illness and frequency of hospitalization. *J. Gerontol.* 18:260-266, 1963.

7. Verwoerdt, A., and Dovenmuehle, R.H. Heart disease and depression. *Geriatrics* 19:856-864, 1964.

8. Miller, C.K. Psychological correlates of coronary artery disease. *Psychosom. Med.* 27:257-265, 1965.

9. Rhodda, B.E., Miller, M.C., and Bruhn, J.G. Prediction of anxiety and depression patterns among coronary patients using a Markov Process Analysis. *Behav. Sci.* 16:482-489, 1971.

10. Bruhn, J.G., Shekelle, R.B., Ostfeld, A.M., and Paul, O. Prospective and retrospective psychological studies of coronary heart disease. *Psychosom. Med.* 31:8-19, 1969.

11. Lebovits, B.Z., Shekelle, R.B., Ostfeld, A.M., and Paul, O. Prospective and retrospective psychological studies of coronary heart disease. *Psychosom. Med.* 29:265-272, 1967.

12. Friedman, M. Behavior pattern and its relationship to coronary artery disease. *Psychosomatics* 8:6-7, Section 2, 1967.

13. Jenkins, C.D., Rosenman, R.H., and Friedman, M. Development of an objective psychological test for the determination of the coronary-prone behavior pattern in employed men. *J. Chron. Dis.* 20:371-379, 1967.

14. Holmes, T.H., and Rahe, R.H. The social readjustment rating scale. *J. Psychosom. Res.* 11:213-218, 1968.

15. Theorell, T., and Rahe, R.H. Psychosocial factors and myocardial infarction. I. An inpatient study in Sweden. *J. Psychosom. Res.* 15:25-31, 1971.

16. Garrity, T.F., and Klein, R.F. A behavioral predictor of survival among heart attack patients. *In*, Palmore, E.B., Ed., *Prediction of Life Span.* Lexington, Mass., Heath Lexington Books, 1971.

17. Bruhn, J.G., Wolf, S., and Philips, B.U. A psychosocial study of surviving male coronary patients and controls followed over nine years. *J. Psychosom. Res.* 15:305-313, 1971.

18. Shapiro, S., Weinblatt, E., Frank, C.W., and Sager, R.V. Social factors in the prognosis of men following first myocardial infarction. *Milbank Mem. Fund Q.* 48:37-50, 1970.

19. Higgins, A.C., and Pooler, W.S. Myocardial infarction and subsequent reemployment in Syracuse, New York. *Am. J. Public Health* 58:312-323, 1968.

20. McPherson, B.D., Paivio, A., Yuhasz, M.S., Rechnitzer, P.A., Pickard, H.A., and Lefcoe, N.M. Psychological effects of an exercise program for post-infarct and normal adult men. *J. Sports Med. Phys. Fitness* 7:95-102, 1967.

21. Naughton, J., Bruhn, J.G., and Lategola, M.T. Effects of physical training on physiologic and behavioral characteristics of cardiac patients. *Arch. Phys. Med. Rehabil.* 49:131-137, 1968.

22. Naughton, J., and Bruhn, J. Emotional stress, physical activity and ischemic heart disease. *DM/Disease-A-Month* July, 1970.

23. Hellerstein, H.K., et al. Active physical reconditioning of coronary patients. *Circulation* 32:22-110, 1965.

24. Brown, T.S. *Physical Activities, Attitudes, and Therapeutic Classification of Coronary Heart Patients.* Fort Worth, Texas Christian University (Institute of Behavioral Research), 1968. (IBR Res. Rep. No. 68-2)

25. New, P.K., Ruscio, R.T., Priest, R.P., Petritsi, D., and George, L.A. The support structure of heart and stroke patients: A study of the role of significant others in patient rehabilitation. *Soc. Sci. Med.* 2:185-200, 1968.

26. Colombotos, J., Elinson, J., and Loewenstein, R. Effect of interviewer's sex on interview responses. *Public Health Rep.* 83:685-690, 1968.

27. *The Influence of Interviewer and Respondent Psychological Behavioral Variables on the Reporting in Household Interviews.* Washington, D.C., U.S. Department of Health, Education, and Welfare, 1968 (Nat. Ctr. for Health Statistics, Ser. 2, No. 26)

28. Mai, F.M.M. Personality and stress in coronary disease. *J. Psychosom. Res.* 12:275-287, 1968.

29. Keith, R.A. Personality and coronary heart disease: A review. *J. Chron. Dis.* 19:1231-1243, 1966.

30. Kahn, R.L., and Cannell, C.F. *The Dynamics of Interviewing.* New York, Wiley, 1957.

31. Adsett, C.A., and Bruhn, J.G. Short-term group psychotherapy for post-myocardial infarction patients and their wives. *Can. Med. Assoc. J.* 99:577-584, 1968.

18

SOCIAL AND PSYCHOLOGICAL FACTORS THAT INFLUENCE THE EFFECTIVENESS OF EXERCISE PROGRAMS

Fred Heinzelmann, Ph.D.

A number of general themes have important implications for the manner in which exercise programs are planned, organized, and administered. These themes address program effectiveness in relation to the following issues:

1. Social and psychological characteristics of the program audience.
2. Social and psychological aspects of program operations.
3. Social and psychological effects of program participation.

Each theme merits attention in terms of those factors that influence voluntary participation in an exercise program; adherence over time; and the kinds of program benefits generated. Special consideration will be given to the body of research and program experience that indicates how these factors influence the effectiveness of an exercise program.

Social and Psychological Characteristics of the Program Audience

In terms of social characteristics and life-style, several studies of middle-aged men have reported a positive relationship between socioeconomic status and voluntary participation in an organized exercise program. In general, the higher the social class (measured in terms of occupation and education), the more likely the men were to participate [1]. These data are consistent with the findings from a number of studies reporting a positive relationship between socioeconomic status and participation in various kinds of voluntary action [2].

With regard to exercise programs, several factors may be instrumental in influencing participation. It may be that persons in the higher social classes recognize and accept more readily the personal need for exercise. A greater level of inactivity consistent with their life-styles may make their risk status more salient for them. Supporting data indicate that men who have coronary-prone characteristics (in terms of elevated blood pressure, body weight, and serum cholesterol levels) are more likely to consider themselves vulnerable to a heart attack than men without such characteristics [3]

In the higher social classes, individuals may also accept the value and benefit of exercise more readily because they believe health status can be influenced by personal health actions—a position less likely to be held by persons in lower social classes. It should be noted that, in general, certain health actions considered to have reached the level of *common sense* (exercise, selective diet, weight control, and control of smoking) are more likely to be viewed as beneficial by persons in the higher social classes than by those in lower social classes [4]. Likewise, persons in the lower social classes more often view themselves as lacking control over events in their life space and environment [5]. This may include a perceived lack of control over various health threats such as heart disease, cancer, and stroke.

Finally, situational factors may play a role. Persons in the higher social classes, (professionals, administrative personnel) may simply have more time available, as well as more flexible schedules, than those in lower social classes who are engaged in occupations requiring a more routine and fixed work role. To the extent that this may be a relevant factor, it highlights the need to establish exercise programs that allow for flexibility in participation, as well as programs that can be conducted within various employment settings.

Various studies have identified several psychological determinants of health behavior and response to different kinds of health programs [6, 7, 8]. These determinants include attitudes and beliefs concerning specific health threats and the actions considered effective in preventing or controlling these threats. In this context, in several studies dealing with participation in exercise programs, positive relationships were found between voluntary *participation* and the following patterns of attitudes and beliefs [3, 9] :

- Perceived vulnerability to a heart attack.
- The perceived benefits of specific health actions including exercise.
- Feelings of control in regard to one's health status.
- Positive attitudes toward physicians and medical research.

With regard to program *adherence*, it was found in one study of an exercise program involving coronary-prone men that the person's attitude toward his job and work environment was an important factor. The person's involvement in his job and dedication to his occupational role was related to program adherence over time [3].

In general, a person's health attitudes and beliefs can influence both his decision to participate in an exercise program and adherence to the program over time. Consequently, some program efforts should be directed toward identifying, and if necessary, influencing the views of potential participants concerning the personal need and benefits of the program proposed. Special attention should be given to the attitudes and beliefs of individuals whose views may not be consistent with program participation.

It is important that program directors take into consideration the variation in the meaning, and response to, physical activity and exercise as a function of life-style. For example, the concepts of physical activity and exercise are not simple and uniform, but rather mean different things to different individuals. Investigators have reported that when persons are asked to define *physical activity*, their statements include different points of reference such as exercise in general; sports or games; manual work; specific exercise such as calisthenics; walking or hiking; and jogging or running [10].

Just as the concept of exercise carries different meanings for individuals, the concept of physical fitness may simply mean the ability to carry out normal daily functions and activities for some, while for others, it means a level of optimal physical and psychological functioning.

The range and diversity in meaning which these concepts convey to individuals may generate a number of different attitudes or reactions. For example:

1. Based on their concept of physical activity and physical fitness, persons may conclude that they are already active or fit, and therefore, need not give additional attention to these issues.

2. Persons may fail to respond positively to a specific exercise program, because a negative attitude toward some form of physical activity or exercise is equated with the meaning of the program being promoted.

In short, it is useful to remember that with regard to physical activity and exercise, persons respond and react in terms of *their* level of understanding and *their* attitudes and beliefs. It is essential, therefore, to provide information that will help individuals become aware of and understand the meaning of terms used in the program. In addition, it is important to clarify the context in which these terms are being used. What kind of physical activity or exercise is being promoted? What kind of setting or specific program is proposed? How is the term physical fitness being used and what does it convey? While this approach will not insure a positive response, it will reduce the possibility that problems in communication become the major barriers to program participation.

Social and Psychological Aspects of Program Operations

The manner in which exercise programs are organized and administered should be examined in terms of various social and psychological consequences. This is important because program operations can influence the decisions which individuals make about program participation, as well as their response to the program over time.

While program recruitment methods may vary, there is considerable evidence suggesting that an approach employing small group discussion and decision-making can be effective in influencing decisions to participate, as well as adherence patterns over time [11, 12]. In one study of an exercise program for middle-aged men, a recruitment method involving small group discussions and decision-making was systematically compared with a large group lecture approach [13]. In general, the small group discussion-decision approach was more effective in influencing the decision to participate. It also had positive effects on program adherence. The findings indicated that the effectiveness of the small group discussion and decision method was *not* limited by the personal and social characteristics of the audience, or by differences in the level of skill, or personal style of the group discussion leaders. In short, this approach was more effective than a lecture approach regardless of the social class and life-style characteristics of the audience.

The use of a small group discussion-decision approach is apparently effective for a number of social and psychological reasons. The active involvement of the participants in the group discussion is likely to increase understanding and learning compared with the more passive reception of information obtained from a lecture. In addition, misunderstandings can be more readily detected and corrected at the time. The small group context also provides an individual with the opportunity to explore and evaluate the benefits and demands of program participation. This establishes the basis for a more realistic form of commitment as soon as a decision has been made. Another critical variable is that individuals make their decisions concerning participation in a group context where their decision is reinforced by the decisions of others.

Other important program components include those making it possible for participants to maintain regular contacts with medical and other program personnel. The social-psychological value of this type of relationship cannot be overemphasized; it makes it possible to provide participants with the feedback, clarification, and support they need and want. Findings from several studies have documented the significant influence of this program component on the level of satisfaction experienced by participants, as well as their adherence over time [14, 15].

In general, several social-psychological guidelines can influence the manner in which exercise programs are organized and implemented.

The *first guideline* deals with the factors that motivate persons to participate in a program and those factors that influence adherence over time.

It is important to emphasize that persons may be motivated to exercise or to participate in a physical activity program for a variety of reasons. While some persons may decide to participate primarily for health reasons (i.e., to enhance their state of health or avoid illness or specific health problems), others may participate because the program makes possible a change of routine, or provides an opportunity for recreation or social contacts. Therefore, when efforts are made to promote exercise or program participation, the focus should be diverse and take into account a variety of motivating factors, whether or not they are health-related, or reflect the views of those persons organizing and/or administering the program.

In promoting effective physical activity programs, it is also useful to remember that factors influencing a person's decision to take part in an exercise program may differ from factors influencing his adherence in the program over time. The factors for motivating participation in an exercise program may be concerned with health, desire for recreation, or a change in routine; while factors such as the organization and leadership of the program, the games aspect, and the camaraderie or social support that is generated may be more instrumental in promoting adherence over time. Several studies have provided evidence highlighting the relevance of these factors [16].

Since the social aspects can play a significant role in promoting program adherence, efforts should be made to insure that exercise programs organized on a group basis are administered in a manner to support rather than impede social development. This is especially important since physical activity and exercise are often viewed as a form of social activity (i.e., persons often prefer to exercise with another or with a group rather than alone) [14]. As a basis for this preference, individuals cite a number of major benefits when physical activity is performed with others. They seem to enjoy exercise more, experience social support, feel a sense of personal commitment to continue, and welcome the opportunity to compare their progress and level of fitness with others. Therefore, organized exercise programs should include opportunities for close interaction among the participants. Group activity should be made available for persons who are interested.

A *second guideline* for program development concerns the role of interpersonal influences with regard to program participation and adherence over time.

In order to promote effective physical activity and exercise programs, the attention should focus not only on the potential participant, but also those to whom the individual relates most directly, and who are, therefore, likely to influence his attitudes and behavior. A man's wife, as well as his friends and colleagues, can play important roles in this sense. It may be useful and productive to direct attention to this broader social network rather than view the individual alone as the focal point in efforts made to influence his behavior. Often the attitude and reaction of those with whom an individual interacts determine whether or not he will participate, as well as influence his pattern of adherence over time. Those persons who serve as *significant others* should be adequately informed about the nature of the program, and be involved in the program on a continuing basis to insure that their reactions provide social support, and reinforce the individual's participation, rather than influence it negatively.

This issue became evident in one study which examined the relationship between the wife's attitude toward the exercise program and her husband's adherence in the 18 months' duration of the program [14] (Fig. 1).

The data indicated clearly that the husband's pattern of adherence in the exercise program was directly related to his wife's attitude toward the program. For example, 80 percent of those men whose spouses had a positive attitude toward the program exhibited good or excellent adherence patterns, contrasted with 40 percent of the men whose spouses' attitudes were neutral or negative. Conversely, only 20 percent of the men whose spouses had a positive attitude toward the program exhibited a fair or poor adherence pattern compared to 60 percent of the men whose wives' attitudes were neutral or negative. The husband's pattern of adherence was apparently influenced as much by the wife's neutral or indifferent attitude as by her negative attitude toward the program. In this context, it is useful to indicate that program social events including both participants and spouses help to create and maintain positive attitudes that support adherence.

In another study of an exercise program conducted within a Federal agency,

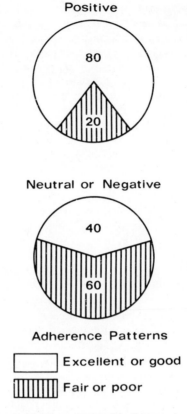

Fig. 1. Relation of wives' attitudes to husbands' adherence in a physical activity program.

the supervisor's attitude toward the program apparently influenced the adherence of employees [15]. The data indicated that when supervisors supported the program with a positive attitude, individuals were more likely to participate regularly.

In summary, issues that have implications for the organization and administration of exercise programs are:

First, as stated previously, motivation to participate in programs may be for various reasons such as health, recreation, and change of routine. Therefore, in promoting participation, the focus should be diverse, and take into consideration a variety of motives whether or not they are health-related or consonant with the views of the persons organizing or administering the program.

Second, the factors influencing a decision to participate may differ from those that influence adherence over time. Since the social aspects of physical activity encourage adherence, attention should be directed to this factor and efforts made to insure that the program is organized and administered to support, rather than impede, the development of social influences.

Third, in promoting exercise programs, it is advantageous to view the target group as comprising the potential participant, as well as those providing a meaningful social network for him, i.e, his family, friends, and possibly work associates. The attitudes and reactions of the persons to whom potential participants relate most directly often determine whether or not they will take part and how well they adhere over time.

Social and Psychological Effects of an Exercise Program

Sedentary individuals who begin exercise may experience a number of beneficial social and psychological effects regarding the major areas of their lives. Investigators have reported that these effects include enhanced work attitudes and performance; more positive feelings of sound health and well being; and better health habits and behavior.

The social-psychological effects of an exercise program were systematically examined in a study of coronary-prone men involving random assignment to an exercise program or to a control group. In general, it was found that participants in the exercise programs reported significantly more effects regarding their work, health, and behavior than did persons in the control groups [14].

For example, with regard to work, program participants often reported important and positive effects on work performance. Typical comments were: "I have a greater capacity to work harder mentally and physically." "I have improved my power of decision and concentration." Differences were also reported in the participants' *attitudes* toward work, with men indicating that they felt more energetic and more productive, and that work seemed less boring (Fig. 2).

Program effects were also observed concerning aspects of personal health. Program participants reported effects of increased stamina and energy, more positive feelings about their health, weight reduction, and greater ability to deal with stress and tension. In all these aspects, participants reported changes more often than did members of the control group (Fig. 3).

Program effects also involved changes in habits and behavior. Participants reported they ate less and were more interested in, and aware of, the importance of weight control than members of the control group. Participants also increased their recreational activities with family and friends. It was clear that physical activity had become a pervasive habit in the life-style of many of the men. Program participants also reported greater changes in patterns of sleep and rest than did members of the control group; they had a need for less sleep, as well as the ability to obtain a sounder and more relaxed sleep. No differences were reported between the exercise and control groups in terms of changes in kinds of food eaten or in smoking behavior. About one-third of the persons in both groups reported eating less fats and starches, and about 20 percent in each group reported they smoked less (Fig. 4).

These findings were replicated in a study of an exercise program conducted in a Federal agency [15], indicating a very strong, positive, and consistent relationship between program adherence and reported program effects. Within each

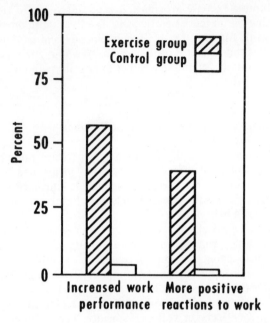

Fig.2. Effect of physical activity program on participants' work situation.

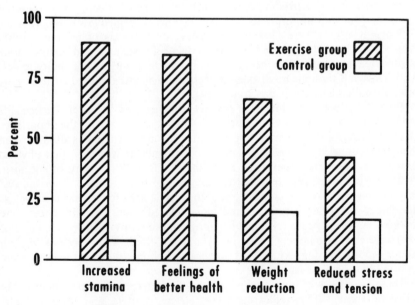

Fig. 3. Effect of physical activity program on participants' health

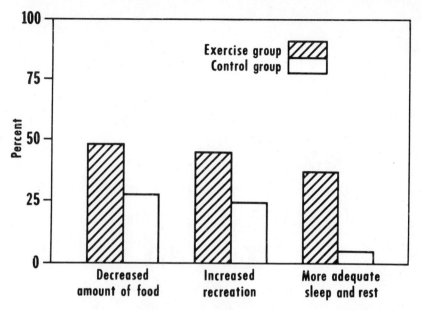

Fig. 4. Effect of physical activity program on participants' habits and behavior.

area relating to work, health, and behavior, program effects were reported most often by those whose adherence level was good, and least often by those whose adherence level was poor (Fig. 5).

It is important to note that the program effects reported by participants were directly related to improvements observed in their cardiovascular functioning based on treadmill performance (TABLE I). Significant differences in measures of cardiovascular improvement were also observed between participants who reported program benefits and those who did not (TABLE II). These findings suggest that improvements in cardiovascular and physiological functioning can influence a person's thoughts and feelings about his state of health, as well as his pattern of health attitudes and behavior.

Exercise may also influence an individual's self-concept and feelings of self-sufficiency and emotional stability [14]. Participants in an exercise program may experience a feeling of accomplishment along with an enhanced sense of control over their lives. Such social-psychological effects in turn can provide support for program adherence.

Participation in exercise programs can also lead to changes or effects in the health attitudes and habits of the spouse, family members, and friends of persons participating in such programs. These changes in others may include a heightened interest in, and greater awareness of, health matters, as well as health behavior changes regarding exercise, diet, and weight control. To the extent such changes occur, they reinforce and support patterns of adherence among persons participating in the exercise programs.

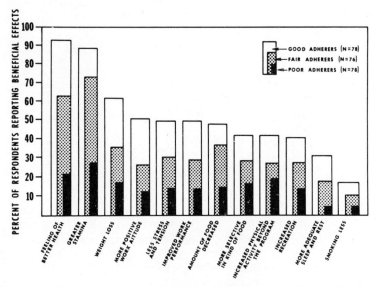

Fig. 5. Total effects of NASA Health Evaluation and Enhancement Program in relation to adherence.

TABLE I

Number of effects reported and mean
changes observed in stress tests parameters

MEAN CHANGE IN STRESS TEST PARAMETERS	NUMBER OF PROGRAM EFFECTS REPORTED*			
	NONE (N=66)	ONE (N=39)	TWO (N=99)	THREE (N=15)
DURATION OF STRESS TEST	1.0 MIN.	1.8 MIN.	2.1 MIN.	3.3 MIN.
TIME REQUIRED TO REACH HEART RATE OF 140 BEATS/MIN	1.8 MIN.	2.6 MIN.	3.4 MIN.	4.3 MIN.
TIME REQUIRED TO REACH HEART RATE OF 150 BEATS/MIN	2.3 MIN.	2.6 MIN.	3.3 MIN.	5.1 MIN.
HEART RATE AT 12 MINUTES	-12.6	-21.1	-20.2	-28.1
HEART RATE AT 15 MINUTES	-12.1	-22.7	-20.8	-25.4
MAXIMUM HEART RATE	-12.5	-22.4	-20.6	-26.4

*The effects reported included feelings of better health; greater stamina; and/or increases in health interest and awareness. A respondent could report effects in any one or all of these areas.

TABLE II

Differences in mean changes observed in stress
test parameters between group reporting a specific
effect and group reporting no effect

	DIFFERENCES IN MEAN CHANGE IN STRESS TEST PARAMETERS					
SPECIFIC EFFECTS	STRESS TEST DURATION (MIN.)	TIME TO REACH 140 BPM (MIN.)	TIME TO REACH 150 BPM (MIN.)	HEART RATE AT 12 MIN. (BPM)	HEART RATE AT 15 MIN. (BPM)	MAXIMUM HEART RATE (BPM)
FEELINGS OF BETTER HEALTH	1.4**	1.36**	1.15**	6.8**	6.1**	6.5**
GREATER STAMINA	.9**	1.31**	.90**	5.9**	6.3**	6.9**
GREATER HEALTH INTEREST & AWARENESS	1.2**	2.01**	2.12**	8.6**	8.6**	10.1**
LESS STRESS AND TENSION	1.1**	1.67**	1.16**	7.3**	6.6**	7.6**
WEIGHT REDUCTION	1.0**	1.44*	1.08**	7.2**	8.5**	7.8**
MORE POSITIVE WORK ATTITUDE	.8*	1.73**	1.44**	6.8**	6.2**	6.2**
IMPROVED WORK PERFORMANCE	.3	.60	.81*	2.4	4.3*	3.3
AMOUNT OF FOOD DECREASED	.7*	1.02**	.63	2.4	3.0	3.5*
MORE SELECTIVE IN KIND OF FOOD	.8*	.47	.23	.3	2.1	2.5
MORE ADEQUATE SLEEP & REST	.6	.92*	1.01*	3.5	2.4	3.1
INCREASED PHYSICAL ACTIVITY BEYOND THE PROGRAM	.9**	.57	.90*	.2	.1	2.3
INCREASED RECREATION	.9*	.57	.63	.6	.9	3.3
SMOKING LESS	.7	.17	.55	.7	.0	2.5

*Indicates a significant difference at the .05 level of confidence between Group reporting an effect & Group reporting no effect.
**Indicates a significant difference at the .01 level of confidence between Group reporting an effect & Group reporting no effect.

In order to promote changes in health interest and action among the network of individuals to whom program participants relate, periodic discussions of the exercise program and its effects should be provided, to include the participant's spouse and family members whenever possible.

In short, participation in an exercise program can generate a dual set of social-psychological effects:

- The program may serve as a catalyst for change in the participant's broader pattern of health behavior, as well as influence his feelings of health and well-being and his self-image.

- The program may also stimulate health behavior change among those with whom participants are in most direct contact. This *ripple effect* can serve in the diffusion of additional program benefits and promote adherence within the program itself.

Summary

The relevance of social and psychological factors should be considered when planning, organizing, and administering exercise programs, which means giving attention to the characteristics of the program audience and the manner in which the program is presented to them. Program operations should also be examined in terms of how they influence voluntary participation and adherence in the program over time. Likewise, in considering the effects of an exercise program, it is important to recognize that participation can influence how a person thinks and feels about himself and his state of health and what he does relative to disease prevention and health enhancement.

Systematic attention to these issues should make it possible to deal more effectively with the broad range of factors that influence program success.

REFERENCES

1. Heinzelmann, F. Attitudes of middle-aged men toward exercise and health. Paper presented at *Annual Meeting of the College of Sports Medicine*, Albuquerque, N.M., May 1970.

2. Smith, D.H., Reddy, R.D., and Baldwin, B.R., Eds. *Voluntary Action Research: 1972*. Lexington, Mass., Heath, 1972.

3. Taylor, H., Remington, R., Buskirk, E., Balke, B., Fox, S., Stamler, J., and Epstein, F. (Steering Committee). *Co-operative Pilot Studies of Physical Activity and Coronary Heart Disease* [data from]. A cooperative study by three participating universities (Univ. Minn. Univ. Wis., and Penn State Univ.). Supported by a U.S. Public Health Service contract, 1968.

4. Hassinger, E.W., and Anderson, T.M. *Information and Beliefs about Heart Disease Held by the Public*. Columbia, University of Missouri, 1964. (Univ. Mo. Agric. Exp. Sta. Res. Bull. 874)

5. Svalastoga, K. Social differentiation. *In*, Faris, R.E., Ed. *Handbook of Modern Sociology*, pp.530-575. Chicago, Rand McNally, 1968.

6. Hochbaum, G.M. *Public Participation in Medical Screening Programs*. Washington, D.C., GPO, 1959. (PHS Pub. No. 572)

7. Rosenstock, I.M. Why people use health services. *Milbank Mem. Fund Q.* 44(3):94-127, 1966.

8. Russell, R.D. Motivational factors as related to health behavioral change. *In*, Veenker, H., Ed. *Synthesis of Research in Selected Areas of Health Instruction*. Washington, D.C., School Health Education Study, 1966.

9. Durbeck, D., et al. The National Aeronautics and Space Administration—U.S. Public Health Service Health Evaluation and Enhancement Program. *Am. J. Cardiol.* 30:784-790, 1972.

10. Heinzelmann, F. Physical fitness: The challenge to the profession as seen by the behavioral scientist. Paper presented at Annual Convention, *American Association for Health, Physical Education and Recreation*. Seattle, Wash., April 1970.

11. Kerrick, J.S., et al. A symposium on lecture versus group discussion. *Int. J. Health Educ.* 10(3):106-129, 1967.

12. Bond, B.W. *Group Discussion–Decision: An Appraisal of Its Use in Health Education.* Minneapolis, Minn., Department of Health, 1956.

13. Heinzelmann, F., and Bagley, R. *An Evaluation of Two Methods of Promoting Behavior Change in a Health Program Context.* Unpublished manuscript, U.S. Public Health Service, 1970.

14. Heinzelmann, F., and Bagley, R. Response to physical activity programs and their effects on health behavior. *Public Health Rep.* 85(10):905-911, 1970.

15. Heinzelmann, F., and Durbeck, D.C. Personal benefits of a health evaluation and enhancement program. *Proceedings, NASA Annual Conference of Clinic Directors, Environmental Health Officials and Medical Program Advisors*, pp.52-79. Cambridge, Mass., October 1970.

16. Heinzelmann, F. Factors influencing response to physical activity programs and the effects of participation on health attitudes and behavior. Paper presented at *National Institute on Executive and Employee Fitness.* St. Louis, June 1969.

17. Ismail, A.H., and Trachtman, L.E., Jogging the imagination. *Psychol. Today* 6(10):78-82, 1973.

19

UNMET NEEDS IN PSYCHOLOGICAL EVALUATION
OF INTERVENTION PROGRAMS

Stanley Fisher, Ed.D.

Psychological Aspects of Rehabilitation

While there may be questions about the significance of psychological factors as a cause of heart disease, there appears to be no question about the significance of the patient's psychological reaction to his illness from the time he is seen in an emergency room, or coronary care unit, to the time he considers returning to work [1]. Clinical observers have long recognized the psychological problems faced by the cardiac patient [2]. An international survey [3], promoted by the International Society of Cardiology's Psychological Aspects Committee, reported that the major psychological problems of the cardiac are anxiety, fear of sudden death, and lack of confidence, as well as his fear of recurrence of heart disease. Psychological factors are ever present and often crucial in all aspects of rehabilitation, including exercise training programs. Professor K. Lange-Andersen [4], in discussing training programs as part of an overall cardiac rehabilitation program, stated that . . . "the most important effect of exercise is psychological rather than physiological." Recently, a number of studies [5, 6, 7, 8] sought to measure the psychological effects of training programs for cardiac patients. This report will summarize these studies, and summarize the unmet needs these studies suggest in the psychological evaluation of intervention programs.

Studies of the Rehabilitation Potential of Individuals with Coronary Heart Disease by Dr. C. Plavsic and his associates in Yugoslavia was published in 1968 [5]. The wide objectives of this project included development of a comprehensive program for cardiac rehabilitation as well as an epidemiological study of risk factors associated with coronary heart disease (CHD). One of their many objectives was to investigate a number of psychological factors and approaches which would facilitate better rehabilitation of patients. Of particular interest to us is the psychological hypothesis that . . . "Systematic personality changes take place in the coronary heart disease patients who have undergone medical treatment for rehabilitation" [5]. To test this hypothesis, 71 patients (68 male, 3 female) whose ages ranged from 27 to 76 years, with an average age of 50, were the subjects. Of these, 73 percent were new CHD cases, while 27 percent had had two, three, or even four attacks. Psychological testing was performed before a patient began rehabilitation treatment and a short time after his return from treatment. Treatment included a regular diet, scheduled resting and sleeping hours, personal discussion with individual patients, and physical activity, which had the most important role. The type of exercise with magnitude of the required effort and duration was determined for each patient individually—with regard to his clinical status, time span following the infarction, his emotional attitude, and other inclinations, i.e., his acceptance of the training program, as he is often apprehensive of movements.

Diagnostic Techniques

The psychological ratings, made pre- and postrehabilitation treatment, were based on six psychological diagnostic techniques:
1. the interview
2. Cornell Index N/4
3. Rosenzweig's picture frustration scale
4. Byrne's scale of repression-sensitization
5. Plutchik's profile index of emotions
6. a multidimensional scale of personality assessment

which the investigators composed for this study.

The results of this investigation were obtained by a comparison of psychological ratings before beginning rehabilitation treatment and again a short time after return from this treatment. Only 16 patients of the sample group of 71 were retested. The investigators found a statistically significant increase on the Cornell Index N/4 of depressive, hypochondriacal, and inhibitory conversion tendencies. They state:

> Without indulging in speculation we may conclude from this that after finishing rehabilitation treatment our patients become more preoccupied with somatic troubles (increased hypochondriacal tendency) and were more worried [5].

It should be noted that Dr. Plavsic and associates [5] did not use a control group. Between the pre- and postpsychological testing approximately 2 months elapsed, suggesting that other change-producing events may have occurred in addition to rehabilitation treatment. Maturation of the heart disease over the passage of time, independent of rehabilitation treatment, may be mistaken for the specific effect of rehabilitation treatment. In addition, personality tests taken for the second time can show positive or negative adjustment, depending on whether the patient has discovered the disguised purpose of the test and is anxious to be perceived in a special way. We can speculate about the part of the treatment that caused the psychological changes. Perhaps discussions with the patient, informing him that he would have to go on a regular diet and have scheduled rest, made him "worry" more about his illness.

Hellerstein and associates [6] studied a group of 656 middle-aged men referred for exercise therapy by their physicians. As part of that study, the group was evaluated psychologically with:

1. the Holzmann Inkblot Test
2. the Minnesota Multiphasic Personality Inventory, and
3. the Rosenman-Friedman taped interview.

Hellerstein reported that at intake "the study subjects had elevation of depression, hysteria, and hypochondriasis scales on the Minnesota Multiphasic Personality Inventory (MMPI)" [6]. After each subject had been studied, a program was formulated to enhance his overall fitness. Physical conditioning was only a part of a comprehensive program which included nutrition, attainment of normal body weight, adequate rest, abstinence from tobacco, and continuation of gainful employment. In addition, each subject was counseled by a study physician, a dietician, and a physical educator. In essence, a specialized program involving exercise, weight reduction, diet, and abstinence from smoking was formulated for each subject with the approval of the referring physician. Of the 656 subjects evaluated, counseled, and given a specialized program, 254 had CHD. Of the 254, 100 were analyzed in greater detail. Seventy-five percent of the 100 subjects adhered to the program.

> The spouses of the subjects were enthusiastic because of the change in the personality and the greater ease of cohabitations, and the increased frequency of sexual activity. The decrease in the scores of the depression and psychosthenic scales was noteworthy [6].

Reactions of Patients

Many subjects insisted that they had more positive attitude to work, felt more energetic, accomplished more, and were less bored. They had increased work output, felt more ambitious, met tense situations better, slept better, and needed less sleep. Hellerstein concluded that in this multifactorial intervention program:

> The changes in the mood, in the functions of the cardiovascular system, in nutrition, body weight, etc., indicate that the training program with its many facets (psychological, nutritional, physical conditioning, and group participation), has produced significant changes in both the cardiovascular and nervous systems [6].

Differences in the needs of patients with CHD required variability in the overall multifactorial training plan, rather than a fixed application of procedures to all patients being studied. Thus, there was a wide array of experimental variables being considered under a single notion called a training program. This oversimplification clouds some of the possible findings. This poses the question: What aspect or combination of aspects included under "a training program" have the greatest influence on the psychological changes reported? For example, Fisher and Hanna [9] in 1931, as well as observations by employment counselors, have long recognized that individuals are depressed when unemployed and show less depression when they return to work. It is possible that patients in this group felt continuation of employment meant that they were not severely ill.

It should be noted that Hellerstein reported that on intake the scales on the MMPI, hypochondriasis, depression, and hysteria were elevated. "In the present study, these psychological scores showed significant improvement after conditioning" [6]. These findings differ from those of Dr. Plavsic [5], which indicated an increase rather than a decrease in depressive, hypochondriacal, and conversion tendencies because of their training programs. One can only speculate about the completely opposite results. Greater weight could be given to the Hellerstein study since there were 75 subjects in his study compared to 16 in the Plavsic group. Although both investigators described their initial large study groups, they did not describe the much smaller group used in the psychological testing part of the studies. In Hellerstein's study, only 75 of the original 656 subjects were used; in the Plavsic study, only 16 of the original 71 patients were used. It is quite possible that the two small groups were unlike their original parent group and unlike each other. This possible difference in the groups may also account for some of the psychological differences reported.

Further Studies

In a study entitled "Rehabilitation of Coronary Patients," Kellerman and coworkers investigated . . . "whether a short rehabilitation program based on physical activities, such as gardening and calisthenics, can improve a patient's capabilities to such an extent that he can return to work even after he has been out of work for years" [7]. Psychological testing before and after rehabilitation in 55 ambulatory cardiac patients involved the use of (1) the Rorshach, (2) draw-a-person, (3) Bender Gestalt, and (4) Rosenzweig's picture frustration test. These investigators found that "there is a marked psychological profit" [7] for the cardiac patient undergoing a physical training rehabilitation program. This "profit" is perceived in the patients' "increase in emotional stability" [7]. They define emotional instability as fear of death, despair for the future, and an acute feeling of instability to maintain the previous position in their family, jobs, and friends. They state, however, that after

> administering many tests, we learned that only a few results are available for research and statistical analysis. They recommend minimizing the use of projective techniques and extending the use of questionnaires [7].

Similar to the studies of Plavsic and Hellerstein, a control group was not used and, again, different psychological tests were employed. In view of Kellerman's comment regarding projective techniques, it is interesting to note that although the other investigators used projective techniques, they did not report or make clear the results of those tests.

Professor Askanas of the Institute of Cardiology of the Medical Academy of Warsaw, Poland, reported on a study entitled, *Investigation into the Effect of Medical Rehabilitation and of Therapeutic Procedure on Vocational Rehabilitation of Patients with Recent Myocardial Infarction*" [8]. As part of this study,

91 rehabilitated cardiacs and 70 nonrehabilitated cardiacs were given a battery of psychological tests four times during their hospitalization. They were tested during the first week of hospitalization; then just before discharge from the hospital, a third time when they were in the sanatoriums; and then 9 months after rehabilitation was completed. The rehabilitated patients, while in the hospital, were given "therapeutic gymnastics" that included:

> respiratory exercises, dynamic exercises of small muscle groups, isometric exercises, deeper respiratory exercises, dynamic exercises of the upper and lower extremities, coordinating dynamic exercises, passive or active verticalization, light resistance exercises of the lower extremities in recumbent position, relaxation exercises, gradual march from 3 to 159 meters, going upstairs to the first floor

over a period of 6 weeks. The control group did not perform these exercises. The experimental group was sent to a sanatorium where reconditioning was accomplished by individual and group gymnastics and walking outdoors at different distances. The control groups did not go to the sanatoriums. The rehabilitated group received psychotherapy; the nonrehabilitated group did not receive psychotherapy. Both groups were given the same psychological tests which included:

1. a modified tapping test
2. Courvé test of concentration and attention
3. a special questionnaire
4. the Thematic apperception test
5. Wartegg's test
6. Cattel's questionnaire
7. Rumbaugh cardiac adjustment scale.

Comparing the two groups, the tests revealed:

> improvement of concentration, psychic energy level, and in anxiety reactions in both groups—the improvement, however, was greater in the rehabilitation groups. The rehabilitation group is also reputed as having a better attitude toward illness, in the sense that more symptoms of acceptance and less of negativism and anxiety appear [8].

In discussing the effectiveness of their rehabilitation program, the authors conclude

> that their attempt to analyze remote effects of rehabilitation did not show significant differences in the somatic state of patients compared, but the period of observation seems to have been too short to draw conclusions. Significant differences were found in the indices of mental adaptation both during hospitalization and one year after admission to the hospital. These differences were in favor of rehabilitated patients. This simultaneously suggests that proper and valuable methods of psychological testing and psychotherapy, which is an integral part of the process of rehabilitation, were applied [8].

Since the major finding in this exercise study appears to be psychological, the question must be asked: Were the psychological changes in the rehabilitated group due to the exercise training received or the psychotherapy received during the course of their hospitalization?

The findings of Dr. Askanas' group appear to support the findings of Dr. Hellerstein and Dr. Kellerman and his group in that there is a reduction in the amount of anxiety due to the exercise program. The two additional findings relating psychic energy level and concentration are due to the kinds of tests used: the tapping test and Courvé's test of concentration. As anxiety is reduced, it is expected that concentration improves, and as psychasthenia is reduced, psychic energy might increase, but this would require substantiation through further research.

Discussion

It would seem, as in all research which assesses change, that it would be most helpful if Plavsic, Hellerstein, and Kellerman had made provision for a control group in their studies, as did Askanas and his group. In view of the small number of subjects used and the lack of a control group, we cannot be sure that the multifaceted training programs influenced the psychological findings reported, or that another factor is causing the increase in "somatic findings" [10] and "worry" in the Plavsic study, the decrease in hypochondriasis, depression, hysteria, and psychasthenia in the Hellerstein study, or the "marked psychological profit" of the Kellerman study.

If psychological evaluations are used to measure the effects of a training program, we should not include variables, such as personal counseling or psychotherapy by psychologists or other personnel within the training program. We should expect that counseling and psychotherapy can change attitudes toward illness, reduce anxiety, and increase "psychic energy level" [11]. Until there are better controlled studies, any one of the activities of a multifactorial training program could account for the psychological changes reported.

Future studies on intervention programs could focus on the number of different variables considered in "a training program" to determine which variable or combinations of variables affect the psychological changes perceived in patients.

Based on findings so far, it would appear that the majority of the reported results have been obtained from psychological questionnaires. Kellerman and associates indicated that the projective personality tests used in their study (Rorschach, Rosenzweig's Picture Frustration Test, and Draw-a-Person Test) do not lend themselves to research and statistical analysis. Kellerman recommends in the future, use of such tests as the Edwards Personal Preference Schedule and the Cattell's 16 Personality Factors. Future research in this area should consider the psychological tests that lent themselves to analysis in those studies reported here:

1. the MMPI, used by Hellerstein and associates;
2. the Cornell Medical Index N/4, used by Plavsic and colleagues;
3. the tapping test;
4. the concentration, used by Askanas and his group.

In addition, future investigations should consider the questionnaire used by Plavsic and Askanas to determine if they can be used to compose a reliable and valid measurement of the psychological variables which have been associated with training programs.

If the major objective of training programs is to return the CHD patient to work, it might be helpful to the patient if he could move from gym-like activities to job activities [10]. This might suggest to the cardiac patient that he is moving closer to the time when he can return to work, and be better adjusted psychologically to do so. Such vocational reconditioning of cardiac patients can best be accomplished in an industrial workshop [11] where work activities can be graded based on known energy levels of activities, and where cardiacs can continue to be supervised medically.

Based on a 14-year longitudinal study of patients, before and after MI, Fisher [12] reported that 81 percent of cardiac patients return to work within 1 year after the onset of their illness. Weinblatt et al [13] found that 9 out of 10 MIs return to work by 18 months. Kellerman and associates [14] report that all subjects who returned to work did so within 1 year, 83 percent within 5 months. These findings suggest that training programs or vocational reconditioning programs concerned with returning patients to work should be concerned with that 20 percent of cardiac patients who do not return to work on their own. In addition, future studies on return to work should include those psychological factors which may distinguish between rapid returnees (3 months or less) and slow returnees (4 months or more). Future psychological studies may indicate that those cardiac patients who are the slow returnees to work would profit most, psychologically, from intervention programs. Such information would be most helpful to those concerned with the vocational rehabilitation of the cardiac patient.

REFERENCES

1. *Psychological Aspects of the Rehabilitation of Cardiovascular Patients.* Report of Working Group convened by Regional Office for Europe of the World Health Organization, 1970. (WHO)

2. Fisher, S. Psychological aspects of rehabilitation. *Acta Cardiol.* Suppl. XIV, 1969.

3. Fisher, S. International survey on the psychological aspects of cardiac rehabilitation. *Scand. J. Rehabil. Med.* 2-3:71-77, 1970.

4. Working Symposium on Cardiology, Vienna, March 1972, Council on Rehabilitation. *International Society of Cardiology, Selecta* 24, p.9, June 1972.

5. Plavsic, C., et al. *Studies of the Rehabilitation Potential of Individuals with Coronary Heart Disease.* Washington, D.C., Department of Health, Education, and Welfare (Social and Rehabilitation Service), 1968. (Report of Project VRA-Yugoslavia 5-66)

6. Hellerstein, H.K. Exercise therapy in coronary heart disease. *In,* De Haas, J.H., et al. *Ischaemic Heart Disease*, pp.406-429. Baltimore, Williams & Wilkins, 1970.

7. Kellerman, J.J., et al. *Rehabilitation of Coronary Patients.* Washington, D.C., Department of Health, Education, and Welfare (Social and Rehabilitation Service), 1968. (Grant No. ISR 17-62)

8. Askanas, S., et al. *Investigation into the Effect of Medical Rehabilitation and of Therapeutic Procedure on Vocational Rehabilitation of Patients with Recent Myocardial*

Infarction. Washington, D.C., Department of Health, Education, and Welfare (Social and Rehabilitation Service), 1969. (Report on SRS-Pol 7-67)

9. Fisher, V.E., and Hanna, J.V. *The Dissatisfied Worker.* New York, Macmillan, 1931.

10. Fisher, S. Vocational reconditioning of the cardiac. *Psychol. Aspects Disabil. Bull.* Vol. 15, No. 1, March 1968.

11. Hockhauser, E. The role of the social agency in a rehabilitation program for the cardiac patient. *Am. Heart J.* 43:743-748, 1952.

12. Fisher, S. Impact of physical disability on vocational activity: work status following myocardial infarction. *Scand. J. Rehabil. Med.* 2-3:65-70, 1970.

13. Weinblatt, E., et al. Return to work and work status following first myocardial infarction. *Am. J. Public Health* 56:169, 1966.

14. Kellerman, J.J., et al. Return to work after myocardial infarction. *Geriatrics* 23:151, 1968.

PART III

Cardiac Rehabilitation

20

THE PRINCIPLES OF
CONDUCTING EXERCISE PROGRAMS

Karl G. Stoedefalke, Ph.D.

```
M A N     I S     C R E A T I V E
  O   O     S   N   O   E   N   E   H   N   I   A   D
  T   N       U   D   N   C   J   R   E   S   A   R   U
  I   C       P   I   T   R   O   O   R   T   B   I   C
  V   O       E   V   R   E   Y   B   A   R   L   A   A
  A   M       R   I   O   A   A   I   P   U   E   B   T
  T   P       V   D   L   T   B   C   E   C     I   I
  I   E       I   U   L   I   L   —   U   T     N   O
  O   T       S   A   E   V   E   A   T   I     T   N
  N   I       E   L   D   E   —   C   I   O     E   A
      T             (   A   E   T   C   N     N   L
      I             E   N   N   I   -     S
      V             X   D   E   V   I     I
      E             E       R   E   M     T
                    R       G     P     Y
                    C       I     R
                    I       Z     O
                    S       I     V
                    E       N     I
                            G     S
                            —     E
                            F     D
                            U
                            N
```

The essence of medical rehabilitation is the reduction and progressive withdrawal of supervision and support. A medical prescription to increase a patient's level of physical activity requires, in most cases, the assistance and supervision of a qualified leader of physical activity.

Before a physical activity specialist accepts a man into an exercise program, a medical examination, physician's referral, and graded exercise stress test are necessary. The graded exercise stress test can be performed on the motor-driven treadmill, bicycle ergometer, or stepping device. An evaluation of the results should be available to the physical educator prior to the participant's accession into the program. In addition, information, on the need-to-know basis, regarding medication or medical problems should be relayed to the physical exercise leader. The exercise prescription is made in conjunction with the participant's personal physician or the physician assigned the medical responsibilities of the program.

Throughout man's educational experiences, he has probably had more classes in physical education than in any other subject. However, research indicates that his level of physical activity decreases as he ages and that he knows little about sport, games, or how to use his body in a safe, enjoyable manner. Very few men at risk have the ability to undertake successfully a self-directed program of physical rehabilitation. In the interest of a patient's personal safety, the physician should recommend a physical exercise program led by competent leaders.

Program Requirements

Aging man at risk has a vested interest in his future. The type of physical activity program in which he participates should have these requirements: (1) medical supervision, (2) method of evaluating performance capabilities, (3) individual exercise prescriptions, (4) enjoyable activity, (5) education, and (6) competent leadership.

Supervision. *Axiom—Supervised Physical Activity Reduces the Frequency of Injury.* In intervention or rehabilitative programs, men demonstrate a wide variety of performance capabilities. They tend to know very little about energy expenditure, pacing themselves in sustained movement, or the selection of activities. Often, man overestimates his ability to perform activity and needs programs in which there is close supervision of his exercise, its intensity and duration.

Methods of evaluating performance capabilities. *Axiom—Physiological Assessment Is a Science.* Before an exercise prescription is written, a graded exercise test should be conducted. Exercise tests minimize the need for skill and motivation. Physiological assessments of aerobic power can be obtained through tests using a stepping device, bicycle ergometer, or motor-driven treadmill. These three methods may be used interchangeably. Intermittent monitoring of the heart rate, arterial blood pressure, and electrocardiogram is required in the testing protocol. Without the exercise test the physical educator can only rely on previous experience. The selection of activities may not be in the best interests of the participant's current state of cardiorespiratory conditioning. The science of physiological assessment is well-established. Assessment must be required of all participants in an exercise program.

Individual. *Axiom—Individually Prescribed Exercise Programs Can Be Quantified and Evaluated.* Each man enters an exercise program with a varied background of physical experiences. Traditional programs where all participants perform the same activity are met with disfavor and negative attitudes. Insofar as possible, a program designed to meet individual needs is desirable. When men have similar performance capabilities, they can be taught to work in pairs or small groups, but each participant must feel that what is being prescribed for him is unique to his abilities.

Education. *Axiom—Learning Influences Behavior.* Education is an ongoing process in an exercise program. Incidental teaching and information on the subjects of posture, respiration, orthopedic problems, or energy expenditure should be included in all activity sessions. Man often is not educated in the cognitive aspects of physical activity. The time spent in education may provide the basis for a lifesaving decision on energy expenditure at a later date.

Enjoyable activity. *Axiom–Man Seeks Pleasure and Avoids Discomfort.* Standard exercise programs have the following format: warmup, calisthenics, game, and cool-down. Aging man tends to dislike calisthenics; not only do they put him in uncompromising positions, but also, calisthenics tend to be dull and boring. If man is to sustain interest in an exercise program, every effort should be made to provide a wide variety of physical activities that are enjoyable.

Program Activities

The exercise leader's responsibility, in addition to leading enjoyable activity, should include activities selected with these characteristics: (1) therapeutic, (2) dynamic, (3) aerobic, (4) programmed at a viable intensity, (5) recreational, (6) noncompetitive, and (7) relaxing to the participant.

Therapeutic. *Axiom–Therapeutic Exercise Improves the Quality of Muscle– Strength, Power, Elasticity, and Endurance.* A previously sedentary man may encounter a variety of orthopedic problems of the trunk and extremities as he engages in physical activity. Furthermore, former orthopedic ligament or joint problems may be aggravated when participating in activities which are contra-indicated. Therefore, the physical activity leader must interview the new participant to establish a medical history for his own use. If, through muscle testing or goniometry, segments require increased levels of muscle strength, routines of therapeutic exercise should be developed. It is known that muscle endurance is gained rapidly when desirable strength levels have been attained.

Attention should be paid to the extremities of the arm and leg when throwing, catching, or kicking sport balls. If the mechanics of these gross motor movements are faulty, the participant could incur injuries or aggravate weak joints. Each individual exercise prescription must contain specific recommendations based on scientific determinations; these determinations include the assessment of muscle strength and the range of motion of a segment.

The participant must be educated to judge whether or not certain activities will be tried or practiced. For example, if a middle-aged participant had a medial ligament instability, jogging with an abducted and everted foot strike could result in pain and discomfort. If, in addition, the participant was asked to foot-dribble a soccer ball with his instep, unnecessary strain would be placed on the medial ligament. The solution to the problem would be to teach the participant to jog with the foot pointed straight ahead and if soccer dribbling is performed, that it be done with the outside portion of the foot. Similar examples would apply to a variety of orthopedic problems: foot, ankle, spine, or upper extremity. Attention to the therapeutic aspects of the exercise program is in the best interest of the participant and the exercise leader must determine the recommended activity as well as the intensity and duration of the therapeutic exercise. Therapeutic exercise of a dynamic type which encourages hyperemia is necessary. Isometric or static exercises should be avoided. Medicine balls, multi-stationed weight machines, or weights moved through a complete range of motion are recommended.

Dynamic aerobic activity. *Axiom—Performance Capability Improves with Exercise Programs Meeting Two or Three Times Weekly, from 20 to 40 Minutes in Duration, and of an Intensity of 60 to 80 Percent of the Test Aerobic Power.* The objective of an intervention and rehabilitation program is to increase the participant's performance capabilities. To meet this objective, the participant should sustain a form of locomotion over a prescribed period of time. The length of the aerobic portion of the exercise program should be at least 20 minutes in duration. During the aerobic portion, the participant sustains his movement through a variety of locomotions—walking, jogging, running, or swimming. This can be done with or without sporting equipment. He must also maintain an acceptable velocity.

The intensity of the aerobic component of the exercise session is determined by selecting a target heart rate and a percentage of the participant's tested aerobic power. Participants move alone, in pairs, or in small groups, keeping in mind that they have their own exercise prescription which may differ from those of other men. Relays and interval work while moving at a prescribed velocity give variation to an otherwise monotonous program. Periodic heart rates of 15-second duration provide the exercise leader and the participant with meaningful information on the intensity of the workload. When the participant exceeds the target heart rate or feels signs of stress, the intensity of the movement is decreased, but the participant continues the activity at a lower level. Increased performance capabilities do occur when the exercise prescription based on treadmill or ergometry testing is established at 60-80 percent of the man's tested maximum aerobic power. With a high-risk population to include postmyocardial infarct subjects, the aerobic prescription must be determined with consideration of the man's state of deconditioning and his adaptation to the work.

Viable intensity. *Axiom—Physiological Adaptation Occurs when the Workload Remains Constant; to Improve a Man's Aerobic Capacity, the Intensity of Training Must be Increased.* Conditioning adult men requires a gentle application of stress which is increased as individual adjustment occurs to a given workload. At the time of accession to a physical exercise program, baseline measures obtained during bicycle ergometry or treadmill testing are the bases for the exercise prescription. The physical activity leader must remember that a superior graded exercise test result does not mean that the participant would be able to comfortably perform exercise of 40-minute duration. The muscular system and its response to stress may impair sustained efforts.

Every effort should be made to gradually introduce the participant to the exercise program. For the safety of the participant, it is recommended that early sessions leave the man feeling that the work accomplished did not tax him to a point of general fatigue, or to the point of feeling uncomfortable. As he adapts to the exercise program, there should be a moderate increase in intensity; this increase would be governed by successive graded exercise tests or heart rate responses to known workloads. Realistic goals of velocity or distance covered should be established. Predetermined end points are also desirable. Intensity can be increased by sustaining a given activity over time (distance), decreasing the rest periods during interval-type work, or increasing the velocity of the pre-scribed work. At all times the subjective feeling of the participant and objective evaluations of the physical activity leader are important.

Recreational. *Axiom—Age Is Not a Deterrent to a Motivated Man in the Learning of New Physical Skills.* It is never too late for aging man to learn a new physical skill, sport, or game. There will be many times when the participant will not be able to attend a specific gymnasium for physical activity. Physical activity must be taken on a regular basis if a training effect is to result. The physical activity leader should teach a variety of activities which the participant can do in his leisure time, either as an individual, with his family, or with friends. Aerobic activities such as walking, jogging, and running require comfortable foot apparel, time, and interest in sustaining human movement. The *scouts pace* of jogging 100 double paces, and walking 100 paces, or of a progressive step-interval work-out can be designed.

In progressive programs the participant walks 10 double steps, jogs 10 double steps, walks 20 double steps, jogs 20 double steps . . . walks 50 steps, jogs 50 steps . . . walks 100 double steps, jogs 100 double steps, and so forth, regressing in intensity until he returns to the initial starting workload of walking and jogging 10 double steps. Other variations may be to jog from one street sign to another (approximate distance of 100 yards), walking one block, and jog again. Other recreational activities would include kicking or throwing various types of sport balls and jogging after them. Cement or brick walls may also be used while throwing or kicking sport balls or long, sustained comfortable walks can be taken anywhere at any time.

The need for physical activity must be imparted through education. It is never too late to learn bicycling, roller-skating, ice-skating, cross-country skiing, rowing, or swimming. Man is a social being and he tends to enjoy these activities with others, but this does not preclude him from undertaking safe, enjoyable activities on his own if he understands the extent to which he can be com-fortably stressed.

Noncompetitive. *Axiom—Man Does Not Always Do What He Wishes To Do—Fortunately!* A high-risk middle-aged man who was previously vigorous in undertaking sports such as paddle-ball, tennis, handball, and community basket-ball, may be required to withdraw from these physically intensive activities. Most often the intensity of the activity and the competitive aspect are dele-terious to the well-being of a high-risk participant. The hard-driving businessman with a variety of responsibilities and constant need for decisionmaking should be provided with activities which are not rehearsals for his full-time occupation.

In the American society there tends to be artificial standards of perfection. For the young, these are excellent goals for which to strive. For the middle-aged man, whose capability has decreased for executing gross motor skills in a fluid and efficient manner, a realistic decision should be made. The activity leader must provide the atmosphere of play for its own sake. It is more important to strike the volleyball than to score the point. It is also more important to play the game than being on the winning side. Too many games players are concerned with the winning point and the winning side rather than playing the game. To strive for perfection is admirable but it relegates the less proficient participant to the role of being the person who is the last out, who cannot serve, or who catches the ball rather than striking it sharply. Rotating members within the team during games or setting premature closures on what is necessary to terminate the activity are methods that the physical activity leader can use to minimize the competitive aspects inherent to any games situation.

Relaxing. *Axiom—The Antithesis of Exercise Is Relaxation.* Programs of physical activity should place stress on a man short of the point of fatigue. This means that controlled and supervised activity should extend the man but not exhaust him. The man likewise should be taught to recognize and make value judgments on the extent of his participation. If a noontime program finds the participant tired in the afternoon and uncomfortable in the evening, he has done too much. Every effort should be made to lead physical activity so that the participant has sufficient reserves available to enjoy leisure time. An exercise program should leave the man feeling comfortably tired as a result of the exercise experience. The adage that *it hurts good* is not applicable to a high-risk adult population.

Participant motivation. *Axiom—Life Is Short but Boredom Lengthens It.* To assure desirable levels of attendance and adherence to a physical activity program, the physical activity leader must be concerned with the attitude and motivation of the participant. Too often negative attitudes toward physical activity are the result of previous unpleasant experiences acquired through exercise. The activity leader must determine, through interview or questionnaire, essential background material on the participant's physical recreation experiences, skills, hobbies, and interest in exercise. Through interview and discussion, the exercise leader is in a position to make intelligent decisions regarding the type of activity the participant would enjoy.

To sustain the motivation of the participant is another problem. Regular attendance and participation are necessary to the training regime. Improved cardiorespiratory responses occur systematically through participation. Every effort must be made to sustain interest and adherence to the exercise commitment. Man's interest tends to wain when activities are routine or boring. The activity leader must provide a variety of sports and games which serve to keep the participant's interest at a high level. Methods of sustaining interest include participant report cards, social events, physician participation, and information dissemination. In other words, the participant should receive maximum feedback on his progress.

Summary

The principles of conducting exercise programs reflect the science and art in current prevention, intervention, and rehabilitative physical activity programs. Man's performance capabilities can be evaluated. Training regimes to improve performance can be written. The art of leading men rests with the phrase, *Man is Creative.* In the text, principles were related to the requirements of the exercise program and criteria for the selection of program activities. The success of the leader rests with his ability to motivate others to perform. His ability to innovate and create new activities is desirable. In the future, it is hoped, physical educators and members of the medical profession will continue to work together as a team.

21

THE USE OF EXERCISE TEST RESULTS
IN VOCATIONAL REHABILITATION OF CARDIAC CLIENTS

Sterling B. Brinkley, M.D.

Attention is directed, in various parts of this volume, to techniques for measuring the abilities (physiological, psychological, and social) of persons disabled by coronary heart disease (CHD), or who are coronary-prone. These measurements help to evaluate a cardiovascular condition, develop a rational treatment, and enhance function. They serve as guides for clinicians, for they help individuals to establish life-styles appropriate to their condition.

Vocational rehabilitation was defined by Corbett Reedy, who emphasized that vocational rehabilitation is goal-oriented; that vocational rehabilitation asks, "Conditioning for what purpose?" and that the purpose of vocational rehabilitation is to help the individual regain the ability to work. We believe that work is an essential ingredient for quality of living. We have seen too many people who quit too soon, *sitting on porches, watching the cars go by.* I have also been impressed by the numbers who die within a year or two after retirement. I have wondered if the stimulus of work did not, in fact, give life itself.

In our industrial, increasingly urban society, vocational rehabilitation is a very complicated process. In the course of a cardiac disability, when should vocational rehabilitation services be provided? What services should be provided, when, and by whom? Studies show that 80 to 90 percent of persons who have had their first myocardial infarction (MI) are back at work 24 months after their infarction. This makes me wonder whether or not the vocational rehabilitation approach could do a better job than is being done presently with the help of many different *hands* and the natural healing process of the body.

It is anticipated that broadscale research studies will answer some of the questions about the role of vocational rehabilitation in serving persons with CHD; I am confident that when these studies are completed, the vocational rehabilitation program will design its services accordingly.

Exercise Tests in Vocational Rehabilitation

In discussing the use of exercise test results in the vocational rehabilitation of cardiac clients, it is important to point out situations when a knowledge of functional capacity of the heart (or the heart and lungs) is critical, or at least helpful, in the vocational rehabilitation process.

When a client has a history of MI and his work skills require relatively heavy exertion for a high portion of his workday, the rehabilitation plan could involve conditioning him to a level sufficiently above the job requirement to enable safe return to the job he held previously. Another approach is to develop a conditioning with modification of some elements of his work activity. For example, there might be substitutions for the highest energy activities, or the use of special equipment to substitute for muscular work, or the development of work-rest schedules. There are various ways to modify the energy requirement of the job itself.

The rehabilitation plan could involve training and conditioning for work at a lower level of energy requirement with vocational training in a different, less arduous occupation, along with counseling, and job placement. The plan of choice would be determined, in large measure, by the results of exercise tests and the desires and motivation of the individual. Testing after physical conditioning would be the most important single way to make this judgment.

In vocational rehabilitation, special attention should be given to stress testing if the individual's job involves the safety of others. Of particular concern are high-risk occupations such as airline pilots, truck drivers, taxi drivers, and those who work in heavy construction also affect the safety of many others. These workers should be carefully evaluated with an appropriate exercise stress test.

In work classification units, the greatest problem of persons who are referred is in the mind rather than in the heart. Exercise testing, testing before certification for return to work, can be used effectively to reassure the individual. Also, the conditioning activities help the individual fearful of sustaining another heart attack to gain confidence that he can safely return to certain occupations. Work settings which have been used to train individuals (work settings in place of exercises in gym or clinic) have a very important role in vocational rehabilitation. Work skills can be developed which reduce the amount of energy that must be used to accomplish a specific task.

In my 20s I was in very good physical condition. When I got on the other end of a crosscut saw with a man in his 60s who did not appear to be in good condition, in short order I was ready to quit and he was ready to take on another young man. He knew *how* to use the saw.

Uses of Exercise Testing

Where else would exercise testing be useful? One of the problems of the disabled is the architectural barrier to normal functioning. When I walk out of New York subways, I am reminded that an individual has to possess a high level of physical fitness to use subways. Public awareness of the energy requirements of subway steps and the exercise capabilities of great numbers of persons using subways would be helpful in removing architectural barriers.

There is ongoing work at the University of Alabama in various types of prostheses for hip disarticulation. The researchers are testing such prostheses in the individual and determining how much energy various activities, such as walking, require. The same approach used to test the condition of an individual can be used to test his ability to use various prostheses and to perform certain activities.

How can the vocational counselor be involved with you in encouraging the use of exercise testing in the areas where you live? He is not in the position of ordering exercise testing for his clients, but may recommend such procedures. He is dependent on his district medical consultant for medical guidance and on the experts in his community. If, in a particular community, the leading cardiologists do not utilize exercise testing, the vocational counselor is in no position to encourage its use. He can work with the American Heart Association or other interested groups in establishing such a program, possibly on an experimental basis, and if necessary, he can refer his client to more distant places for exercise testing. Basically, leadership in such areas depends on the medical profession, and the vocational rehabilitation program is always willing and able to assist.

In future programs, assessment of disability and assessment of potential for rehabilitation will be critical. Under the House of Representatives Bill, HR-1, the welfare bill, there may be categories termed *incapacity* as well as *disability*, where individuals will need screening for the ability to perform various activities involved in work. Incorporation of some exercise testing principles could be a very important and necessary part of this screening.

22

EARLY AMBULATION OF POST-MYOCARDIAL INFARCTION PATIENTS

A. EARLY ACTIVITY AFTER MYOCARDIAL INFARCTION

Joseph Acker, Jr., M.D.

Traditionally, the patient with an acute myocardial infarction (MI) was treated by severely restricting his activities. Prolonged bed rest reduced the work load for the heart while it was healing. During bed rest, there was increased risk of embolization; deconditioning of the whole patient occurred; and the patient's tendency to become an invalid was enhanced.

In 1952, Levine and Lown [1] reported the results of early armchair treatment of the MI patient. They demonstrated a 23 percent reduction in cardiac output after the patient was lifted from his bed to a chair. Though safe and practical, their recommendations were not readily accepted.

Saltin et al [2] studied the effects of prolonged bed rest followed by heavy training in a group of five young normal subjects. The most striking effect of 20 days of bed rest was a significant decrease in maximum oxygen intake, stroke volume, and cardiac output. The maximum oxygen intake decreased from 3.3 l/min in the control study to 2.4 l/min after prolonged bed rest. The stroke volume decreased approximately 30 percent and cardiac output 15 percent during submaximal upright exercise. The heart rate at a comparable workload increased from 145 to 180 beats per minute. After 50 days of twice daily rigorous physical training all parameters exceeded the control state.

Level of Activity

Brock et al [3] demonstrated marked enhancement of exercise capacity after supervised physical reconditioning programs for cardiac patients which began 3 to 4 weeks post-MI. Wenger [4] adapted her program to prevent the effects of deconditioning and to institute early reconditioning during phases I and II of the hospital stay, and phase III, home convalescence.

Our experience indicates that early activity after MI safely neutralizes the adverse effects usually associated with prolonged bed rest or "slow ambulation."

In our community hospital (St. Mary's Memorial Hospital), using facilities available to most medium-size cities, the emphasis has been on early ambulation, prevention of psychological problems, and education of the patient and his family.

When the patient is free of pain or complications of his MI, direction of his physical activities is begun. The physician may order successive increases in the patient's activities (and energy expenditure) by employing an Activity Level Order Sheet (TABLE I). Only one of the in-hospital activities requires more than 2 to 2½ METS[1] of energy expenditure. The use of bedpan or bedside commode requires 4 and 3 METS. These Activity Level Order Sheets are placed on each chart while the patient is in the Coronary Care Unit (CCU) or the Cardiac Rehabilitation Unit (CRU). The rate of ambulation depends upon the severity of the MI and the conservatism of the individual physician. The uncomplicated patient may progress from one activity level to the next on successive days, and occasionally may skip a level. Thus by the 9th or 10th day the patient with an uncomplicated MI may begin walking in the hall for 5 minutes, four times daily.

---

[1] The approximate energy requirement of sitting quietly in a chair.

TABLE I

Activity Level Order Sheet

(St. Mary's Memorial Hospital, Knoxville, Tenn.)

Stage	Level of Activity	METS [1]	Daily Living Activities	METS [1]
I.	Complete bed rest	1	May turn self	1
			Watch TV & Radio	
			Complete bath (when stable)	1
II.	Complete bed rest	1	May be shaved	1
			Feed self	1
			Lift onto bedside commode	3
			or bedpan	4
			(specify bedside commode or bedpan on doctor's orders)	
III.	Complete bed rest	1	Read newspaper	1
			Wash face and hands	2
			and brush teeth	2
IV.	Dangle feet 5 minutes – T.I.D.	1	Shave self	2
			Make up face	2
			Comb hair	2
			Up on bedside commode	3
V.	Dangle feet 10 minutes – T.I.D.		Same	
VI.	In bedside chair 10 minutes – T.I.D.	1	Same	
VII.	Up in chair 15 minutes – T.I.D.	1	Begin partial bath	2
VIII.	Up in chair 15 minutes – Q.I.D. Walk 1-2 minutes in room each time up	1 2	Progressive bath Bathroom privileges if bath- room adjoining–if not, bathroom in wheelchair	2 2
IX.	Walk in hall 5 minutes each time up	2	Self-care Dressing, undressing, etc.	2
X.	Up ad lib	2	Same	

---

[1] METS – Metabolic Equivalent – one MET· is tne approximate energy expenditure while sitting quietly in a chair.

Contraindications

At the other extreme, a patient with extensive damage or impairment may stay at a very low level of activity for several days. The severity may be gauged by the presence of shock, heart failure, persistent arrhythmias, or markedly elevated serum enzyme levels. Shock will have been corrected before activity is permitted. Controlled heart failure and persistent, but stable, arrhythmias are relative contraindications to progressive physical activity. It may take the more severely ill patient as long as 2 to 3 weeks to progress to activity level X. During this period, they are limited to sitting in the bedside chair or moving to the bathroom. We advocate early use of the chair and bedside commode, with higher levels such as walking being delayed in such patients.

TABLE II

Adverse response to increased activity

Chest pain
Dyspnea
Heart rate above 110
ST-T abnormality
Significant arrhythmia
Systolic blood pressure decrease in excess of 20 mm

Precautions for increasing activities are depicted in TABLE II. The most important symptoms are chest pain, undue dyspnea, or a feeling of weakness. Aside from the general appearance of the patient, a heart rate of 110 beats per minute is the most important objective indication of an adverse response. If any one of these occur, the physician should be more cautious in increasing activity levels.

Prior to discharge from the hospital, the patient is instructed in an exercise program which will eventually require 3½ to 4 METS of energy expenditure before he returns to work. Within a week after arriving home, he is encouraged to walk in the yard, and then down the street. He exercises 2 to 3 times a day. By gradually increasing the distance he walks each time, the average uneventful, angina-free, uncomplicated cardiac patient can walk a mile at his own comfortable pace within 4 to 6 weeks post-MI. He can then increase his distance to develop more endurance. The speed of walking is assessed by measuring the time required to cover a given distance, and a gradual increase in speed to 3 to 3½ miles per hour is reached by the average patient before he returns to work. During this period, adverse responses such as angina pectoris, undue fatigue, marked dyspnea, or heart rate response beyond 115 beats per minute indicate the need to decrease the walking speed or distance or both. Most patients need additional encouragement. This, and evaluation of a possible adverse response, can be performed by observing the patient while walking in the office, on stairs, over steps, on a bicycle ergometer, or on a treadmill.

This program of early activity [5], together with education of the patient and his family and special attention to psychological problems has resulted in an 11.6 percent increase in return to former employment in a group of 75 MI patients treated in our unit from July 1, 1969 through June 30, 1970. The average hospital stay was decreased by 3.6 days and the convalescence period was reduced an average of 21 days.

Summary

A program of supervised early activity for the postmyocardial infarction patient is described. Emphasis on an orderly, progressive increase in level of energy expenditure is stressed. This program resulted in 90 percent of the patients returning to their former or slightly modified employment. This program can be used in any community hospital, regardless of size.

REFERENCES

1. Levine, S.A., and Lown, B. Armchair treatment of acute coronary thrombosis. *J.A.M.A.* 148:1365, 1952.

2. Saltin, B., Blonquist, G., Mitchell, J.H., Johnson, R.L., Jr., Wildenthal, K., and Chapman, C.B. Response to exercise after bed rest and after training. *Circulation* Suppl. VII: 37-38, 1968.

3. Brock, L.L. Personal Communication.

4. Wenger, N.C. The use of exercise in the rehabilitation of patients after myocardial infarction. *J.S.C. Med. Assoc.* Vol. 65 Suppl. 1:66-68, 1969.

5. Acker, J.E., Jr. The cardiac rehabilitation unit: experiences with a program of early activation. *Circulation* 44: Suppl. 2:119, Oct. 1971.

B. EARLY RECONDITIONING
FOR POST-MYOCARDIAL INFARCTION PATIENTS:
SPALDING REHABILITATION CENTER

Loring Brock, M.D.

Spalding Rehabilitation Center is located in the center of the Midtown Hospital district of Denver, Colorado. There are four large general hospitals and one children's hospital in the area. Its cardiac rehabilitation program is an outgrowth of the Work Evaluation Unit of the Colorado Heart Association.

The principles used to develop the program were:

1. The experience of the Work Evaluation Unit indicated that many patients had a cardiac capacity to return to work, but failed to do so. The data indicated that motivational and fitness factors were not remedial at this late date. We were thus persuaded, in 1966, to develop an early intervention program using techniques familiar to the Work Evaluation Unit, which were applied in a preventive and therapeutic approach.

2. Studies reported by Naughton et al [1a], Gottheiner [1], Brunner [2], Kellermann [3], and Hellerstein [4] indicated that many cardiac patients could perform regular exercise and subsequently improve (TABLES I and II).

3. Studies reported by Gelfand [5], Philadelphia Work Evaluation Unit, indicated that psychological and motivational factors were the primary reasons that patients with otherwise adequate cardiopulmonary function did not return to work.

4. Saltin and Mitchell [6] reported that the functional capacity of normal subjects confined to bed rest for 3 weeks decreased approximately 33 percent. Frick [7], Varnouskas [8], and others reported hemodynamic improvement attending physical reconditioning of the cardiac patient. Recent work by Amsterdam [9] indicated that training reduced sympathetic activity in response to exercise.

These observations were used to develop a rehabilitation approach in a community setting. Patients were referred either during their convalescence from myocardial infarction (MI) or as out-patients 4 weeks or more after the MI. The major thrust of the program has been in the out-patient area. By applying the

TABLE I

One-year followup in two comparable groups of
postmyocardial infarction patients [2]

	Active reconditioning	Without active reconditioning
Number of patients	64	65
Recurrent MI	4	9
Fatalities	2	7
Anginal pains on effort	0	30

TABLE II

Physical working capacity of actively rehabilitated and nonrehabilitated coronary patients (age group 40 to 60) [3]

Category	Physical working capacity (watts/min)	Percent of normal
Healthy	112.5	100
Actively rehabilitated		
Before rehabilitation	64.1	57
After rehabilitation	93.3	83
"Self-rehabilitated"	81.0	72

previous principles, it was feasible to reduce the patients' anxiety and loss of fitness, hence to enhance the motivational, as well as the physiological capacity of patients to return to work or to attain other rehabilitation goals. Since loss of fitness and confidence reinforce each other during the second and third month following an infarct, the timing of the program's initiation 4 weeks after an MI was not arbitrary. Although physicians provide rehabilitation in their offices, it is usually insufficient due to the patients' infrequent visits and inadequate time spent with them, insufficient facilities and expertise in the areas of social, psychological, vocational, and dietary needs. Our programs were more successful when wives were involved in the rehabilitation process. Group psychotherapy among the patients also enhanced the program.

Methods

First visit. History of an acute event, risk factors, continuing symptoms, complications, medications, and previous exercise experience are documented.

Examination of the cardiovascular system for enlargement, gallop rhythms, arrhythmias, murmurs, evidence of fluid retention, hyperlipidemia, premature vascular aging, a resting electrocardiogram and chest x-ray, serum cholesterol and triglycerides are performed.

Second visit. Exercise tolerance is determined for low-level exercise, on a motor-driven treadmill, with the onset of angina pectoris (AP), arrhythmia, major ECG changes, dyspnea, or predetermined heart rate approximating 65 percent of the age—adjusted maximum serving as end points. The mean level of tolerated exercise during this period is 2 mph on a 7.5 percent grade or an oxygen consumption of about 13 ml/kg body weight (4 METS).

Third visit. Exercise tolerance is determined with a bicycle ergometer using similar end points. The blood pressure response on the bicycle is likely to be higher than on the treadmill. The average workload attained by patients at this time was 332 kpm/min (O_2 intake 13/ml/kg/min). Social services and vocational counseling are initiated. When data on blood lipids are received, appropriate dietary prescription counseling is begun, if indicated.

Fourth through twenty-eighth visits. Exercise in a gym (TABLE III) is conducted 3 times a week for 1 hour between 9:30 A.M. and 12 noon under the supervision of a physical therapist or exercise physiologist. Each patient has a daily prescription sheet based on his previous treatment session and any change in symptoms between the two sessions is noted. The patient is taught to count his heart rate after each exercise modality. The heart rate response, in part, influences the prescription that is developed for the following day.

Twenty-ninth visit. The patient is retested on the treadmill to the same workload he achieved originally and thereafter. The workload is increased periodically until he reaches the heart rate approximating 75 to 80 percent of his age—adjusted maximum—unless he develops symptoms or other abnormal signs.

Thirtieth visit. The patient returns for a bicycle test similar to the third visit and a chest x-ray; resting ECG and blood lipids are remeasured. He has another interview with the vocational, social, and dietary counselors.

When the data are accumulated, the patient meets with the director to review the entire program experience for his continuing exercise prescription, as well as for other risk factor modification advice. He is evaluated 6 months later in a similar fashion.

During the course of the program, the patient and the spouse meet with the director and dietitian to discuss the nature of his illness, the treatment, and the secondary intervention. Those patients who wish to continue in the program are permitted to do so.

Results

One hundred and twenty-six patients were evaluated during 2½ years. Eleven were rejected for reasons which included congestive heart failure, psychosis, or an unwillingness to cooperate. The average age of the group was 52; eight were women and the remainder men (TABLE IV).

TABLE III

Spalding Rehabilitation Center
EXERCISE RECORD

NAME ___Peterson, Don___   DATE ___November 1, 1971___

RESTING PULSE ___84___   RESTING BLOOD PRESSURE ___128/80___

| EXERCISE | WORKLOAD | | | ml/kg | HEART RATE RESPONSES | | |
	Duration (min)	Ex. Rate	METS	$\dot{V}_{O_2}$	Immediate	Increase	3' Rate
Calisthenics	4	#12,14, 20,29			100	16	84
Treadmill	4½	3 mph 7½%	6	21	120	36	84
Pulleys	4	4 wts × 2			108	24	84
Bicycle	5	600 kgm	6	19	108	24	84
Dumbbells	2½	20 lbs × 2 60 cpm			100	16	84
Rowing	4	12/m			100	16	84
Barbell	2½	45# @ 6/m			112	24	84
Steps	3½	16" @ 12/m	5.5	18	108	24	84
Other							

General symptoms and signs: None   Weigh out: 175   Total exercise time (min): 30

In 88 percent, the diagnosis on entry to the study was MI; 4 percent had AP; 4 percent post-bypass coronary surgery; and the remaining 4 percent a combination of other diagnoses. The patients, referred by 70 different physicians, were treated for their acute illnesses at 18 different hospitals.

Significant complications had occurred during the acute hospital phase of illness 46 times in 40 patients. These complications included five cardiac arrests; five insertions of cardiac pacemakers; 13 episodes of congestive heart failure; 11 episodes of significant arrhythmias, and two episodes of cardiogenic shock.

Complications. There were no complications in the gym sessions (TABLE V). One patient developed an infarct during the day between sessions. One patient

TABLE IV

Cardiac reconditioning–SRC

Patients

Total in program	114
Average age (years)	52
Myocardial infarct	89
Angina pectoris	4
Bypass	2
Arrythmia	1
Psychophysiological reaction	1
Cardiac neurosis	3
Hypertensive HTD	1
RHD	1
ASD	1
Not accepted	11

TABLE V

Cardiac reconditioning–SRC
Complications after program in 73 patients with MI

Cumulative months observation: 959
Cumulative years observation: 80

Complications	*Number*	*Incidence/Year*
Death (cardiac)	2	2.5%
Re-infarction	2	2.5%

developed a cardiac arrest after finishing the program, which occurred while waiting for a scheduled appointment with the director. His heart was defibrillated; he was hospitalized; coronary arteriography was performed; and subsequently, coronary bypass surgery was performed. He returned to the program 4 weeks after surgery, completed a second 8-week program, and subsequently returned to full-time employment. Three patients developed incipient myocardial insufficiency while in the program; only two showed significant congestive phenomena. Six patients had selective coronary arteriography during the course of the program because of persistent symptoms of AP, excessive tachycardia, gallop rhythm, or arrhythmias. Coronary venous bypass surgery was performed on three patients during their participation in the program. During the 2-year followup period, four others developed recurrent MIs. Two of these subjects died and two recovered and returned to the program.

Employment status. Ten patients retired prior to suffering MIs; three retired after having sustained an MI; and three were within a year of regular retirement. Eighty-four patients returned to work, almost all to the same jobs; two remained unemployed; two were in training with Vocational Rehabilitation; one in a sheltered workshop. The remainder are currently in the program.

Physiologic data. The physiologic data are summarized in TABLES VI-X.

TABLE VI

Cardiac reconditioning—SRC (70)

OXYGEN CONSUMPTION ($\dot{V}_{O_2}$)

	Pretraining	Posttraining
Treadmill		
Total ml/min	999	1688
Range	474-1650	510-2585
Increase	— —	69%
ml/kgm bw/min	13	22.2
Range	6-24.5	7-28
Increase	— —	70%
Bicycle		
Total ml/min	960	1387
Range	600-1500	900-1950
Increase	— —	44%
ml/kgm bw/min	12.9	18.4
Range	8.3-20	13.4-25
Increase	— —	42%

TABLE VII

Cardiac reconditioning—SRC (70)

OXYGEN CONSUMPTION CHANGE ($\dot{V}_{O_2}$)

		− −10-0%	0 Unchanged	+ 0-9%	+ 10-24%	+ 25-49%	+ 50-99%	+ 100-up
Treadmill	no. pts.	0	1	2	7	18	31	11
Bicycle Ergometer	no. pts.	0	0	1	5	30	30	4

TABLE VIII

Cardiac reconditioning—SRC (70)

BICYCLE ERGOMETER

Workload kpm/min	Pretraining	Posttraining
Mean	332.19	545.15
Range	150-600	300-825

Percent increase: 64%

Workload Changes (kpm/min)

NUMBER OF PATIENTS	− −10-0%	0 Unchanged	+ 0-9%	+ 10-24%	+ 25-49%	+ 50-99%	+ 100-up
	0	5	0	7	14	25	19

TABLE IX

Heart rate responses to treadmill and bicycle ergometer—SRC

	Pretraining	Posttraining	% change
BICYCLE ERGOMETER			
Maximum	104	119.5	+13.3%
% age adj. max.	63	71.4	+ 8.4%
Increase over resting	28.4	45.5	+61.0%
TREADMILL			
Maximum	103.2	122.1	+18.0%
% age adj. max.	63.3	73.2	+10.0%
Increase over resting	28.1	47.02	+64.0%
TREADMILL AT 2MPH, 7½% GRADE	101	94.3	− 6.9%

TABLE X

Cardiac reconditioning (70)

O_2 Pulse Determinations

	Pretraining	Posttraining
Mean $\triangle \dot{V}_{O_2}$ (ml/kg/min)	9.3	18.7
Mean $\triangle HR$	31.79	51.04
Mean $\triangle O_2$ pulse	.292	.366

Improvement: 25.4%
$\triangle$: Increase over resting

Summary

Most patients participating in the program have made an excellent recovery and exhibit return of confidence. Graded exercise tests on the treadmill before and after the 8-week treatment period (TABLE VI) indicated a 70-percent increased O_2 consumption after the treatment. This represents the increased workload. Less increase was noted on the bicycle ergometer. TABLE VII reveals that 60 percent were increased by at least 50 percent and 16 percent increased their O_2 intake by at least 100 percent. TABLE VIII reveals a mean increase of 213 kpm (64 percent) in workload on the bicycle ergometer. TABLE IX depicts the mean changes in heart rate in testing before and after the program, which, on the average, were 103 and 121 beats/min respectively, 4 and 12 weeks after the MI. On the average level of 2 mph, 7½ percent grade test before and after treatment, a decreased heart rate of 6.9 percent was noted.

TABLES X and XI reveal the oxygen pulse as represented by the increased O_2 intake and heart rate. It was noted that approximately 25 percent improvement in O_2 transport or related heart rate occurred. All patients resettled in a satisfactory vocational or retirement way of life. There were no significant complications during the performance of the program although three individuals

TABLE XI

Cardiac reconditioning (70)

O_2 Pulse Determinations

	Pretraining	Posttraining
Mean $\triangle \dot{V}_{O_2}$ (total—ML)	702	1412
Mean $\triangle$ HR	31.79	51.04
Mean O_2 pulse	22.08	27.68

Improvement: 25.4%

exhibited insufficient myocardial or coronary reserve for long-term participation in the program. In general, patients who evidenced poor ventricular function due to coronary insufficiency and were amenable to surgical intervention or to drug therapy, did return to the program after appropriate therapy. Former patients who suffered recurrent episodes of MI returned to the program for subsequent treatment.

This type of program requires close rapport between the referring physician and the medical director, and between the patient and the team members working with him.

Initially, financing was arranged by the Colorado Heart Association and the Spalding Rehabilitation Center. A portion of the patient's participation is now financed through third party coverage. Survival of this type of program eventually depends upon broad insurance coverage for a large sector of the population.

The local heart associations cannot be expected to subsidize such programs indefinitely. Additional support for programs will probably require other forms of activity such as preventive large-scale screening and detection programs, standard stress testing to detect heart disease, disability evaluation, and programs for exercise prescription testing.

REFERENCES

1. Gottheiner, V. Long-range strenuous sports training for cardiac reconditioning and rehabilitation. *Am. J. Cardiol.* 22:426, 1968.

1a. Naughton, J., Lategola, M., and Shaubaur, K. A physical rehabilitation program for cardiac patients. *Am. J. Med. Sci.* 242:545, 1966.

2. Brunner, D., and Meskulam, N. Prevention of recurrent myocardial infarction by physical exercise. *Isr. J. Med. Sci.* 5:783, 1969.

3. Kellerman, J., Modan, B., Levy, M., et al. Return to work after myocardial infarction: Comparative study of rehabilitated and non-rehabilitated patients. *Geriatrics* 23:151-156, 1968.

4. Hellerstein, H. Exercise therapy in coronary disease. *Bull. N.Y. Acad. Med.* 44:1028, 1968.

5. Gelfand, D. Cardiac Work Classification Unit of Southeastern Pennsylvania (Philadelphia): *Work and the Heart*, pp. 322-329. Scranton, Pa., Harper & Row (Hoeber), 1959.

6. Saltin, B., Mitchell, J., Blomquist, G., et al. Response to exercise after bedrest and after training. *Circulation* 38: (Suppl. VII), November 1968.

7. Frick, G. The effect of physical training in manifest ischemic heart disease. *Circulation* Vol. XL, No. 4 (October, 1969).

8. Varnauskas, E., Bergman, H., et al. Hemodynamic effects of physical training in coronary patients. *Lancet* 2:8, 1966.

9. Amsterdam, E. What's New in Myocardial Infarction, presented at Snowmass at Aspen, *American College of Cardiology*, January, 1972. (In press)

C. EARLY AMBULATION AFTER MYOCARDIAL INFARCTION: GRADY MEMORIAL HOSPITAL– EMORY UNIVERSITY SCHOOL OF MEDICINE

Nanette K. Wenger, M.D.

The advent of the Coronary Care Unit (CCU) substantially decreased the mortality rate of patients hospitalized for myocardial infarction (MI); the emphasis of rehabilitation programming is an enhanced quality of life for the increasing number of patients who survive MI. This chapter considers one aspect of the rehabilitation effort: a carefully supervised, gradually progressive, early intervention physical activity program.

The immediate objective of a physical activity program is to decrease the physical and psychologic disabilities associated with MI, i.e., to overcome the deleterious or *deconditioning* effects of prolonged bed rest and to decrease the anxiety and depression associated with MI by a systematic, progressive plan for return toward normal living. Both epidemiologic data and uncontrolled observations suggest possible long-term beneficial effects of a physical activity program on the natural history of coronary heart disease (CHD) including a reduction in the incidence of and the mortality from recurrent MI [1].

Bed Rest

There is also increasing documentation that prolonged, strict bed rest, long the traditional therapy for MI patients [2], is associated with deleterious physiologic changes. Prolonged bed rest results in diminution of the physical work capacity. Even healthy young adults, kept at strict bed rest for 3 weeks, sustain a decrease of 20 to 25 percent in their maximal oxygen intake, a good index of the aerobic work capacity [3]. The *deconditioning* effects of extended strict bed rest also include an increased heart rate response to effort and a decreased adaptability to change in posture, manifested primarily by orthostatic hypotension. These may, in part, be due to a diminution of the circulating blood volume, which may decrease by as much as a liter after 4 weeks of bed rest [4].

Patients with congestive heart failure, whose circulating blood volume is not depleted, do not manifest this decreased adaptability to postural change after prolonged bed rest [5]. The plasma volume decreases to a greater extent than the red blood cell mass and the increased blood viscosity, coupled with venous stasis, may predispose the patient to thromboembolic phenomena. Other deleterious effects of bed rest include a decrease in the lung volume and vital capacity, a decreased serum protein concentration, a negative nitrogen and calcium balance, and a decrease in the contractile strength of the muscles by as much as 10 to 15 percent for each week of physical inactivity [6].

Physical Activity Program

During the past 6 years, over 2,000 patients hospitalized for an acute coronary event or definite MI at Grady Memorial Hospital and the Emory University School of Medicine participated in a supervised, early intervention physical activity program. This 14-step series of progressively increasing physical activity levels involves three areas: actual exercises, activities of daily living, particularly self-care; and educational and recreational activities [7]. A patient is eligible for the rehabilitation program when his clinical condition stabilizes and he is free of the major complications of MI (heart failure, shock, persistent or recurrent chest pain, or significant arrhythmia).

The early phases of the program are often begun while the patient is in the CCU. Physical activities are permitted which require a low-level oxygen demand. These include self-care (feeding, sharing, and the use of a bedside commode), and supervised active and passive movements of the upper and lower extremities. The latter movements are designed to decrease venous stasis and to maintain muscle tone. Systematic progressive ambulation affords the patient tangible and realistic reassurance, and it is associated with a decrease in the level of anxiety commonly encountered in the first days of hospitalization [8]. The patient progresses initially to chair rest, then to walks in the room, and later to walks in the hospital corridor. He is usually allowed to climb a flight of steps prior to discharge from the hospital. The various physical activities are interspersed with rest periods, and physical activity is avoided immediately after meals when the patient is not in a near-basal state. Isometric exercises are avoided because of the increased workload they impose on the left ventricle, with the danger of provoking arrhythmias. Patient and family education programs and diversional activities parallel the graded physical activities. Provision of information and education for the patient and family and a progressive ambulation program constitute the structured plan for the return of the patient toward normal living. This education and physical activity help allay the depression which characteristically appears during the third or fourth day after MI, and which may persist for days or weeks [9]. The inpatient program is designed to enable the patient to attain the activity level required for self-care by the time he returns home, generally at 2 to 3 weeks [10].

The *homecoming depression* of post-MI patients, as described by investigators at the Massachusetts General Hospital, is triggered by the patient's awareness of weakness and fatigue upon returning home; it can be minimized or averted by an in-hospital physical activity program [11]. The early ambulation program merges into an outpatient program which is designed initially to increase endurance and permit the patient to return to work, and which later attempts to enhance cardiovascular function with more intensive exercise levels.

The physician determines the progression of physical activity levels, but the program can be implemented by nurses, therapists, and/or trained technologists and technicians.

During in-hospital physical activity, the patient is observed for breathlessness or chest pain; for heart rate and blood pressure response; and for ECG changes. The occurrence of chest pain or dyspnea, an increase in the heart rate to over 120 beats per minute, increased ST segment displacement on the ECG, the occurrence of significant arrhythmias, or a decrease in systolic blood pressure greater than 20 mm Hg below the control measurement indicate that a patient's response is disproportionate to the effort. In such situations, the level of physical activity is decreased for the patient.

Following these guidelines, an early intervention inpatient physical activity program appears to be safe. Only one patient in more than 2,000 had an episode of ventricular fibrillation. This occurred in a young man with second MI during passive range of motion exercises while still in the CCU. He was successfully resuscitated. No other episode of cardiac arrest, evidence of recurrent MI, sudden death, or other major catastrophe has occurred directly associated with or immediately related to the cardiac conditioning exercises.

The first 500 patients entered in the program had an average age of 58; about 50 percent had experienced prior angina pectoris, and about 40 percent prior MI. More than one-third reported a family history of CHD and over 50 percent were cigarette smokers. Forty percent had hypertension and 25 percent diabetes mellitus. Over one-third of the patients had ECG evidence of transmural MI and 50 percent had serial ST-T ECG changes of MI, with or without abnormal elevations of the serum enzyme levels. In 15 percent of the patients, the diagnosis of MI was based solely on the clinical history.

Our experience with an early intervention physical activity program has highlighted the increasing acceptance of the safety and advantages of early ambulation for the patient with uncomplicated MI, and has identified a number of areas where more information is needed.

We know that an early intervention physical activity program is feasible. A number of cardiovascular centers and community hospitals currently conduct supervised early ambulation programs. The known energy cost of specific activities appears comparable for apparently normal individuals and for patients with clinical evidence of CHD. They can guide the design of an early ambulation program. The documented deconditioning effects of bed rest provide a scientific basis for the implementation of physical activity programs. We also know that *apparently* increased physical activities, such as chair rest versus bed rest and the use of a bedside commode versus the use of a bedpan, actually involve a decreased oxygen cost for patients [13]. Knowledge of the physiologic response to isometric exercise warrants its exclusion from physical activity programs for patients with MI [14].

The available data [12, 15, 16, 17] appear to indicate that an early intervention physical activity program is safe, and that it is not associated with an increase in life-threatening arrhythmias, in recurrent MI, or in sudden death. Data from other studies also indicate that the anxiety and depression scores on standard psychologic tests [18] are reduced as a result of such programs. Saphenous vein thrombosis and thrombophlebitis are apparently decreased.

Areas for Further Study

Some problems which still require study include: (a) the assessment of the deleterious results of the *deconditioning* effects of extended bed rest for the patient with uncomplicated acute MI; (b) the immediate effect of early ambulation on non-life-threatening arrhythmias, and the long-term effect on left ventricular function; (c) the effectiveness of early intervention physical activity programs in preventing recurrent MI or sudden cardiac death, or in altering the total mortality from MI; (d) its effect on the patients' earlier and/or increased return to work, improvement in functional performance, and eventual psychologic status; and (e) the increased value, or possibly increased danger, of early ambulation programs for specific subgroups of patients after MI. The answers to these questions and their critical evaluation by well-designed, controlled studies are required to further refine management of patients with MI.

REFERENCES

1. Fox, S.M., III, Naughton, J.P., and Gorman, P.A. Physical activity and cardiovascular health, I. Potential for prevention of coronary heart disease and possible mechanisms, II. The exercise prescription: intensity and duration, III. The exercise prescription: frequency and type of activity. *Mod. Concepts Cardiovasc. Dis.* 41:17-30, 1972.

. 2. Duke, M. Bed rest in acute myocardial infarction. A study of physician practices. *Am. Heart J.* 82:486-491, 1971.

3. Saltin, B., Blomqvist, G., Mitchell, J.H., Johnson, R.L., Wildenthal, K., and Chapman, C.B. Response to exercise after bed rest and training. *Circulation* 38 (Suppl. 7):1-78, 1968.

4. Miller, P.B., Johnson, R.L., and Lamb, L.E. Effects of four weeks of absolute bed rest on circulatory functions in man. *Aerospace Med.* 35:1194-1200, 1964.

5. Fareeduddin, K., and Abelmann, W.H. Impaired orthostatic tolerance after bed rest in patients with myocardial infarction. *N. Engl. J. Med.* 280:345-350, 1969.

6. Bonner, C.D. Rehabilitation instead of bed rest? *Geriatrics* 24:109-118, 1969.

7. Wenger, N.K., Gilbert, C.A., and Siegel, W. Symposium: The use of physical activity in the rehabilitation of patients after myocardial infarction. *Southern Med. J.* 63:891-897, 1970.

8. Cassem, N.H., and Hackett, T.P. Psychiatric consultation in a coronary care unit. *Ann. Intern. Med.* 75:9-14, 1971.

9. Hackett, T.P., and Cassem, N.H. The psychological adaptation of myocardial infarction patients to convalescence. *In*, Naughton, J., and Hellerstein, H., Eds. *Exercise Testing and Exercise Training in Coronary Heart Disease.* New York, Academic, 1973.

10. Wenger, N.K., Hellerstein, H.K., Blackburn, H., and Castranova, S.J. Uncomplicated myocardial infarction. Current physician practice in patient management. *J.A.M.A.* In press.

11. Wishnie, H.A., Hackett, T.P., and Cassem, N.H. Psychological hazards of convalescence following myocardial infarction. *J.A.M.A.* 215:1292-1296, 1971.

12. Wenger, N.K., Gilbert, C.A., and Skorapa, M.Z. Cardiac conditioning after myocardial infarction. An early intervention program. *Cardiac Rehabil.* 2:17-22, 1971.

13. Benton, J.G., Brown, H., and Rusk, H.A. Energy expended by patients on the bedpan and bedside commode. *J.A.M.A.* 144:1443-1447, 1950.

14. Nutter, D.O., Schlant, R.C., and Hurst, J.W. Isometric exercise and the cardiovascular system. *Mod. Concepts Cardiovasc. Dis.* 41:11-15, 1972.

15. Groden, B.M. The management of myocardial infarction. A controlled study of the effects of early mobilization. *Cardiac Rehabil.* 1:13-16, 1971.

16. Harpur, J.E., Kellett, R.J., Conner, W.T., Galbraith, H.-J.B., Hamilton, M., Murray, J.J., Swallow, J.H., and Rose, G.A. Controlled trial of early mobilisation and discharge from hospital in uncomplicated myocardial infarction. *Lancet* 2:1331-1334, 1971.

17. Royston, G.R. Short stay hospital treatment and rapid rehabilitation of cases of myocardial infarction in a district hospital. *Br. Heart J.* 34:526-532, 1972.

18. Hellerstein, H.K. Exercise therapy in coronary disease. *Bull. N.Y. Acad. Med.* 44:1028-1047, 1968.

D. EARLY AMBULATION OF POST-MYOCARDIAL INFARCTION PATIENTS: MONTEFIORE HOSPITAL

Lenore R. Zohman, M.D.

When the Montefiore Hospital Cardiac Rehabilitation Program began in 1964, medical practice in New York City permitted the patient to sit in a chair during the second week after myocardial infarction (MI) and to begin limited ambulation during the third week. Compared to the Newman program reported in 1948, this was considered early ambulation, since at that time, the patient was allowed only to perform supervised walking for 3 to 5 minutes twice a day during the fourth week of recovery [1]. At the inception of the Montefiore Program, it was common practice [2] to monitor the patient's electrocardiogram (ECG) when there was any question of the advisability of an activity.

Torkelson reported in 1958 that exercise tolerance tests were performed on a treadmill during the seventh week post-MI by patients whose ambulation was increased in the fifth and sixth weeks [3]. The Wenger program instituted at Grady Memorial Hospital in Atlanta in 1967 was using essentially the same methods, and added a greater experience with monitored early ambulation of post-MI patients in a city hospital compared to our smaller experience in a private hospital [4]. More recently, Groden in Scotland reported a controlled study on the effects of early activation, mobilizing one group of post-MI patients in 15 days and the other in 25 days [5]. He demonstrated that there was no significant difference in the frequency of arrhythmia, further episodes of pain, the development of ventricular aneurysm, psychological disturbances, or mortality rates in the early mobilized group. Further, Hakkila in Finland compared a group of post-MI patients who were mobilized within the first few days using light physical exercise, with a control group given the conventional treatment, and found no difference in serum enzymes, ECG changes, or heart volumes between the groups [6].

Early ambulation was designed to prevent the *evil sequelae of bed rest* [7], namely, thromboembolism and deconditioning; to offer psychological benefit to patients and possibly favorably influence their return to work; and be helpful in releasing heavily utilized hospital beds.

The Setting for Cardiac Rehabilitation at Montefiore Hospital and Medical Center

The Montefiore Program was oriented to:

1. Serve patients hospitalized in a voluntary hospital contrasted to city patients in Dr. Wenger's program or to veterans in Dr. Torkelson's group.

2. Be administered in accordance with the current American health care system, contrasted to the programs of Groden or Hakkila carried out in Europe.

3. Be conducted in a rehabilitation rather than a cardiology setting, and offer *early ambulation* as only one facet of a comprehensive cardiac rehabilitation effort. The referring internist or cardiologist maintained direction of the definitive medical management of the patient while the rehabilitation residents and physiatrists were responsible for activity programming (physical, psychosocial, and vocational).

Patient Selection

Any patient referred by a physician was accepted in the program provided the following criteria were satisfied:

1. That he require a multidisciplinary approach to care, rather than management by only a physician and nurse.

2. That the physician permitted his transfer to the Rehabilitation In-Patient Service.

Patients were recruited through announcements on the availability of the program to attending physicians and house staff of Montefiore and Morrisania Hospitals, through meetings with groups of hospital-based physicians, such as the Health Insurance Plan (HIP) physicians, and through contacts between the rehabilitation residents and other house officers.

Principles

Two principles guided the program: *equi-caloric* matching and radio-monitoring. The equi-caloric concept consists of calorically matching activities prescribed by rehabilitation medicine physicians to the permissible caloric limits recommended by the cardiologists. Traditional orders for bed rest, self-care activities, sitting in a chair, or ambulation, issued by the cardiologist, were converted to caloric values determined by the work of Passmore and Durnin (TABLE I) [8]. Lists of the caloric values of self-care activities were provided to the nurses [9]. Lists of the caloric values of various calisthenics were provided to the physical therapists who supervised the reconditioning exercises [10]. Patients were usually ambulated and begun on reconditioning exercises during the second week post-MI.

TABLE I

Equicaloric matching—patient S.S. early convalescent period

Cardiologist allows (Cals/min)		Physiatrist matches (Cals/min)	
1.2	Sitting	1.2	Leather lacing
1.4	Eating	1.5	Passive exercise of extremities
1.4	Conversation on phone	1.7	Active exercise to upper limbs
2.5	Washing own hands and face	2.0	Active exercise to lower limbs
3.6	Walking 2.5 mph	3.6	Graded calisthenics to 3.6

Equicaloric matching—patient S.S. late convalescent period

Cardiologist allows (Cals/min)		Physiatrist matches (Cals/min)
3.6	Bedside commode	Weaving, overhead loom
3.6	Walking 2.5 mph	Graded calisthenics to 3.6 (to ex. #20)
4.2	Showering	Graded calisthenics to 4.2 (to ex. #25)
5.2	Walking downstairs	Conducting office business with secretary in hospital room

The second principle was monitoring the electrocardiogram via radio-telemetry. Initially, the RKG 100 radiotelemetry apparatus was used. Either the Gulton telemetry or the Holter Avionics magnetic tape monitoring system were employed later. Finally, a do-it-yourself telemetry apparatus was used. It was constructed by one of the house officers, for $16, using his FM radio [11]. When a new activity was prescribed, on-line monitoring was performed so that activity could be interrupted if detrimental ECG changes occurred. Thereafter, the patient was monitored with the Holter Avionics magnetic tape system for several hours, and the tracing reviewed and compared with his diary of activities for the day. For the monitoring, a true unipolar was used rather than a bipolar lead, to avoid postural alterations in the ST segments [12]. The lead selected was the one with the tallest R wave, or that lead which might be expected to show ischemic changes because of its proximity to the infarcted area.

As soon as the caloric level was determined by the physicians, paramedical staff developed activity programs of self-care and calisthenics within the patient's specified level of physical tolerance. Each new ·activity, including showering, stair climbing, recreational pursuits, visiting hours, and stress interviews, was monitored.

Results

Twenty-eight patients (19 men and 9 women) participated in the initial program. Their average age was 56. Fifteen were private patients and 13 were service cases. The average length of stay in the hospital was 52.9 days, approximately evenly divided between stays on the medicine service and on the rehabilitation service. These patients were generally considered poor risks because of their health status. Eight of the 28 continued receiving treatment for cardiac decompensation, four required digitalis, and 10 required nitroglycerin to relieve angina subsequent to infarction. Of the 28 patients six had died at the time of our first published report [13]. One patient died in intractable heart failure while on the service. Three died of MI within 6 months of having participated in the program; one suffered a cardiovascular accident (CVA); and another died of a renal tumor. However, seven of the 28 patients returned to their prior level of activity or work within 2 months of infarction, or within 1 month of discharge; six had returned to full-time employment within 17 days of discharge; and one, age 77, who was retired prior to illness, returned to his former level of activity. The remaining 15 patients returned to work more than a month after discharge.

In a followup study at the end of 4 years of the program, 57 patients (42 men and 15 women) had been treated on the rehabilitation inpatient service [14]. Of the total group, eight patients had died since the beginning of the program; 1.8 percent dying on the service and 14 percent dying within 1.5 years of infarction. Of the survivors, 31 returned to work or retraining; 12 assumed the same full-time job they had prior to hospitalization; 17 resumed the previous job with modification of required physical activity; and two were retrained for other types of employment by the State Vocational Agency. Eighteen of the 49 survivors did not return to work and 10 patients were over 65 years old. Only two patients, who were medically capable of reemployment, did not return to work because of social factors. The others remained dependent in their homes due to a concomitant medical illness such as CVA, rather than the cardiac disease per se.

Pros and Cons of the Cardiac Rehabilitation Program at Montefiore Hospital

The most positive effect of this inpatient program was the provision of restorative services to individuals who, due to the complexities of their readjustment to community life, could not be appropriately managed in a medical inpatient program. The team approach considered the medical, psychological, vocational, and social factors involved in returning to work and community living. This approach helped restore these individuals to premorbid levels of function, not attainable by medical management alone. Patient morale and satisfaction were very high. In addition, although the hospital course was prolonged, many patients returned to work earlier after the infarction than had been the previous general experience in work evaluation units or in private practice [15].

Restorative Program Difficulties

Difficulties encountered in providing an early ambulation and comprehensive restoration program for cardiac patients on a rehabilitation medicine service included questions of professional competence, and cost.

Despite acknowledgment of the theoretic value of a cardiac rehabilitation program, some cardiologists were reluctant to transfer even the patient with marked psycho-social-vocational problems to a rehabilitation inpatient service at 10 to 14 days post-MI. They were concerned that, even if the physiatrist was knowledgeable in the interpretation of the ECG, he was not trained to provide medical management for the patient, particularly in an emergency situation. Further, they stressed that the rehabilitation nurses and paramedical staff were not accustomed to handling acute cardiac emergencies.

The physiatrists and paramedical staffs raised similar objections. They were remote from cardiologic practice; ill-prepared for reading ECGs; and uneasy about taking the responsibility for acute cardiac care which was not within their usual area of expertise. It was necessary to provide a refresher course to the physiatrists and rehabilitation medicine residents in exercise electrocardiography and management of acute cardiac emergencies. The nursing and therapy staffs reviewed the management of cardiac arrest.

Rehabilitation residents became part of the hospital's cardiac arrest team in rotation with the medical residents. The rehabilitation residents assumed a night call rotation with backup by the attending physiatrists. Initially, as a cardiologist on the rehabilitation service, I provided liaison to the referring cardiologists and internists, and assumed the overall patient responsibility. Later, as the staff demonstrated its competence I served only as a consultant to the physiatrists. After these readjustments were accomplished, cardiologists began to refer their patients for inpatient cardiac rehabilitation on a regular basis.

The cost of the program was often prohibitive. Hospitalization insurance would not reimburse the additional stay on Rehabilitation Medicine if the stay was for rehabilitative care alone. Many of our patients had complicated medical problems which required prolonged hospitalization in addition to their complicated rehabilitation problems, so that third-party payments did cover the additional cost of hospitalization. In a few instances, however, when claims initially approved were reviewed in retrospect, they were disapproved and patients were sometimes faced with hospital bills of thousands of dollars to be paid out-of-pocket.

Team meetings were also expensive. A 2-hour meeting, at which four patients were discussed, usually involved a cardiologist, physiatrist, physical therapist, occupational therapist, psychologist, nurse, and vocational counselor. It was possible to provide such comprehensive service to cardiac patients only because the team was already operating for the neuromuscularly disabled on the rehabilitation service.

Lastly, the Loeb Center for Nursing and Rehabilitation, an extended care facility occupying two floors at Montefiore Hospital, raised additional problems regarding cost. The per diem rate at the Loeb Center was considerably below that of the medical or rehabilitation service in the hospital proper, even though the Loeb Center was part of the same building as the Rehabilitation Medicine Service. Therefore, many convalescent MI patients who required more than the care of the physician and the nurse were referred for extended care to the Loeb Center. These patients might have profited from the cardiac rehabilitation program. Hence, there was competition for placement of the complicated post-MI patient. To compound the matter, once a patient was transferred to the Loeb Center, and subsequently required cardiac rehabilitation care, he could not be transferred to Rehabilitation Medicine without having to pay, because of the third-party payment system in New York, the entire remaining bill out-of-pocket. Under such circumstances, the patient was returned to the Medicine Service. He could then be relocated, although not transferred, to the Rehabilitation Medicine floor to continue his medical care, or the hospital would not be reimbursed by the third-party carrier. This situation created conflict within the house staff in terms of who would provide patient coverage.

Summary

The experience with early ambulation as part of a comprehensive cardiac rehabilitation program at Montefiore Hospital in New York City is reviewed. The principles of equi-caloric matching and radiomonitoring of the electrocardiogram guided the program. Patients were provided with a supervised and monitored environment in which they experienced physical and/or emotional stresses prior to experiencing these same stresses outside the hospital. Simple, early demonstration of physical capacities in a setting which is comfortable and safe for the patient seems to permit a more satisfactory and permanent readjustment to the illness, convalescence, and resumption of normal activities in the community.

REFERENCES

1. Newman, L.B., Wasserman, R.R., and Borden, C. Productive living for those with heart disease: The role of phys. medicine and rehabilitation. *Arch. Phys. Med. Rehabil.* 37:137, 1956.

2. Cain, H.D., Frasher, W.G., and Stivelman, R. Graded activity program for safe return to self-care after myocardial infarction. *J.A.M.A.* 177:111, 1961.

3. Torkelson, Leif O. Rehabilitation of the patient with acute myocardial infarction. *J. Chronic Dis.* 17:685, 1964.

4. Wenger, N.K., Gilbert, C.A., and Skorapa, M.Z. Cardiac conditioning after myocardial infarction. *Cardiac Rehabil.* 2:17, 1971.

5. Groden, B.M. The management of myocardial infarction. *Cardiac Rehabil.* 1:13, 1971.

6. Hakkila, J. Finds working ability works. *Chronic Dis. Mgmt.* 6:1, Jan. 1972.

7. Dock, W. The evil sequelae of complete bed rest. *J.A.M.A.* 125:1083, 1944.

8. Passmore, R., and Durnin, J.V.G.A. Human energy expenditure. *Physiol. Rev.* 35:801, 1955.

9. Zohman, L.R., and Tobis, J.S. *Cardiac Rehabilitation*, pp. 46-47. New York, Grune & Stratton, 1970.

10. Weiss, R.A., and Karpovich P. Energy cost of exercise for convalescents. *Arch. Phys. Med. Rehabil.* 28:447, 1947.

11. Fasceneldi, F.A. Electrocardiography by do-it-yourself radiotelemetry. *N. Engl. J. Med.* 273:1076, 1965.

12. Lachman, A.B., Semler, H.J., and Gustafson, R.H. Postural ST-T wave changes in the radioelectrocardiogram simulating myocardial ischemia. *Circulation* 31:557, 1965.

13. Tobis, J.S., and Zohman, L.R. A rehabilitation program for inpatients with recent myocardial infarction. *Arch. Phys. Med. Rehabil.* 49:443, 1968.

14. Tobis, J.S., and Zohman, L.R. Follow-up study of cardiac patients on a rehabilitation service. *Arch. Phys. Med. Rehabil.* 51:286, 1970.

15. Clark, R.J. Experience of the cardiac work classification unit in Boston, Mass. *In,* Rosenbaum, F.F., and Belknap, E.L., Eds. *Work and the Heart.* New York, Hoeber, 1959.

23

THE EFFECTS OF ACUTE AND CHRONIC EXERCISE
ON CARDIAC PATIENTS

John Naughton, M.D.

Rehabilitation for patients with coronary heart disease (CHD) manifested by myocardial infarction (MI) begins with the onset of the clinically manifested impairment. It begins with a patient's admission to a coronary care unit (CCU), and is defined as the process whereby a cardiac patient is *restored to* and *maintained at* his optimal physiological, psychologic, vocational, and social status. Implicit in the process is the restoration of those measures which will *prevent* progression of the underlying disease and the development of additional impairment [1]. The optimally achieved status may be at the patient's original level or at a newly adjusted level commensurate with the severity of his cardiac condition.

Stages of Cardiac Rehabilitation

The rehabilitative process for MI patients includes these stages:

Stage 1 - Coronary Care Unit (CCU)
Stage 2 - Cardiac Rehabilitation Unit (CRU)
Stage 3 - Convalescence
Stage 4 - Recovery.

Stages 1 and 2 are reviewed elsewhere in this volume [2, 3, 4, 5]. In general, the uncomplicated patient is cared for in the CCU for 3 to 5 days, and is transferred to a secondary unit for the remainder of his hospital stay. Low-level physical activity and routine activities of daily living (shaving, washing, and eating) are instituted in accordance with a patient's physical tolerance as early as

Supported in part by Grant RT-9 (C-5) from the Social and Rehabilitation Service, Department of Health, Education, and Welfare is feasible, and in many CRUs formalized education of the patient and his family is included in the process.

Convalescence begins with a patient's discharge from the hospital and ends when he returns either to work or to his usual life pursuits. The latter is determined in large part by the patient's physical and emotional status and by the physical and emotional demands of the job. The average, uncomplicated patient with a clerical or sedentary job returns to work from 6 to 10 weeks post-MI whereas patients with more stressful occupations usually return between 8 and 14 weeks post-MI. The return to work is determined by a number of variables, including the patient's attitudes toward the job and/or his employer, whether or not he has adequate compensation for a longer convalescent period, and by the presence or absence of symptoms. Asymptomatic patients are usually ready to return to work sooner than are those patients who experience recurring episodes of chest pain, exertional fatigue, dyspnea, or palpitations.

Physical activity during Stage 3 usually includes a regimen of mild calisthenics designed to increase flexibility and to induce muscular relaxation and short walks. The spouse often acts as the patient's monitor. Ideally, she is taught to measure the heart rate at the radial pulse while the patient is hospitalized, so that she can measure it before and after each new form of physical activity performed at home. The patient is instructed to use the presence or absence of symptoms as his guideline for too much or too little physical exertion, and the spouse is given a prescribed peak heart rate level as a guideline not to be exceeded. Should she detect new dysrhythmias, she is instructed to contact the physician. By 6 weeks, many post-MI patients are able to negotiate a total distance of 2.0 miles a day in 45 to 75 minutes. Some patients will perform this activity in distances of one-eighth to one-quarter of a mile, 4 to 8 times a day, while others will accomplish it with a continuous mile-long walk in the morning and again in the evening.

By the time the patient is prepared to return to work he is encouraged to have established a specified regimen for his pattern of life-style, and should have resumed most, if not all, of the so-called routine activities of daily living.

Recovery. (Stage 4) begins with a patient's return to work. Prior to entering this phase, each patient is evaluated by his physician to determine his level of physiologic, psychologic, and social adjustment and to advise him concerning vocational and recreational adaptation. Thus, this evaluation is rather extensive and often includes:

1. Appropriate cardiovascular history
2. Physical examination
3. Standard ECG and chest x-ray
4. Serum lipids
5. Psychosocial evaluation
6. Work capacity test.

History. The patient's symptoms since discharge from the hospital are reviewed. The physician evaluates those psychological reactions which commonly result from an MI, which are anxiety, depression, and loss of self-esteem; he directs particular attention to the cardiovascular history for evidence of undue fatigue, chest pain, exertional and/or nocturnal dyspnea, and palpitations. The patient's historical functional status is rated according to the criteria of the New York Heart Association (NYHA) [6].

Physical examination. The patient's mood and reactions to questions of relevance are observed and noted. The cardiovascular examination includes observing the neck veins for distension and pulsations; recording the heart size, and extra or paradoxical precordial impulses; the presence or absence of murmurs or abnormal heart sounds (ventricular (S3) or atrial (S4) gallops), the examination for hepatic enlargement and engorgement; and the presence or absence of peripheral edema.

Laboratory. The laboratory evaluation includes a standard ECG, upright PA chest x-ray, measurements of the hematocrit, serum cholesterol, and triglyceride concentrations, and a 2-hour postprandial blood glucose.

Psychosocial evaluation. Many aspects of the psychosocial evaluation are part of the history and physical examination. The physician who evaluates a patient with a healed MI need not perform detailed psychiatric or sociological interview or testing. Rather, he focuses attention on those goals in the psychosocial sphere which are important to total recovery and rehabilitation. These include his current and proposed adjustment to the job, family, and sexual activity; the need for medication; modification of life-style; and physical and recreational activity.

In most instances each patient will make appropriate adjustments commensurate with his state of recovery and well-being. Counsel and guidance may be all that is required for many patients. Should the patient require more intensive counseling, the physician may wish to enlist a social worker, clinical psychologist, or psychiatrist depending on the severity of the problem.

Physiologic evaluation. If the results of the patient's history and physical examination indicate that his cardiovascular condition has stabilized, if the ECG is stable, and if the heart size is not enlarging on chest x-ray, the patient may then perform a standardized multistage exercise test. In this instance, the exercise test is not a diagnostic procedure, but is an evaluative procedure designed to determine the patient's adaptation to various levels of physical stress, measure his capacity for physical work, and provide an objective measurement on which to base a work and/or exercise prescription.

A work capacity test is contraindicated for patients who are in overt congestive heart failure, or whose baseline evaluation at rest indicates that they have not yet recovered. Obviously, some patients will require other types of intervention (diagnostic, surgical, pharmacological, or electrical) prior to entering a long-term rehabilitation program, while for others the convalescent phase will simply be appropriately extended rather than accentuated.

The Work Capacity Test

In our laboratory, the following procedure is employed:

A patient reports to the laboratory after either an overnight fast or 2 hours postprandially. His skin is cleansed with acetone at the left midclavicular line of the 5th intercostal space and 2.0 cm to the right of the sternum in the 2nd intercostal space. The prepared skin area is coated with electrode paste, and an electrode is applied firmly to each area. The resultant ECG lead approximates precordial V_5, and is identified as CM_5. The ECG is recorded by hard wire (direct cable).

The patient is placed at supine rest for 5 minutes. In the fifth minute, a single lead ECG, a phonocardiogram, and a carotid pulse contour are recorded simultaneously on photographic paper at a speed of 100 mm/sec, and blood pressure and heart rate are measured and recorded.

The patient then stands in a resting and relaxed posture for 5 minutes; blood pressure, heart rate, and ECG are recorded during the fifth minute. He is instructed in the technique of performing treadmill exercise and begins walking on a level grade at a speed of 2.0 mph for 3 minutes. This is followed by a 3-minute period of rest. If the blood pressure, heart rate, ECG, and symptomatic response are satisfactory, he begins walking at a speed of 2.0 mph on a slope of 3.5 percent. The speed is maintained while the slope of treadmill bed is elevated in increments of 3.5 percent every 2 minutes. Should a patient complete a walk on a 17.5 percent grade without attaining a specified end point (symptoms, ECG changes, or heart rate level), the slope of the treadmill bed is lowered to 12.5 percent and the speed is increased to 3.0 mph. Thereafter, the speed is maintained and the slope of the treadmill bed is elevated in 2.5 percent increments every 2 minutes.

In this procedure, the initial workload approximates twice the external O_2 intake of supine rest, and each additional energy requirement increases the O_2 threshold an additional increment above that of rest, i.e., 2, 3, 4, and so forth times the work or O_2 requirement of rest. Thus, each workload is translated into METS, and the work capacity is so defined. For example, a patient who becomes limited at a speed of a 2.0 mph on a 10.5 percent grade has a work capacity of 14.0 ml O_2/kg/min or 4 METS. The test is of a continuous design, but can be modified easily to an intermittent procedure. In the latter circumstance, the workload should be maintained for at least 3 rather than 2 minutes to insure the achievement of a near-steady state performance. The test is terminated either when the patient becomes symptomatic (chest pain, dyspnea, fatigue, or palpitations), develops signs of cold sweat, pallor, or ataxia, achieves a predetermined age-adjusted heart rate level, or develops significant ECG changes. Blood pressure, heart rate, and ECG are recorded during the last 30 seconds of each workload.

Immediately after walking he assumes the supine position and the ECG, phonocardiogram, and carotid pulse contour are recorded simultaneously within the initial minute of recovery. Blood pressure, heart rate, and ECG are recorded in the 5th minute of recovery, and if the patient has recovered the procedure is terminated.

The systolic time intervals, i.e., pre-ejection period (PEP), left ventricular ejection time (LVET), and total electromechanical systole (QS2) are measured from the simultaneously recorded ECG, PCG, and CPC. Each value represents the mean of 10 consecutively recorded complexes. The LVET and QS2 are corrected for heart rate and the adjusted values are referred to as LVETc and QS2c. The product of blood pressure and heart rate is calculated for each physiologic state to determine the systolic time tension index (STTI).

The first work capacity evaluation is usually terminated either for the above reasons or at a heart rate level which approximates 70 percent of the age-predicted maximum heart rate. At subsequent evaluations, the test is usually terminated at 85 percent of the age-predicted maximum heart rate level if no other indications for terminating the test have occurred.

Responses to Acute Exercise

A multistage exercise test provides the physician with a comprehensive physiologic appraisal of the patient's adaptation to graded physical stress and an objective measure of his functional capacity.

The normal physiologic responses to graded exercise are discussed and reviewed elsewhere in this volume. Many investigators have reported that the character of blood pressure, heart rate, cardiac output, ECG, and respiratory gas exchange responses in many patients with healed MIs are comparable, at submaximal workloads, to those of otherwise healthy, sedentary, middle-aged men [7, 8]. Certainly, it has been our experience that many patients with uncomplicated courses have had similar physiologic profiles both at rest and during exercise. In fact, the peak O_2 intakes often differ insignificantly. Therefore, it is appropriate to state that following healing there are many identifiable CHD patients who cannot be distinguished physiologically from many healthy subjects. It is obviously these patients who are candidates for participation in medically supervised exercise programs.

On the other hand, many CHD patients with healed MIs are not so fortunate. A graded exercise test will help the physician characterize their mode of physiologic adaptations and rate their physiologic functional class. We have seen a number of varied adaptations in post-MI patients over the years. In most instances a reduction in work capacity (peak O_2 intake) and abnormal blood pressure, heart rate, and ECG responses correlate quite well. However, there has been an occasional instance where a patient has achieved a relatively high O_2 intake threshold (7 to 9 METS) with a stable ECG and heart rate response, and yet has had an inappropriate blood pressure response. This abnormal response has generally taken two forms: the first is characterized by a minimal increase in systolic blood pressure and a modest increase in diastolic blood pressure, and the second by elevations of both systolic and diastolic blood pressure (Fig. 1). In both situations the net effect is either no change or a slight decrease in pulse pressure. This response is interpreted as representing an inadequate myocardial adaptation, and therefore, indicative indirectly of myocardial dysfunction. Although we have not observed enough patients in a well-designed manner, these patients eventually experienced sudden cardiac death.

It was this abnormal blood pressure response that stimulated us to apply the measurement of the phases of systoles to the exercise test procedure. Weissler

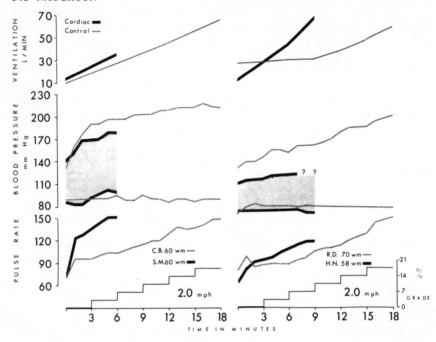

Fig. 1. The pulse rate, blood pressure, and ventilatory adjustments of four subjects are depicted. The adaptive responses of S.M. (cardiac patient) are compared with those of C.B. (healthy subject) and of H.N. (cardiac patient) with R.D. (healthy subject). C.B. and R.D. achieved O_2 requirements of 7 METS (2.0 mph, 17.5 percent grade) without evidence of physiologic impairment whereas S.M.'s performance capacity was limited to 3 METS (Functional Class III) and H.N.'s to 4 METS (Functional Class III). Both had inappropriate physiological adaptations to these very low workloads, and were considered ineligible for an exercise training program.

and colleagues reported their value in evaluating myocardial function in the resting state [9], thus, it seemed that they might provide indirect evidence of the character of the myocardial response to acute exercise. Although studied by only a few investigators in a similar manner so far, their contribution to the acute exercise evaluation has been helpful.

In our laboratory, the normal mean values for PEP are 104 ± 21 mm/sec and LVETc 413 ± 18 mm/sec. The mean values do not differ significantly at supine rest for patients with uncomplicated healed MIs and presumably healthy controls. On the other hand, in patients with definite cardiac impairment, the PEP at rest is significantly longer and the LVETc significantly shorter than in the other subject groups. The PEP response to acute stress does not differentiate healthy subjects from cardiac patients nor physically active subjects from sedentary subjects [10]. The LVETc response does provide apparently significant information. In healthy, sedentary subjects the LVETc response to acute exercise is characterized either by no change or minimal change; in healthy, physically active subjects by significant decrease in duration; and in cardiac patients by prolongation. The latter relates to the significance of impairment, and is interpreted as indicating the presence of myocardial dysfunction [11].

The stress ECG is another important indication of adaptation. Similar to the situation of patients with angina pectoris, many patients with healed MI will develop ischemic changes during physical stress. However, exercise-induced dysrhythmias are more common. Should they occur, the patient should be treated pharmacologically prior to entering a physical activity program.

Lastly, physiologic functional class can be determined with a stress test [12]. Most healed, uncomplicated patients will achieve thresholds of from 5 to 8 METS before terminating a stress test. These patients are classified as functional class II (5 METS) or I (6 METS or greater) and can be entered into a physical activity program. Most patients whose performance capacity is below 4 METS should probably be treated medically, and reevaluated 3 months later to determine their acceptance for an exercise program.

In summary, many patients with healed MIs will adapt to physical stress in a manner comparable to presumably healthy middle-aged men. These patients can be entered into a medically supervised exercise program. Those patients whose exercise test is complicated by an abnormal blood pressure, heart rate, ECG, LVETc, and/or functional capacity response should be followed, treated medically and pharmacologically, and reevaluated at a later date to establish their ability to tolerate and participate in a medically supervised exercise program.

Exercise Programs

Those patients who satisfactorily complete the evaluation described can be entered into programs of regular, graduated, physical activity. An exercise prescription is developed [13], given to the patient, and sent to the referring physician. Preferably, exercise programs should be conducted under medical supervision in a facility equipped and manned to administer emergency care. There is obviously a deficiency of properly trained manpower and of equipped community facilities in the United States to implement this ideal for the vast numbers of new MI survivors each year. Thus, for many patients, an individualized home prescription is required, and the patient's spouse is taught the necessary precautions.

In our experience, most patients prefer group programs where the physical activity is varied to include individual and group exercises. Patients either learn or relearn to perform a regimen of calisthenics, intermittent walking and jogging, and to play games. Volleyball provided the greatest stimulus for participation because it was not physically exhausting, permitted each patient an opportunity to play at his level of capability, and at the same time, provided a healthy competitive spirit which promoted individual and group interaction. The type and variety of activities is obviously determined by the quality of the facility and the number of patients in a group at any one time.

Ideally, each patient is monitored with a telemetered ECG at intervals of 4 to 6 weeks to determine his heart rate and ECG adaptations to the program. This evaluation complements the standardized treadmill evaluation, and makes repeated treadmill evaluations less imminent. The testing is recommended if it is apparent that the level of the exercise program is inadequate to promote an additional training effect or if it is apparent or suspected that additional deterioration in the quality of cardiovascular integrity has occurred. In the latter circumstance the exercise prescription may have to be redesigned at a lower level of intensity or withdrawn altogether as a therapy.

In one 5-year experience with a group of cardiac patients, I found that a frequency of 3 times per week for a duration of 50 to 60 min/session was a practical program promoting regular adherence and attendance. The early dropout rate in a volunteer study is quite high, as indicated in other studies [14]. Those patients who remained for 3 months or longer usually stayed. It should be emphasized that those patients whose previous life experience never included a regimen of any type of physical activity had the highest dropout rate [15]; those who were physically active as youngsters had the best adherence; and cooperation in terms of risk factor modification was easily maintained throughout the first year post-MI. All patients tended to relax more and be less health conscious after a year of survival.

Thus far, exercise programs have been relatively safe. We recorded one death in a 5-year experience [16]. This fatality was totally unexpected by the professional staff, but apparently had been predicted as a possibility by the other patients because he was the one individual least able to change his overall lifestyle pattern. The incident came as a shock, however, and for the next several weeks the group was extremely cooperative and automatically reset the intensity of the activity. Subsequently, they reequilibrated and continued to increase their activity levels. No one dropped out as a result of this experience. In fact, they became more cohesive and tended to reinforce their own belief that this form of therapy was that most required for their well-being.

Effects of Chronic Exercise

The history of regular chronic exercise programs for cardiac patients is very short. Hellerstein [17] reported the earliest experience in the United States. There has been a large number of subsequent reports from centers throughout the United States, Europe, Israel, and Canada. Some programs have been of a short duration in terms of weeks while others have followed patients for several years. Regardless of the type of program employed, the results have been amazingly similar. Among the reported effects are:

1. *Increased physical working capacity*

In our experience, most patients following recovery have a performance capacity which ranges from 5 to 8 METS with a mean of 6 METS. Following 3 to 6 months, these values have usually increased to a low of 7 and a high of

10 METS, and after 1 year most patients exceed 9 METS and many achieve thresholds of 11 and 12 METS.

2. *Decreased systolic blood pressure at rest and comparable levels of submaximal work*

Although not all investigators have measured systolic blood pressure throughout exercise, those who did have reported significant reductions at rest and throughout submaximal exercise. The peak systolic blood pressure achieved is usually near identical before and after physical training.

3. *Decreased heart rate levels at rest and at submaximal exercise*

Similarly, the heart rate level at rest and submaximal exercise is reduced.

4. *Decreased myocardial O_2 work at rest and submaximal exercise*

The systolic blood pressure-heart rate product is significantly reduced and thus indicates that myocardial O_2 requirements under these conditions have been lowered. This is a desired physiological effect.

5. *Evidence of altered myocardial performance*

Crews and Aldinger [18] have reported specific effects related to physical training in animals. In man there is still a requirement to demonstrate definitive effects on the myocardial contractile state. Although not a prospective study, Whitsett and Naughton [10] did report significant postexercise shortening of the LVETc in training post-MI patients and prolongations in the untrained patients. It is probable that these findings indicate enhancement of the myocardial contractile process as a result of the training.

6. *Altered life-style*

Physically conditioned patients are more likely to alter those conditions which promote the development and/or aggravation of CHD risk factors than are the patients who remain sedentary. The active patients usually stop smoking, maintain more normal weight, sleep better, drink less alcoholic beverages, and require less medication.

Obviously, not every patient responds to physical activity. We have observed several patients who report an improved state of well-being but who have not increased their work capacity or modified the character of their physiologic adaptations to graded exercise. However, the usual uncomplicated patient with functional Class I or II status has usually responded favorably.

In conclusion, Burch's admonition that it is sometimes possible to rehabilitate a patient and not his heart should be borne in mind [19].

REFERENCES

1. Parmley, L.F., Jr., Ed. Proceedings of the national workshop on exercise in the prevention, and the evaluation, in the treatment of heart disease, 104 pp. *J. S.C. Med. Assoc.* Suppl. to vol. 65, Dec. 1969.

2. Acker, J., Jr. Early activity after myocardial infarction. *In*, Naughton, J., and Hellerstein, H.K., Eds. *Exercise Testing and Exercise Training in Coronary Heart Disease*. New York, Academic, 1973.

3. Brock, L. Early reconditioning for postmyocardial infarction patients: Spalding Rehabilitation Center. *In*, Naughton, J., and Hellerstein, H.K., Eds. *Exercise Testing and Exercise Training in Coronary Heart Disease*. New York, Academic, 1973.

4. Wenger, N.K. Early ambulation after myocardial infarction. Grady Memorial Hospital—Emory University School of Medicine. *In*, Naughton, J., and Hellerstein, H.K., Eds. *Exercise Testing and Exercise Training in Coronary Heart Disease*. New York, Academic, 1973.

5. Zohman, L.R. Early ambulation of postmyocardial infarction patients: Montefiore Hospital. *In*, Naughton, J., and Hellerstein, H.K., Eds. *Exercise Testing and Exercise Training in Coronary Heart Disease*. New York, Academic, 1973.

6. Criteria Committee of New York Heart Association. *Diseases of the Heart and Blood Vessels: Nomenclature and Criteria for Diagnoses*, 6th ed., pp. 112-113. Boston, Little Brown, 1953.

7. Naughton, J., Shanbour, K., Armstrong, R., McCoy, J., and Lategola, M.T. Cardiovascular responses to exercise following myocardial infarction. *Arch. Intern. Med.* 117:541, 1966.

8. Chapman, C., and Fraser, R. Cardiovascular responses to exercise in patients with healed myocardial infarction. *Circulation* 9:347, 1954.

9. Weissler, A.M., Harris, W.S., and Schoenfeld, C.D. Systolic time intervals in heart failure in man. *Circulation* 37:149-159, 1968.

10. Whitsett, T.L., and Naughton, J. The effects of systolic time intervals in sedentary and active individuals and rehabilitated patients with heart disease. *Am. J. Cardiol.* 27:352, 1971.

11. Pouget, J., Harris, W., Mayron, B., and Naughton, J. Abnormal responses of the systolic time intervals to exercise in patients with angina pectoris. *Circulation* 43:289, 1971.

12. Patterson, J.A., Naughton, J., Pietras, R.J., and Gunnar, R.M. Treadmill exercise in assessment of the functional capacity of cardiac patients with cardiac disease. *Am. J. Cardiol.* 30:757, 1972.

13. Hellerstein, H.K., et al. Principles of exercise prescription. *In*, Naughton, J., and Hellerstein, H.K., Eds. *Exercise Testing and Exercise Training in Coronary Heart Disease*. New York, Academic, 1973.

14. Sanne, H., Elmfeldt, D., and Wilhelmsen, L. Preventive effect of physical training after a myocardial infarction. *In*, Tibblih, G., Ed. *Preventive Cardiology*, pp. 154-160. [Halsted Press] New York, Wiley, 1972.

15. Naughton, J., Bruhn, J.G., and Lategola, M.T. Effects of physical training on physiologic and behavioral characteristics of cardiac patients. *Arch. Phys. Med. Rehabil.* 49:131, 1968.

16. Naughton, J., Lategola, M.T., and Shanbour, K. A physical rehabilitation program for cardiac patients. A progress report. *Am. J. Med. Sci.* 252:545, 1966.

17. Hellerstein, H.K., Hirsch, E.Z., Cumler, W., Allen, L., Palster, S., and Zucker, N. Reconditioning of the coronary patient: A preliminary report. *In*, Likoff, W., and Moyer, J.H., Eds. *Coronary Heart Disease*, pp. 448-454. New York, Grune & Stratton, 1963.

18. Crews, J., and Aldinger, E.E. Effects of chronic exercise on myocardial function. *Am. Heart J.* 74:536, 1967.

19. Burch, G., and DePasquale, N. Potentials and limitations of patients after myocardial infarction. *Am. Heart J.* 72:830, 1966.

24

LONG-TERM ACTIVITY PROGRAMS FOR CORONARY PATIENTS

J. E. Merriman, M.D., F.R.C.P. (C)

Introduction

Exercise training programs for patients with coronary artery disease are being instituted with increasing frequency in all parts of the world. The main emphasis has been only on exercise training in some centers, while in others the exercise training has been an integral part of an overall rehabilitation program [1-39]. Most rehabilitation programs for patients with coronary artery disease have as their goal the modification of diet, the achievement of ideal body weight, the cessation of smoking, and the improvement in physical fitness.

Physical activity and the epidemiology of coronary artery disease was discussed by Keys [40], who stated, " . . . so the claim that exercise helps to prevent coronary heart disease continues to be unproven. Increasing exercise for our more sedentary men is probably socially and psychologically desirable. Whether such increased activity will effect the incidence and mortality of heart disease can only be decided from the results of large scale trials—that have not yet been inaugurated."

In a recent review on physical activity in the prevention of coronary heart disease, Fox, Naughton, and Haskell [11] stated that "data suggests, but falls short of proving, that an increase in habitual physical activity is beneficial." They continued, "more studies are urgently needed, particularly concerning whether increased physical activity will contribute to cardiovascular and general health enhancement, increased total human performance, and a vigorous creative society."

Several *short-term* studies have shown certain changes in cardiopulmonary fitness after a period of training [1, 2, 3, 5, 6, 10, 14, 15, 19, 22, 23, 25, 32, 33, 34, 36]. In these studies, the preexercise values served as the control.

The important question that needs an answer is: "Do long-term activity programs for coronary patients improve the quality of life, do they decrease the incidence of myocardial infarction, and do they prolong life?" There is a paucity of long-term studies in which matched controls have been used. In many rehabilitation programs the patient is defatted, deweighted, desmoked, and made fit. In these studies, if an improved mortality is demonstrated, is the evidence such that we can attribute improvement to improved physical fitness?

The published results from the majority of centers with long-term activity programs for patients with coronary artery disease have been reviewed [1-39]. Some of the factors which should be considered in reviewing long-term activity programs will be discussed in the following sections of this chapter.

Assessing an Exercise Activity Program

Factors that merit consideration in assessing an exercise activity program are:

Specificity of exercise. Was exercise activity to be the sole variable or was exercise to be an integral part of an overall rehabilitation program? Were there indications that a similar group of nonexercising control patients would be similarly studied and followed?

Age of patient. Evidence does not suggest that age is a specific limiting factor in an exercise activity program. Usually, patients are less than 65 years of age.

Testing methods. Several excellent reviews on this subject should be consulted [41, 42, 43].

Fitness evaluation. In the majority of cases, the maximal oxygen intake has been used as an index of cardiopulmonary fitness. Since there are at least three energy sources for exercise, it is important to distinguish between improved performance on the fitness test and an improvement in the maximum oxygen intake as directly measured.

Criteria for acceptance. It is important to determine what has motivated the patient to become interested in an exercise activity program. This becomes an important consideration relevant to adherence to the program and reasons for dropouts. In a well-controlled research study on activity, what is to be done about the patient who was selected for the exercise program but does not believe in exercise?

Criteria for nonacceptance. Exercise, like any drug, has its indications and contraindications. Briefly, there are cardiac, medical, orthopedic, and other contraindications to an exercise training program. If a patient has significant hypertension or frequent ventricular premature beats, it is wise to defer starting the patient on an exercise program until these problems are under adequate medical control. Patients with diabetes and chronic obstructive lung disease should similarly have these problems stabilized before starting an exercise program, if at all. Orthopedic problems may be a highly important limiting factor.

Prescription for exercise. On the basis of the exercise test, a precise prescription for exercise training should be given. This is usually provided by the physician and will include, at least, advice about the use of prophylactic nitroglycerin and the intensity, frequency, and duration of exercise. In some centers, the prescription for exercise is intuitively given by a physician or qualified technician.

Intensity of training. For those subjects not limited by angina, is the target heart rate assigned and is this based on a percentage of maximum oxygen intake? What percentage is used? Better than 60 percent? Is there any indication that the individual exceeds this intensity?

Supervision. Is the activity program under the supervision of a physician or a physical educator? Are methods and techniques available to ensure that the patient has been following his prescription for exercise? In the patient with ventricular premature beats at rest or during exercise, are there facilities for monitoring during the actual exercise training? Is the patient with angina obtaining the maximum benefit from prophylactic nitroglycerin? Are periodic checks made of the exercise blood pressure in the patient with hypertension?

Facilities. In evaluating long-term results, it is important to know which facilities are available. Are a gymnasium and a track included, or is the exercise training conducted in a laboratory using either a bicycle ergometer or a treadmill?

Type of training. Is it an endurance-type training? Is use made of calisthenics and recreational games such as volleyball?

Complications. To assess the results of an exercise activity program, it is important to note the incidence of complications. The noncardiac complications are usually orthopedic in type. Their incidence can be decreased with the use of proper gym equipment such as track shoes, also by a well-planned training and conditioning program. Bruce [44] has reviewed the problem of cardiac emergencies during exercise training programs.

Adherence to program. If the number of *poor attenders* or dropouts is significant, the reasons should be noted, which may include lack of motivation, scheduling problems, or social or medical factors.

Short-term Exercise Program

In numerous studies, definite physiologic changes have been shown after the commencement of an exercise training program. In these studies each patient is his own control. After a period of exercise training, there is increased maximal oxygen intake, decrease in heart rate for the same workload, increase in stroke output, and decrease in minute ventilation volume for the same oxygen intake. The degree of improvement depends primarily upon the initial level of fitness.

It is my impression that a short-term exercise program produces such a feeling of well-being in the patient that he is motivated to maintain his improved fitness.

Long-term Effects

When patients on an exercise training program have been studied more than a year later, many of the changes noted above are again demonstrated. Most investigators agree that the major improvement occurs during the early months of the training program. There then follows a further slight increase in maximal oxygen intake.

In the objective assessment of the short-term effects, the patient's initial study serves as the control observation. For the long-term evaluation, a well designed pair-matched study is needed. One of the pair would be enrolled in the exercise training program and his matched control would have the same spectrum of coronary risk factors but would not be on an exercise rehabilitation program.

This author's contention is that there are few, if any, published series that meet the above criteria and that could answer these three questions:

1. Do patients on a supervised exercise training program live longer when compared to their control?
2. Are there fewer coronary events in these patients on an exercise training program?
3. If there is any difference between the exercise and the control group, what is the significant factor? Is it physiologic or psychologic?

Training Program—Saskatoon

The Saskatoon Training Program was instituted in February, 1970. The aim of this research study was to answer the questions listed above and to test the hypothesis that a supervised exercise training program has a beneficial effect on the natural history of coronary artery disease. Each patient on the program was pair-matched according to age, diagnosis, serum cholesterol level, blood pressure, and smoking history. The patients are frequently checked to ensure that they do not knowingly change their diet, weight, or smoking pattern. Exercise is to be the only *known* variable. Each patient had his coronary risk factors assessed before starting the program which included an exercise-tolerance test. An exercise prescription was written by the cardiologist and the target heart rate assigned. The exercise training program is supervised with a physician and a physical educator always in attendance.

An exercise training program must be practical, or the patients will not attend and the dropout rate will be high. In our program, the patient may leave his office, drive to the laboratory, park, change into his gym clothes, and carry out his exercise prescription in full; then change, shower, have a snack, and be back to the office in approximately 75 minutes.

The training program is centered in a hospital gymnasium. The patients comment that they feel safer exercising in a hospital environment than in a nonmedical setting.

An active ingredient of a successful exercise training program is that the patients have fun. If an activity program is boring, the subject will usually find an excuse to prevent him from attending. The patients are given 3-4 minutes of calisthenics and advised to do similar exercises at home. We use volleyball as an enjoyable warmup. Ideally, it should be possible to provide variation in the recreational activity and still remain within the limits of prescribed exercise.

The intense phase of the exercise prescription is based on walking and jogging. Similar to the warmup phase, there is always a cool-down phase in a successful exercise prescription.

It has been stated by many that exercise is the best antitension *drug* available. Our psychiatrists tend to support this observation. The professional staff on the exercise training program must have a real concern for the participants, primarily as individuals, and only secondarily as coronary artery disease cases.

Summary

The published literature on long-term activity programs for patients with coronary artery disease has been reviewed. Short- and long-term studies have been compared and their deficiencies outlined. The factors which should be assessed in evaluating an exercise activity program have been discussed.

A review of the literature indicates that three questions have not yet been answered:

1. Do patients on a supervised exercise training program live longer when compared to their pair-matched control?
2. Are there fewer coronary events in these patients on an exercise training program?
3. If there is a difference between the exercise and the control group, what is the significant factor? Is it physiologic or psychologic?

The Saskatoon Program, which is an attempt to answer these questions, has been described.

REFERENCES

1. Barry, A.J., Daly, J.W., Pruett, E.D.R., Steinmetz, J.R., Birkhead, N.C., and Rodahl, K. Effects of physical training in patients who have had myocardial infarction. *Am. J. Cardiol.* 17:1-8, 1966.

2. Boyer, J.L., and Kasch, F.W. Exercise therapy in hypertensive men. *J.A.M.A.* 211:1668-1671, 1970.

3. Bruce, R.A., and McDonough, J.R. Coronary disease and exercise. *Tex. Med.* 65:73-77, 1969.

4. Brunner, D., and Meshulam, N. Prevention of recurrent myocardial infarction by physical exercise. *Isr. J. Med. Sci.* 5:783-785, 1969.

5. Clausen, J.P., and Trap-Jensen, J. Effects of training on the distribution of cardiac output in patients with coronary artery disease. *Circulation* 42:611-624, 1970.

6. Detry, J.M.R., Rousseau, M., Vandenbroucke, G., Kusumi, F., Brasseur, L.A., and Bruce, R.A. Increased arteriovenous oxygen difference after physical training in coronary heart disease. *Circulation* 44:109-118, 1971.

7. Dorossiev, D., Pertchev, I., Nikov, A., and Tzolov, A. Limiting factors for physical training after myocardial infarction. *Cor Vasa* 13:18-24, 1971.

8. Enselberg, C.D. Appraisal and reappraisal of cardiac therapy. Physical activity and coronary heart disease. *Am. Heart J.* 80:137-141, 1970.

9. Fejfar, Z., and Pisa, Z. Ischaemic Heart Disease. *Cor Vasa* 13:1-17, 1971.

10. Fletcher, G.F., and Cantwell, J.D. *Exercise in the Management of Coronary Heart Disease. A Guide for the Practicing Physician.* Springfield, Ill., Thomas, 1971.

11. Fox, S.M., III, Naughton, J.P., and Haskell, W.L. Physical activity and the prevention of coronary heart disease. *Ann. Clin. Res.* 3:404-432, 1971.

12. Fox, S.M., III, Naughton, J.P., and Gorman, P.A. Physical activity and cardiovascular health: I. Potential for prevention of coronary heart disease and possible mechanisms. II. The exercise prescription: intensity and duration. III. The exercise prescription: frequency and type of activity. *Mod. Concepts Cardiovasc. Dis.* 41:17-30, 1972.

13. Gottheiner, V. Long-range strenuous sports training for cardiac reconditioning and rehabilitation. *Am. J. Cardiol.* 22:426-435, 1968.

14. Hakkila, J., and Rinne, H. Rehabilitation of patients with myocardial infarction and patients with heart surgery. *Rep. Inst. Occup. Health* (Helsinki), No. 30, 1965.

15. Hanson, J.S., Tabakin, B.S., Levy, A.M., and Nedde, W. Long-term physical training and cardiovascular dynamics in middle-aged men. *Circulation* 38:783-799, 1968.

16. Heller, E.M. Practical graded exercise program after myocardial infarction. *Arch. Phys. Med. Rehabil.* 50:655-662, 1969.

17. Hellerstein, H.K. Exercise therapy in coronary disease. *Bull. N.Y. Acad. Med.* 44:1028-1047, 1968.

18. Katila, M., and Frick, M.H. A two-year circulatory follow-up of physical training after myocardial infarction. *Acta Med. Scand.* 187:95-100, 1970.

19. Kattus, A.A., Alvaro, A., and MacAlpin, R.N. Treadmill exercise tests for capacity and adaptation in angina pectoris. *J. Occup. Med.* 10:627-635, 1968.

20. Kavanagh, T., Shephard, R.J., Doney, H., and Pandit, V. Intensive exercise in coronary rehabilitation. *Med. Sci. Sports* 5:34-39, 1973.

21. Kellermann, J.J. Cardiac rehabilitation. What has been done and what should be done! Report of an international survey. *Acta Cardiol.* 14:61-68, 1970.

22. Klassen, G.A., Woodhouse, S.P., Hathirat, S., and Johnson, A.L. The effect of physical training of post-myocardial infarction patients: A controlled study. *Can. Med. Assoc. J.* 107:632, 1972.

23. Lovell, R.H., and Verghese, A. Haemodynamic effects of physical training in coronary patients. *Br. Med. J.* 3:327-330, 1967.

24. Lukomsky, P.E., and Cazov, E.I. Prophylaxis of ischaemic heart disease. *Bull. Int. Soc. Cardiol.* Special Issue, April 1972.

25. Mann, G.V., Garrett, H.L., Farhi, A., Murray, H., and Billings, F.T. Exercise to prevent coronary heart disease. *Am. J. Med.* 46:12-27, 1969.

26. Merriman, J.E. The physiological effects of physical activity in cardiac patients. *Acta Cardiol.* Suppl. 14:39-46, 1970.

27. Miller, M.G., and Brewer, J. Factors influencing the rehabilitation of the patient with ischaemic heart disease. *Med. J. Aust.* 1:410-416, 1969.

28. Nye, E.R., and Wood, P.G. Exercise and the patient with ischaemic heart disease. *N. Z. Med. J.* 70:31-34, 1969.

29. Pyfer, H.R., and Doane, B.L. Cardiac arrest during exercise training *J.A.M.A.* 210:101-102, 1969.

30. Radke, J.D., Hellerstein, H.K., Salzman, S.H., Maistelman, H.M., and Ricklin, R. The quantitative effects of physical conditioning on the exercise electrocardiogram of subjects with arteriosclerotic heart disease and normal subjects. *In*, Brunner, D. and Jokl, E., Eds. *Physical Activity and Aging.* Medicine and Sport Series, Vol. 4, pp. 168-194. Baltimore, University Park Press, 1970.

31. Rechnitzer, P.A., Pickard, H.A., Paivio, A.U., Yuhasz, M.S., and Cunningham, D. Long-term follow-up study of survival and recurrence rates following myocardial infarction in exercising and control subjects. *Circulation* 45:853-857, 1972.

32. Redwood, D.R., Rosing, D.R., and Epstein, S.E. Circulatory and symptomatic effects of physical training in patients with coronary artery disease and angina pectoris. *N. Engl. J. Med.* 286:959-965, 1972.

33. Rudd, J.L., and Day, W.C. A physical fitness program: community aspects. *Am. Correct. Ther. J.* 22:148-151, 1968.

34. Sloman, G., Pitt, A., Hirsch, E.Z., and Donaldson, A. The effect of a graded physical training programme on the physical working capacity of patients with heart disease. *Med. J. Aust.* 1:4-7, 1965.

35. Tobis, J.S., and Zohman, L.R. Follow-up study of cardiac patients on a rehabilitation service. *Arch. Phys. Med. Rehabil.* 51:286-90, 1970.

36. Varnauskas, E., Bjorntorp, P., Fahlen, M., Prerovsky, I., and Stenberg, J. Effects of physical training on exercise blood flow and enzymatic activity in skeletal muscle. *Cardiovasc. Res.* 4:418-422, 1970.

37. Wenger, N.K., Gilbert, C.A., and Siegel, W. Symposium: The use of physical activity in the rehabilitation of patients after myocardial infarction. *South. Med. J.* 63:891-897, 1970.

38. Whitsett, T.L., and Naughton, J. The effect of exercise on systolic time intervals in sedentary and active individuals and rehabilitated patients with heart disease. *Am. J. Cardiol.* 27:352-358, 1971.

39. Evaluation of Rehabilitation Programmes for Patients with Myocardial Infarction. *W.H.O. Rep. – Work. Group*, Bordeaux, 1970. (Doc. Euro 8206(5))

40. Keys, A. Physical activity and the epidemiology of coronary heart disease. *In*, Brunner, D., and Jokl, E., Eds. *Physical Activity and Aging*. Medicine and Sports Series, Vol. 4, pp. 250-266. Baltimore, University Park Press, 1970.

41. Physical Exercise Committee. *Physician's Handbook for Evaluation of Cardiovascular and Physical Fitness*. Nashville, Tennessee Heart Association, 1971.

42. Committee on Exercise. *Exercise Testing and Training of Apparently Healthy Individuals: A Handbook for Physicians*. New York, American Heart Association, 1972.

43. Andersen, K.L., Shephard, R.J., Denolin, H., Varnauskas, E., and Masironi, R. *Fundamentals of Exercise Testing*. Geneva, W.H.O., 1971.

44. Bruce, R.A., and Kluge, W. Defibrillatory treatment of exertional cardiac arrest in coronary disease. *J.A.M.A.* 216:653-658, 1971.

25

PREVENTION AND CONTROL OF
CARDIOVASCULAR COMPLICATIONS

Robert A. Bruce, M.D. FACC, FACP, FRSM

From time to time the question is asked: Why isn't there more evidence of standardization of testing and training procedures? Although obviously standardization is needed, it cannot be achieved until a variety of approaches are explored. It would be a mistaken effort if all investigators performed these procedures in precisely the same way. A *diversity of approaches* and the exchange of information such as occurs at these meetings enables us to sort out the particular objectives, methods, and criteria which best serve the real needs of our patients. Indeed, our knowledge and understanding are advanced by opportunities to discuss a variety of approaches to the common problems.

Circulatory Responses of the Heart to Isometric Exercise

Although many aspects of safety precautions have been cited, two aspects should be discussed in depth. The first relates to isometric exertion, particularly with arm work, which, as noted by the industrial physiologist, is a more common problem on the job. Accordingly, observations of a study conducted with colleagues in Edinburgh [1] should be cited. In order to control muscle temperature, the forearm was immersed in a water bath at 34° C for 20 minutes. Maximal voluntary contraction and its reproducibility were then defined just as many of you performed a handgrip test with a dynamometer. Next, 30 percent of maximal contraction was maintained to the limits of fatigue and onset of ischemic pain which finally resulted in sudden release. During this time, more proximal-muscle contractions of the upper arm, shoulder girdle, and back were recruited. Color photographs also documented cutaneous flushing of the head and neck; in some subjects this was very marked. In this instance, I could maintain this state of contraction, which initally seemed easy, for only 3-1/3 minutes. During this time, my heart rate and blood pressure increased from 72 to 90 beats/min and from 115/80 to 185/110 mm Hg. Immediately on release, heart rate decreased to 72 again as pressure dropped to 110/75 mm Hg. (The minor change in rate but striking changes in systolic and diastolic pressure are noteworthy.) Because of the excessive pressor response, it is easy to overload an ischemic left ventricle; indeed, this form of testing is clinically hazardous. Another point is that, if the same state of contraction is resumed after only 10 minutes and then after 3 minutes of rest (which are too short for adequate metabolic recovery), the heart rate and pressor changes are measured to the same peaks, but the duration of the contraction is shortened (Fig. 1). A subject may experience the subjective effects of this phenomenon as he carries his luggage to the airport. Thus, isometric exertion is more stressful than dynamic work, and it is proportional to the maximal strength of the muscles used.

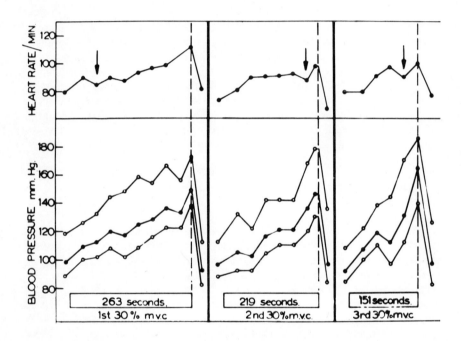

Fig. 1. Heart rate and pressor changes measured to the same peaks [1].

The second aspect that needs to be discussed is the effect of ambient heat. When work is performed in the heat, an additional circulatory stress lower work capacity even though $\dot{V}_{O_2}$ max is not affected. Normally, exercise reduce visceral blood flow and increases blood flow to the working skeletal muscle (Fig. 2). When the same exertion is performed at 110° F instead of 70-75° F

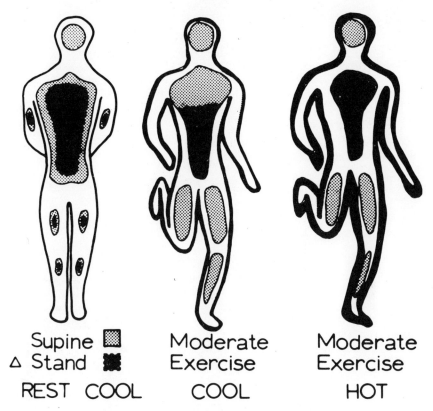

Supine ▦
△ Stand ✖
REST COOL

Moderate
Exercise
COOL

Moderate
Exercise
HOT

Fig. 2. Exercise and blood flow to skeletal muscles.

cutaneous blood flow is greatly increased to facilitate heart dissipation. When maximal exertion is approached, the crunch is applied and something must be sacrificed. The body sacrifices cutaneous circulation in order to meet metabolic requirements of working muscles, and consequently the core temperature may quickly rise to 104° F [2]. This is important in industry when workers are exposed to heat stress, and it is important in those parts of the world where work is performed in hot and humid climates. Similarly, testing procedures should not be unduly prolonged to the point that individuals develop a significant endogenous heat load. In terms of cardiac rehabilitation it is essential that the customary levels of training exercises be reduced under adverse environmental conditions of excessive heat and/or humidity. Individuals who are well trained, however, acquire heat acclimatization, and the trained instructor may not appreciate the additional burden imposed upon his untrained cardiac patient exercising in the heat.

General Hazards

Physicians and physical educators defined reasonable guidelines in 1958 [3]. Undesirable manifestations of exhausting exertion included: (1) cardiorespiratory symptoms persisting for more than 10 minutes; (2) fatigue for more than 2 hours; and (3) restless sleep and fatigue the next day.

More specifically for cardiac patients, there are risks to training which include:

Incidental musculoskeletal complications for the sedentary person who initially attempts calisthenics too strenuous

Prolonged fatigue with no improvement on successive training sessions

Progressive clinical manifestations of angina pectoris (AP) or pre-infarction angina

Exertional cardiac arrest.

The last complication is more common after several weeks of training [4]. It is usually unpredictable, but occasionally transient and subtle symptoms resembling transient ischemic attacks from arrhythmias may be noted. It is important to teach patients to note changes in symptoms, also changes in signs or behavior of their fellow patients. When either occurs, the supervisor should be informed before exercise training is continued.

In the clinical experiences of the Cardiopulmonary Research Institute (CAPRI) Program in Seattle, up to March 1972, there were nine cases of myocardial infarction (MI) in 190 CHD patients who completed 3 months of training.[1] Only one occurred after the first 3 months during a training session, the other eight during everyday activities, including resting at home. In comparison with 180 survivors of MI reported by Peterson [5], the overall expected number of cardiovascular deaths for the CAPRI Program when age-adjusted would be 21.9 (TABLE I). Yet, during this period there have been only six deaths after the initial training program among those participating in physical training, or a ratio of observed to expected of 0.276. This includes the youngest patient of 34 years with a history of prior MI and AP for months until relieved by physical training. He died suddenly while water-skiing on vacation. With neither a physician nor a defibrillator available he could not be resuscitated. Autopsy revealed extensive arteriosclerosis of the coronary vessels, old myocardial scars, but no acute infarction. Several months before, this patient was studied hemodynamically during upright bicycle exercise. At 75-watts workload, he suddenly developed supraventricular tachycardia and bundle branch block. Concomitantly, stroke volume, systolic blood pressure, and cardiac output decreased (TABLE II), as pulmonary arterial blood pressure rose. On this occasion, the tachyarrhythmia disappeared spontaneously when the exertion was stopped. In relation to his fatal arrhythmia, it seems likely that

---

[1] Personal communication of Dr. Howard Pyfer, Executive Director.

TABLE I

Clinical experience in men with coronary heart disease
(angina and/or prior myocardial infarction) who participated in
Physical Training Program sponsored by CAPRI, Seattle, May 1968 through February 1972

Age Group Years	Men Trained	Morbidity		CV Mortality		
		Cardiac Arrest[1]	Myocardial Infarction[2]	Observed	Expected	Ratio
30-39	13	1	0	1[3]	0	
40-49	62	0	2	1	7.75	.129
50-59	84	3	4	2	5.51	.362
60-69	36	1	3	2	8.65	.226
Altogether	195	5	9	6	21.91	.274
Rates		2.6%	4.6%	3.1%	11.2%	

[1] All occurred after initial 12-week training program; no evolving MI, detectable residual anoxic encephalopathy, and no fatalities as a result of immediate defibrillation of ventricles with a single shock.

[2] Only 1 MI occurred during training sessions, 3 others in everyday life during first 12 weeks and 5 thereafter; only 2 were initial infarctions, 7 were recurrent attacks.

[3] Sudden cardiac death several months after training program during whole-body isometric exertion of water-skiing while on vacation.

Data, courtesy of Dr. Howard Pyfer, Executive Director, Cardiopulmonary Res. Inst., Seattle

Data, courtesy of Dr. Donald Peterson, based on followup experience of 180 patients admitted to 4 hospitals in this community and discharged alive; average survival of fatal cases was 8 months. (personal communication)

TABLE II

Patient (D.A.) at age 34 with old MI and angina (dated 3/19/70)

Load watts	$\dot{V}_{O_2}$ ml/min	HR beats/min	C.O. l/min	S.V. ml/min	B.P. sys/dias	P.A.P. mm Hg
Rest	351	74	6.3	84	122/70 88	15
25	810	95	9.1	96	156/72 104	23
50	1138	116	10.9	94	160/72 104	31
75	(1403)	(140)	(13.3)[1]	..	..	..

[1] Expected values

water-skiing represented the extreme degree of whole-body isometric exercise, which must have imposed an enormous pressure afterload on an ischemic myocardium. His is the second case that has come to my attention of sudden cardiac death in a CHD patient while water-skiing.

Precautionary Requirements for Safety in Training

Given these considerations, there are several fundamentals to ensure safety in training.

A medically supervised program is preferable to unsupervised "do-it-yourself" approaches. This should include a preliminary clinical examination, an exercise test, and individualized training prescriptions. To be effective, training intensity must approach 70 percent $\dot{V}_{0_2}$max as measured or reliably estimated; the physician can do little more than tell the patient to work up to the *onset of symptoms*. It requires several minutes at a time, about 3 times a week for several weeks to increase $\dot{V}_{0_2}$max and secondarily reduce the relative aerobic requirement and circulatory stress on the heart at submaximal workloads.

Training regimens should be individualized. CAPRI experience has demonstrated that up to 10 levels of activity are required; each can be performed simultaneously by as many as 50 patients at a time, with a physical educator and a physician in attendance. Patients must be instructed how to *warm up*, to continue just long enough, and to *cool down* again. Heat stress from hot showers and saunas after training is to be avoided.

Monitoring heart rate is helpful, but recovery values are always less than those of peak exertion. Most importantly, the *failure of heart rate to slow* during the *same* level of submaximal exercise after a month or more of effective training is cause for concern. This may be the first sign of progressive coronary vascular disease. Frequent brief checks of the precordial ECG (which can be done within 10 seconds by applying defibrillator paddles and observing the oscilliscope or recording paper) often reveal new changes for the first time.

Continued surveillance is important even for the patient who becomes asymptomatic and no longer requires medication. Such patients may become overconfident under the delusion that they no longer have heart disease, which happened to the patient who died while water-skiing.

The loss of symptoms with effective physical training represents a reduction in the relative aerobic requirements below the threshold for symptoms (Fig. 3). This results from the substantial increase in $\dot{V}_{0_2}$ max and not from a fall in absolute level of $\dot{V}_{0_2}$max. Because $\dot{V}_{0_2}$max is greater, the *relative* aerobic requirement or percent of $\dot{V}_{0_2}$max is lower. An extreme example is that of a patient who had severe AP on walking a short distance, but who lost all symptoms and for more than 2 years has been able to jog a mile 3 times weekly without any medication. The patient and the noncritical physician may suspect cure of CHD, but examination of the precordial ECG during exercise testing still reveals marked changes which persist for at least 12 minutes after cessation of exercise (Fig. 3).

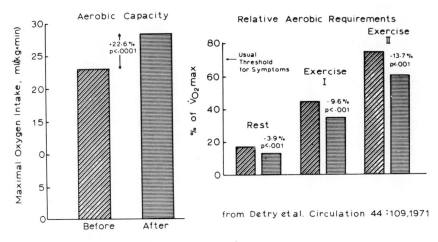

Fig. 3. Effects of physical training of coronary patients.

Other precautions include onset of acute illness, especially symptoms of minor MI, and overdosage with cardiac drugs, especially digitalis, diuretics and/or propranolol. Under these conditions training should be postponed or, if in progress, interrupted temporarily until the untoward effects of overtreatment are dissipated.

Advantages of Exercise Training

Clinically, physical training is feasible; if nothing else, the number of adherents exceeds the number of dropouts. Furthermore, the majority learn the value of maintaining the training regimen indefinitely. There are infrequent risks of MI and sudden exertional cardiac arrest, which makes medical screening and supervision highly desirable. The available evidence, without the benefit of controlled studies, strongly suggests that morbidity and mortality are *less* in the participants. There is, however, a real need for a well-designed study, with random allocation of patients and at least 5 years of followup, to define the differences quantitatively and reliably, and to exclude the possibility of unrecognized bias in the selection of patients who are trained and those who are used as *controls* for trainees.

Physiologically, training increases $\dot{V}_{O_2}$ max, probably because the skeletal muscles of cardiac patients are not diseased and mitochondrial and enzymatic changes can be induced. Heart rate and systolic blood pressure of the trained

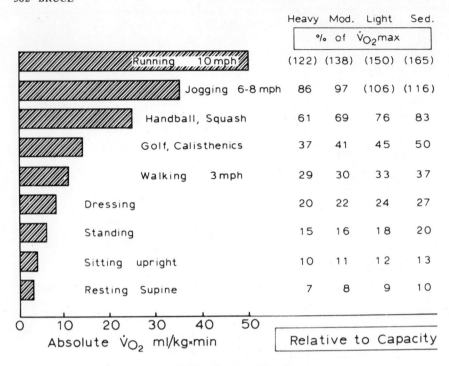

	Heavy	Mod.	Light	Sed.
	% of $\dot{V}_{O_2}$max			
Running 10 mph	(122)	(138)	(150)	(165)
Jogging 6-8 mph	86	97	(106)	(116)
Handball, Squash	61	69	76	83
Golf, Calisthenics	37	41	45	50
Walking 3 mph	29	30	33	37
Dressing	20	22	24	27
Standing	15	16	18	20
Sitting upright	10	11	12	13
Resting Supine	7	8	9	10

Absolute $\dot{V}_{O_2}$ ml/kg·min

Relative to Capacity

Fig. 4. Aerobic requirements in relation to activity status
(healthy, middle-aged men, 52.2 ± 7.2 years).

individual, whether a normal subject or a cardiac patient, usually are somewhat lower for any given level of submaximal exertion. Accordingly, the ischemic myocardium is spared slightly, rather than the restricted coronary blood flow significantly increased.

Psychologically, patients feel better with less clinical evidence of anxiety and depression. There are calculated risks to training, but with proper selection and supervision, especially emergency facilities for defibrillation for the rare occasions that require it, the benefits exceed the risks. Nevertheless, not all patients can be improved with physical training (actually, only about five out of every six patients). The sixth patient, as yet individually unpredictable, will not improve or even exhibit progression of clinical manifestations. He is the patient more likely to need revascularization of the myocardium by the steadily improving surgical techniques. Even then, maximal benefit may not be achieved until physical training is an adjunct to management during the convalescent phase.

Summary

There are many aspects to prevention and control of complications. There is need for physical educators to realize the importance of relative aerobic requirements. Training activities must be adjusted to the capacity of individual patients and not to that of the healthy and often younger members of the training staff. Even in healthy middle-aged men there are appreciable differences in relative aerobic requirements, according to habitual activity status, for ordinary activities (Fig. 4).

REFERENCES

1. Bruce, R.A., et al. The effects of digoxin on fatiguing static and dynamic exercise in man. *Clin. Sci.* 34:29, 1968.

2. Rowell, L.B., et al. Reductions in cardiac output, central blood volume and stroke volume with thermal stress in normal men during exercise. *J. Clin. Invest.* 45:1801, 1966.

3. AMA/AAHPER Report. Exercise and Fitness. *J.A.M.A.* 166:1744, 1958.

4. Bruce, R.A., and Kluge, W. Defibrillatory treatment of exertional cardiac arrest in coronary disease. *J.A.M.A.* 216:653, 1971.

5. Peterson, D.R., and Chinn, N. Survival after intensive coronary care: A method for evaluating therapeutic intervention. *Northwest Med.* 52:1335, 1969.

26

ASPECTS OF COMMUNITY EXERCISE PROGRAMS

A. ECONOMIC ASPECTS OF
CARDIAC REHABILITATION PROGRAMS

Howard R. Pyfer, M.D. and *Belvin L. Doane*

The advent of physical reconditioning programs for patients with cardio-pulmonary disease requires sound financial organization for continued effective service. Initially, some of these programs received financial support in the form of grants from foundations and government sources. As the programs moved from a position of research and study to one of health care delivery, grant support was reduced, and it was apparent that the programs had to become self-supporting. It seems prudent, therefore, to plan for this eventuality from the beginning. It is sad to see a program, which is providing a vital service, succumb to poor financial planning.

The Cardio-Pulmonary Rehabilitation Programs, organized in the State of Washington by the Cardio-Pulmonary Research Institute (CAPRI), a nonprofit corporation, received partial funding in 1969 from the Washington/Alaska Regional Medical Program to develop answers to basic organizational problems. The financial aspects of these programs received a great deal of attention from the outset, since those involved wished to provide ongoing service to patients in the Seattle area.

Issues requiring solutions included:
1. Initial expense involved in developing a program;
2. Guidelines that a community should evaluate when studying the feasibility of developing a program;
3. Optimal class sizes and other factors based on cost; determining a realistic fee schedule to provide enough revenue for self-support; and
4. The role of health insurance companies in such a program.

The goal was to develop a prototype program which could be implemented in any community meeting certain criteria. The organization included a central office which assumed most of the administration, leaving the local staff free to concentrate on the actual task of rehabilitation. The central office functions included: billing, processing insurance claims, purchasing, accounting, quality control, and preparation and production of forms. The following discussion is based on this style of management.

Initial Investment

A specific investment of funds is necessary to establish a new rehabilitation unit. Certain required instrumentation and equipment is critical to the proper operation of the unit. Its reliability must be very high; it must be portable; and must be on hand at all times. The equipment investment will approximate $9,500, plus or minus 15 percent, depending upon the source of supply and other factors (Appendix A).

Another initial investment is the cost of training the physicians and physical educators supervising the program. This cost, depending upon the qualifications of the individuals involved, travel, and compensation levels, ranges from $2,000 to $3,000.

Administrative costs, also incurred during the startup phase, include personnel to coordinate the setup of facilities, and publicity for the development of support. Costs for this phase are estimated between $3,000 and $4,000.

When participants are identified, tested, and enrolled, the program is ready for operation. Costs incurred immediately include rental of facilities, salaries for physical supervisors, and compensation for doctors who maintain an overall cognizance of the program. The initial investment must be repaid so that additional units may be established to satisfy a critical need. A prorated amortized portion of the investment cost can and should be charged to the operation of the unit. Inasmuch as the central CAPRI office provided fee-schedule support, quality control, bookkeeping, billing, and negotiation of cooperation with the insurance companies and other funding organizations, some prorated cost of the central operation was allocated to the operating unit (Appendix B).

Based upon the experience of operating CAPRI, we know that receipts from billings lag the mailing of the billings by 1½ to 2 months. Therefore, a new unit should have an operating reserve of approximately $5,000 in order to meet its operation payroll, pay its rent and other operating costs, and provide for the billing services needed for collection. A lesser amount may necessitate physicians in the program contributing time and deferring payment to other personnel, as well as delayed payment of rent and other costs (Appendix C).

Summary of Initial Costs

Equipment and supplies	$9,500
Training	$2,000-$3,000
Administrative costs	$3,000-$4,000
First year deficit	$5,000
Total	$19,500-$21,000

For maximum security, a contingency fund of 15 percent should be planned; this would approximate $3,000, bringing the total required to $22,500-$24,500.

Financial Guidlines

The development of a self-supporting program requires the projection of all costs and the establishment of a fee schedule to produce the necessary revenue. Appendix B shows a projection of the expenses and income for a new program in the first year of operation. These operations are based on the Seattle experience during 4½ years with certain assumptions applied:

1. New program in a new community.
2. Ten participants in original group.
3. No additional participants in second month.
4. Five new participants added each month beginning with the third month.
5. Attrition per experience model.
6. Fees per current schedule:
   Rate A: 0-3 months $ 4.50/session
   Rate B: 3-12 months $ 4.00/session
   Rate C: 12+ months $25.00/month
7. Participants tested at entry, 3 months, 12 months, and annual intervals thereafter.
8. Tests require 1/2 hour of physician time and 1 hour of physical director time.
9. Activity sessions 3 times/week for 45 minutes. One hour gym time and physician time and 2½ hours physical supervisor time allowed per session.
10. Average attendance per experience:
    Group A: 0-3 months   attend 10 times/month = 80 percent
    Group B: 3-12 months   attend 9 times/month = 72 percent
    Group C: 12+ months   attend 8 times/month = 64 percent
11. Program operates 150 sessions/year exclusive of national holidays. An average of 12½ sessions/month used for planning.
12. Physical directors' tasks include: Testing, mounting and typing test records; setup and pickup of test and exercise equipment; record maintenance; liaison with patients; and coordination with central office.
13. Physicians' duties include: Medical supervision of program; initial and continuing evaluation of each patient; testing and counseling of patients; and emergency medical treatments.

Programs of rehabilitation have been organized in the past with volunteer leadership. It is our observation that such arrangements usually are satisfactory only for a short-term operation. Payment for service rendered is a preferred way of assuring commitment to the tasks to be performed.

A primary aim of the Seattle programs was to improve the cost effectiveness of the physicians involved. Through the use of specially trained paramedical personnel, this has been attained to a great extent. The physician/physical educator team approach makes it possible to supervise a class size of 50 patients efficiently.

Payment for the physical facilities was organized on a flat fee plus participant volume basis. Appendix D describes the rationale and the costs used for planning.

Fee Structure

Based on a program with 40 active participants and the experienced attrition rate previously mentioned, the income and expense will break even at the following fee structure:

Initial 12 weeks — $4.50/session

Subsequent sessions to first year — $4.00/session

Subsequent sessions beyond first year — $25.00/month

The different rates are based on the amount of direct attention usually required for a patient in the program. Initially, the patient requires a great deal of counseling and care; this decreases as the patient better understands the rehabilitation process, his symptoms diminish, and physical condition improves.

The cost of testing has been determined and the following schedule established: maximal exercise tolerance test—$48.00; resting 12-lead ECG—$15.00; timed vital capacity—$5.00.

Coverage by Health Insurance Companies

To make rehabilitation financially feasible for the largest possible number of patients, coverage of costs by health insurance companies is a necessity. A major difficulty is the institutional rigidity in many insurance companies. Since the service is new (the method of delivery is not via hospital or physician's office) and for a host of other vague assumptions, most insurance companies are quite reluctant to provide coverage.

After 2 years of negotiations, a majority of the carriers in the Northwest assumed a positive stance with regard to reimbursing all or a portion of the costs. Factors important to insurance companies are:

1. Billing as a medical service, making actual physician supervision imperative.
2. Charges must be accounted for on a per service basis.
3. The organization billing for the services needs medical orientation. Organizations such as YMCAs and community centers do not meet this requirement. The Cardio-Pulmonary Research Institute, a private nonprofit corporation with medical orientation, contracts with community organizations for their facilities. This appears to satisfy the requirements of the insurance carriers.
4. The programs cannot be funded for research. If research is part of the overall purpose, it must be a clearly separate function from patient care.

Summary

The magnitude of CHD and pulmonary diseases has received major attention. The cost to our society is staggering. Programs of physical rehabilitation offer a logical method for enhancing the lives of the stricken and returning them to productive activity. To be effective and economical, it seems wise to organize these programs as group programs on a communitywide basis. Specially trained teams of medical and paramedical personnel then have greater impact on the problem.

Good financial planning will keep costs low, quality high, and insure the long-term success of the program.

APPENDIX A

Initial Equipment and Supplies

Sphygmomanometer	$ 60
Stethoscope	25
Pulmonary function apparatus	275
Examination table	200
Work table & chair	80
Stop watch	25
Equipment storage cabinet	110
ECG mounter	150
ECG recorders (2)	1,900
Bicycle ergometer	200
Treadmill	2,730
Metronome	15
Oscilloscope	300
Power & signal cables	75
Defibrillation equipment	2,750
Oxygen equipment	65
Medical supplies (emergency)	100
Testing supplies	200
Portable equipment cart	200
Electric clock—modified	20
Patient & emergency files	15
Instruction charts	25
Total	$9,520

Costs are approximate but within normal ranges. With the exception of the bicycle ergometer, defibrillator, and pulmonary function apparatus, the brand of equipment to be purchased will depend on cost, quality, and preference of the local staff. The defibrillator, ergometer, and pulmonary function apparatus have unique features essential to the quality and/or standardization of the program.

APPENDIX B

Expenses (month)	1	2	3	4	5	6
Personnel						
Med. sup–therapy	$ 312	313	312	313	312	313
Med. sup.–testing	125	–	175	67	125	125
Phys. Sup.	200	200	200	200	200	200
Total personnel	637	513	687	580	637	638
Facilities	185	179	209	257	257	281
Supplies	95	18	133	81	119	127
Equipment						
Maint. reserve	40	40	40	40	40	40
Replacement reserve	119	119	119	119	119	119
Insurance						
Equipment	30	30	30	30	30	30
Liability	20	20	25	40	40	50
Subtotal	1,126	919	1,243	1,147	1,242	1,285
Training reserve	99	99	99	99	99	99
Administrative allocation	450	450	450	450	450	450
Expansion reserve	150	150	150	150	150	150
Total operating costs	$1,825	1,618	1,942	1,846	1,941	1,984
Cumulative operating costs	$1,825	3,443	5,385	7,231	9,172	11,156
Income						
Earned revenue	1,130	405	1,582	1,267	1,607	1,751
Less 10% uncollectable	113	40	158	126	160	175
Net revenue	1,017	365	1,424	1,141	1,447	1,576
Cumulative revenue	1,017	1,382	2,806	3,947	5,394	6,970
Surplus-(deficit)	$(808)	(1,253)	(518)	(705)	(494)	(408)
Cumulative surplus-(deficit)	$(808)	(2,061)	(2,579)	(3,284)	(3,778)	(4,186)

Expenses (month)	7	8	9	10	11	12	1st Year
Personnel							
Med. sup.–therapy	312	313	312	313	312	313	3,750
Med. sup.–testing	125	125	125	125	125	175	1,417
Phys. Sup.	200	200	200	200	200	200	2,400
Total personnel	637	638	637	638	637	687	7,566
Facilities	299	317	329	347	359	347	3,366
Supplies	133	139	143	149	151	179	1,467
Equipment							
Maint. reserve	40	40	40	40	40	40	480
Replacement reserve	119	119	119	119	119	119	1,428
Insurance							
Equipment	30	30	30	30	30	30	360
Liability	57	65	73	81	85	81	637
Subtotal	1,315	1,348	1,371	1,404	1,421	1,483	15,304
Training reserve	99	99	99	99	99	99	1,188
Administrative allocation	450	450	450	450	450	450	5,400
Expansion reserve	150	150	150	150	150	150	1,800
Total operating costs	2,014	2,047	2,070	2,103	2,120	2,182	23,692
Cumulative operating costs	13,170	15,217	17,287	19,390	21,510	23,692	23,692
Income							
Earned revenue	1,859	1,967	2,039	2,147	2,219	2,419	20,392
Less 10% uncollectable	185	196	203	214	221	241	2,032
Net revenue	1,674	1,771	1,836	1,933	1,998	2,178	18,360
Cumulative revenue	8,644	10,415	12,251	14,184	16,182	18,360	18,360
Surplus-(deficit)	(340)	(276)	(234)	(170)	(122)	4	(5,332)
Cumulative surplus-(deficit)	(4,526)	(4,802)	(5,036)	(5,206)	(5,328)	(5,332)	(5,332)

Appendix B cont.

Expenses (month)	13	14	15	16	17	18
Personnel						
Med. sup—therapy	312	313	312	313	312	313
Med. sup.—testing	125	150	150	150	150	150
Phys. Sup.	200	200	200	200	200	200
Total personnel	637	663	662	663	662	663
Facilities	383	383	395	401	413	425
Supplies	161	176	180	182	186	190
Equipment						
Maint. reserve	40	40	40	40	40	40
Replacement reserve	119	119	119	119	119	119
Insurance						
Equipment	30	30	30	30	30	30
Liability	91	91	95	97	101	105
Subtotal	1,461	1,502	1,521	1,532	1,551	1,572
Training reserve	99	99	99	99	99	99
Administrative allocation	450	450	450	450	450	450
Expansion reserve	150	150	150	150	150	150
Total operating costs	2,160	2,201	2,220	2,231	2,250	2,271
Cumulative operating costs	25,852	28,053	30,273	32,504	34,754	37,025
Income						
Earned revenue	2,283	2,415	2,403	2,451	2,467	2,499
Less 10% uncollectable	228	241	240	245	246	250
Net revenue	2,055	2,178	2,163	2,206	2,221	2,250
Cumulative revenue	20,415	22,593	24,756	26,962	29,183	31,433
Surplus-(deficit)	105	(23)	(57)	(25)	(29)	(21)
Cumulative surplus-(deficit)	(5,437)	(5,460)	(5,517)	(5,542)	(5,571)	(5,592)

Expenses (month)	19	20	21	22	23	24	2nd Year
Personnel							
Med. sup.—therapy	312	313	312	313	312	313	7,500
Med. sup.—testing	150	150	150	150	150	150	3,192
Phys. Sup.	200	200	200	200	200	200	4,800
Total personnel	662	663	662	663	662	663	15,491
Facilities	431	431	449	454	460	454	8,445
Supplies	192	192	198	200	202	200	3,726
Equipment							
Maint. reserve	40	40	40	40	40	40	960
Replacement reserve	119	119	119	119	119	119	2,856
Insurance							
Equipment	30	30	30	30	30	30	720
Liability	107	107	113	115	117	115	1,891
Subtotal	1,581	1,582	1,611	1,621	1,630	1,621	34,089
Training reserve	99	99	99	99	99	99	2,376
Administrative allocation	450	450	450	450	450	450	10,800
Expansion reserve	150	150	150	150	150	150	3,600
Total operating costs	2,280	2,281	2,310	2,320	2,329	2,320	50,865
Cumulative operating costs	39,305	41,586	43,896	46,216	48,545	50,865	50,865
Income							
Earned revenue	2,531	2,547	2,547	2,595	2,627	2,595	50,356
Less 10% uncollectable	254	254	254	259	262	259	5,022
Net revenue	2,278	2,293	2,293	2,336	2,365	2,336	45,334
Cumulative revenue	33,711	36,004	38,297	40,633	42,998	45,334	45,334
Surplus-(deficit)	(2)	12	(17)	16	36	16	5,691
Cumulative surplus-(deficit)	(5,504)	(5,606)	(5,623)	(5,639)	(5,675)	(5,691)	5,691

APPENDIX C

Projected Billings vs. Costs—First Two Years of Operation*

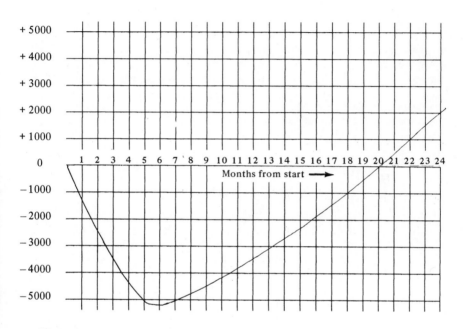

*For cash flow slide 2 months

APPENDIX D

Facilities Rental

Gym Costs

Based on typical membership costs—i.e., YMCA Businessmen's Club at $120 per year.

This fee covers all costs of usage, including space, attendance, physical department staff, and administrative functions. Usage will be typically several times a week at concentrated times—i.e., noon, 5:00 p.m., etc.

CAPRI proposes to use unpopular times and to not include physical staff and administrative costs since these are covered separately. Therefore, an appropriate rental would be about 60% of the "Club" fee or about $6 per enrolled man a month.

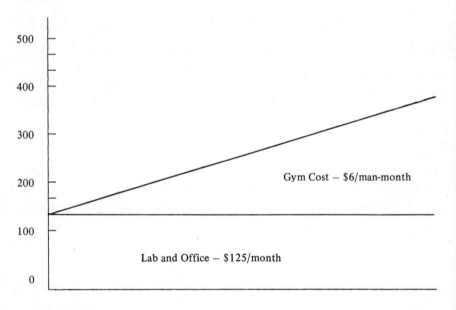

Planning Cost

$125/month plus $6/enrolled man/month.

B. ECONOMIC ASPECTS OF A STRESS TESTING AND EXERCISE TRAINING PROGRAM

Lenore R. Zohman, M.D.

Background

The cardiopulmonary program at Montefiore Hospital, New York City, was initiated with support from the Public Health Service and the Social and Rehabilitation Service at a budget level of approximately $156,000. By January 1971, cardiopulmonary rehabilitation had developed into a self-sufficient clinical program. Although other services were provided as part of the original program, the exercise stress testing and exercise training programs were the most useful to the practicing physicians. Further, stress testing and exercise training programs were necessary to provide continuing care to the patients who previously participated in the study groups. The available clinical services included exercise stress testing, exercise prescription, and the supervision of exercise training programs.

A national survey conducted in 1970, by the Department of Community Programs, American Heart Association, revealed that 87 programs were available for cardiac patients throughout the United States. Approximately 30 programs did appropriate exercise stress testing to evaluate participants. Only two programs available in the New York area. provided monitored testing before prescription of exercise. One was limited to the employees of an insurance company who exercised at indoor company facilities, and the second was conducted in a smaller Brooklyn hospital where the patients exercised individually on calibrated bicycles but not in a gymnasium. Since a comprehensive testing and training facility was not located in the New York area, the Cardiopulmonary Rehabilitation Section, Montefiore Hospital, assumed this role. The testing station was hospital-based (at Montefiore), referring patients to one of three training facilities: the West Side YMCA, Manhattan; the Hubshman Cardiac Rehabilitation Center, Bronx,; and The Manhattan Beach Jewish Center, Brooklyn. Three additional training facilities (Scarsdale, New York; Manhasset, New York; and Trenton, New Jersey) are in the planning stages.

After one year of operation, questionnaires were sent to participants in the program. The data presented were gathered from the results of 349 questionnaires and from actual workload and income statistics.

Patient Referral

The house staff and attending physicians at Montefiore and Morrisania Hospitals were informed that the Cardiopulmonary Research Program provided a clinical program on a fee-for-service basis. Private physicians, who had referred patients to research studies in the past, were contacted directly. The physical directors of the three training facilities listed previously were advised of the change from a research to clinical program. The director of the Montefiore unit spoke to groups of physicians about exercise stress testing and exercise prescription. Medical news media representatives were present at many of these presentations and information was disseminated through the medical press. Subsequently, the new service, considered of public interest, was described on television news broadcasts. Thereafter, a 1/2-hour documentary film about exercise stress testing and exercise training to promote physical fitness and decrease the likelihood of coronary heart disease (CHD) was prepared by a local television station. This documentary was telecast at least three times. Even if patients heard about the program and were self-referred, referrals were accepted only from physicians. The patient might select a personal physician from a panel of physicians if he did not have his own doctor. All patients were returned to their physicians according to the practices set forth in Fig. 1.

The responses to a questionnaire distributed at the end of the first year indicated that 40.7 percent of the patients were referred by their personal physicians, whereas 59.3 percent of the patients initiated the referral themselves on the advice of friends, other patients, because they had learned of the service from television programs, newspaper or magazine articles, or through the staff of the training facilities. Medical clearance was obtained from the patient's private physician. Only 6.5 percent of the physicians did not want their patients to have an exercise stress test. They changed their minds, however, after the director of the unit clarified the test procedures and policies.

Approximately 20 new physicians referred patients to the unit for the first time each month, and five physicians, who had sent patients previously, referred other patients each month.

Patient Eligibility

The antecedent research projects involved only patients with healed myocardial infarctions (MI) or with angina pectoris (AP). The new clinical program accepted these patients, as well as those requiring (1) diagnostic stress testing, (2) evaluation of physical performance with or without a ventricular pacemaker, (3) pre- and post-operative coronary vein bypass graft surgery, (4) enrollment in a rehabilitation program as chronic pulmonary disease patients, and (5) physical performance information as part of a work evaluation program. Deconditioned older adults also were accepted into the program.

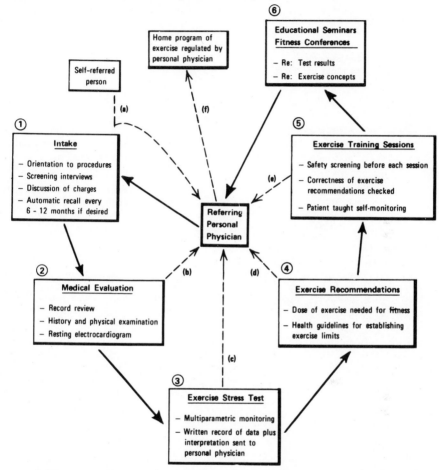

Note: Solid arrows indicate the usual patient routing. Dotted arrows indicate options open to referring physician. Further explanations given in text.

Fig. 1. Relationship of the testing-training station to the personal physician.

OPTIONS OPEN TO REFERRING PERSONAL PHYSICIAN

1-6 Physician may elect to have patient proceed through usual routing, including automatic recall.

a. No self-referred patient is accepted without the knowledge and concurrence of the physician.

b. After medical evaluation, the patient may be rejected for exercise stress testing and referred back to the private physician for further medical evaluation or therapy.

c. The referring physician may want the exercise stress test information for diagnostic purposes only and may not request an exercise program. Patient then returns directly to private physician.

d. The exercise recommendations may be used by the physician to regulate an exercise program for his patient at another training facility (not one affiliated with the testing station).

e. The physician may wish to make all explanations to his patient and bypass the Educational Seminars. Materials useful for discussing programming with patients are provided to physicians on request.

f. The physician may use the results of the exercise stress test to prescribe a home exercise program for his patient.

Procedures

Secretaries were trained to record the medical history from the patient's physician and to make him aware of the different types of programs.

> A program for post-MI patients for reconditioning and increasing physical fitness (the *post-cardiac class*; a program of monitored individualized exercise for AP patients (individualized exercise); a program of breathing training, Bird respirator treatment, and physical conditioning for chronic pulmonary disease patients (Pulmonary Rehabilitation Program); a reconditioning program for older adults (Older Adult group exercise program); a work assessment program for post-MI or other patients (simulated job monitoring and on-the-job monitoring).

In the Work Physiology Unit, Montefiore Hospital, a central testing station was established. Either a bicycle ergometer or a treadmill test was performed in a controlled environment room. The test was either continuous or intermittent, depending upon the physical condition of the patient. The more seriously ill patients performed intermittent tests. All tests were submaximal, proceeding to the end point of either 85 percent of the maximum age-predicted heart rate, or the appearance of symptoms, signs, or detrimental ECG changes. The tests were multistage with monitoring of workload, ECG for heart rate and configuration, blood pressure, and oxygen consumption.

Detailed consent forms patterned after the American Heart Association model were used. A DC defibrillator was operational during testing despite the availability of a complete cardiac arrest emergency team within the hospital. Medical, as well as paramedical personnel, were taught to use the defibrillator and the entire staff, including secretaries, was taught to administer cardiopulmonary resuscitation.

The referring physician received a report of the cardiovascular history and physical examination, the data and interpretation of the stress test, and an exercise prescription for the patient.[1] Both the patient's limits and his recommended activity level were provided. In addition, literature listing the caloric expenditures of the various recreational activities, and describing how to use the target heart rate, were included in duplicate for the physician's use. Telephone contact with the head of the unit permitted clarification of unclear reports. If a

---

[1] If requested.

patient's doctor agreed, a copy of the data and interpretation was sent to the physical director of the facility the patient wished to attend. The physician also was given the option of having a physician member of the laboratory staff explain the test results and the recommendations to the patient. Fewer than one-fourth of the physicians queried wanted test results explained by a laboratory physician. Lastly, group meetings, with an invitation to all patients to attend, were held every 3 or 4 months for general explanations of data and progress.

At all three training stations, the *post-cardiac* classes were held three times a week. The activities consisted of alternating patterns of calisthenics and run/ walk sequences regulated by the target heart rate recommendation (TABLE I, at end of chapter). Individualized bicycle exercise, when prescribed, was performed under the supervision of a nurse specialist or physiologist at the Hubshman Center only. The pulmonary program (also available at the Hubshman Center only) included treatment with the Bird respirator, breathing training, oxygen breathing during exercise, and reconditioning exercise for those with very severe respiratory insufficiency. The older adult classes, conducted twice a week, included special low-level exercises geared to an older population and dietary counseling. Whenever facilities permitted (the Hubshman Center and the West Side YMCA), the classes were not limited to men. Job monitoring was based only at the Hubshman Center which is adjacent to the hospital. The jobs were simulated in hospital industry. On occasion, a nurse specialist, using portable telemetry and dataphone equipment, went to the place of employment and telephoned the ECG back to the hospital where it was observed for several hours.

The Training Stations

The three training stations differed somewhat. The Hubshman Cardiac Rehabilitation Center, Bronx, is affiliated with the Musholu-Montefiore Community Center adjacent to the Montefiore Hospital. This facility is equipped with 8-channel ECG telemetry and a complete cardiac resuscitation unit. It is staffed by a nurse trained in coronary care and an exercise physiologist. It is, therefore, less like a public recreational facility than are the stations at the West Side YMCA and the Manhattan Beach Jewish Center. It has a much smaller gymnasium, 19.5 × 28 ft, since only very incapacitated patients use this facility rather than the more remote training stations.

The West Side YMCA has a gym, 60 × 40 ft, with a 24-laps-to-the-mile running track. Initially, three physical educators were trained in the techniques of cardiopulmonary resuscitation, the recognition of cardiac symptoms, and the specific exercises, patterned after the Cureton program, cardiac patients were to perform. Subsequently, the YMCA hired an exercise physiologist, who began exercise stress testing of normal individuals in collaboration with the Montefiore Program. Because the YMCA testing station existed, more complete resuscitation measures, such as a defibrillator and an emergency drug box were made available.

The Manhattan Beach Jewish Center has a large gymnasium, 70 X 70 ft, containing a 20-laps-to-the-mile track. The physical educators in all the facilities maintain close contact with the Montefiore Testing Station and discuss any questions concerning interpretation of the reports received. The basic exercise patterns administered are very similar. The physical education staff is trained in closed chest cardiac massage and mouth-to-mouth resuscitation.

Job Descriptions and Staffing Patterns

The Montefiore Hospital-based testing station employs one full-time cardiologist to coordinate the activities and two part-time cardiologists who serve 3 hrs/week. The cardiologists screen patients, eliminating those who demonstrate contraindications to testing or training such as acute systemic illnesses, the possibility of recent cardiac damage, ventricular aneurysm, uncontrolled hypertension, or congestive heart failure. The cardiologist monitors the stress test after interpretation of the resting ECG. Upon receiving the data, he provides guidelines for an exercise program if this is indicated, or reports the diagnostic considerations if this is the reason for referral. He frequently discusses the results with the referring physician, and with the referring physician's approval, discusses the results with the patient. He also works with the physiologist if an exercise prescription is to be prepared.

The physiologist participates in the testing with the physician and prepares the exercise prescription based on the stress test results. He teaches the physical education instructors at the training facilities to understand the exercise prescription and to provide appropriate exercises conforming to the suggested guidelines.

The cardiopulmonary technician works with the cardiologist and physiologist during testing, and performs the gas analysis and resulting calculations. She is responsible for all data handling and compilations, as well as test preparations.

At the Hubshman Center training station, exercise classes and breathing training are supervised, and often the ECG is monitored by a nurse specialist while the exercise programs are conducted by the physiologist.

Two secretaries support this operation. One makes the appointments, handles the referrals from physicians, and provides information to patients. She maintains a recall system for followup and types patient reports. The second secretary is responsible for billings to patients and third parties and for compilation of statistics about caseload and income.

Because of heavy workloads, vacation schedules, and staffing problems, each individual is trained to assume a dual role. The cardiologist also learned to prepare exercise prescriptions, sometimes substituting for the physiologist. If the cardiologists were not present during monitoring, the nurse specialist (trained in the coronary care unit) could interpret the exercise ECG. The physiologist assumed the technician role by performing gas analysis and calculations, and the technician was taught to prepare some of the simpler exercise recommendations. The secretaries were able to record resting ECGs and to mount these correctly in the technician's absence. Either a secretary or the nurse could assist in making various recordings during the stress testing procedure.

Financial Data: Testing Station (Montefiore Hospital) and Hubshman Training Station

The charge for an exercise stress test is $155. This includes a $75 stress test fee, $30 for resting ECG (Montefiore usual charge) and a $50 professional consultation fee. For 10 in a group, $1.50/class session is charged ($15 collected per session). For 12 sessions/month, $180 accrued. Patients were monitored with ECG telemetry once a month. The total fee for this service is $250 for 10 patients.

Individual supervised bicycle exercise is provided at $5/session, and is recommended only for those patients with AP or those who require rapid increments in workloads for faster attainment of fitness before beginning a group maintenance program. Each patient is seen three times weekly at a charge of $60 per month.

The pulmonary patients paid $20/session for the individualized breathing training, Bird respirator treatment, and exercise classes. The monthly cost per patient was $240.

Older adults initially required individualized attention and were treated in the same manner as AP patients (individual sessions). They were later transferred to a group maintenance exercise class for older adults.

Hypothetical monthly income approximated the following:

50 stress tests at $155 each	$ 7,750/month
10 group exercisers (cardiac class)	180/month
10 group exercisers (older adult class)	180/month
20 ECG telemetered monitorings at $25 each	500/month
5 individual cardiac exercisers at $60/month	300/month
5 individual older adult exercisers at $60/month	300/month
8 pulmonary patients at $20/session	1,920/month
	$11,130/month

or a yearly potential income of $133,560.

Realization of this projected income presumes a high collection rate. Although a collection rate approaching 90 percent was obtained transiently by asking patients to pay out-of-pocket rather than waiting for reimbursement, the collection rate through the year was only 50 percent during some months.

The income is sufficient[1], however, to cover the salaries of the staff. Total salaries for the full-time cardiologist, nurse, two part-time cardiologists, exercise physiologist, technician, and two secretaries were $95,000. Fringe benefits amount to $19,000 (20 percent) and several thousand dollars were required for supplies and repairs.

---

[1] If assured third party payments are treated as received income.

The questionnaire study revealed that in New York, various types of health insurance reimburse the patient more than half the bill in only a third of the cases. Less than half the bill was reimbursed to the patient by third-party payments in 20 percent of the cases, and an additional 20 percent of patients received no reimbursement whatsoever.

Training Program Financial Arrangements (West Side YMCA, Manhattan Beach Jewish Center)

No fees are charged for the two exercise training programs, either for training their instructors or for supervising patient participation. Membership fees are required of the patients and paid directly to the training facilities. The only understanding with the training facilities is that if they wish to participate as a training station under the imprimatur of Montefiore Hospital, the patients accepted in the training program must be tested at the Montefiore station before entering the program. In this way, there is uniformity of test procedures and a single source of supervision and responsibility.

Satisfaction With the Program

Although an exercise stress testing and training program is capable of generating a large income, it is also a very expensive program. The current staffing patterns and procedures permit the number of tests to increase substantially before an increase in staff is required. In addition, it is possible with automated equipment to shorten the duration of a test, and to perform and supervise two tests simultaneously. Staff satisfaction and morale are high. The attitudes of patients to the test procedures and cost are also of interest. Among the patients, 89.9 percent felt that the test procedure was done professionally and went well, although in a few instances, the exercise was more difficult than had been anticipated. Some of the patients (7.7 percent) indicated that the procedure was rather hectic and prolonged. The patients' major dissatisfaction concerned communication of test results. Although 25.5 percent were satisfied with the explanation of test results and recommendations given by their own doctors, and 24.7 percent were satisfied with the explanation given by the laboratory physician, 11.5 percent required both physicians to explain the test results. In the remainder, the patients felt that test results were not explained adequately and that the recommendations were not clear. Twenty percent of the patients felt that the fees were excessive for the service rendered. However, 52.9 percent of the responders indicated that the fee was justified because of the special service entailed, but 22.7 percent considered it difficult to pay such a high fee.

Discussion: Programmatic Aspects

Results indicate that a program of exercise stress testing, exercise prescription, and exercise training can be made operational and financially solvent within one year. However, a word of caution is appropriate. The concepts involved in performance testing for diagnosis or to guide the therapy of cardiac patients are relatively new. There is a risk of serious cardiac event occurring in 1:10,000 tests. This may not be justified in every case. Since this risk does exist, it must be minimized. The patient must be adequately informed and appropriate emergency care must be readily available. It is crucial, therefore, to urge proceeding with caution and knowledge. Needless deaths or morbidity related to improper patient selection, incorrect or haphazard performance of procedures by improperly trained, inexperienced, or unprepared individuals, and failure of physicians to support, supervise, and control the training programs will cast an undeserved shadow on an extremely important, useful diagnostic and therapeutic tool.

At the present time, it is most convenient to perform exercise testing and training programs within a hospital, thus avoiding the necessity for state licensure. The program should have one central, responsible person as director who is appropriately trained in cardiology and exercise physiology. The success of the program depends on the competence and reputation of the director. Not every physician nor every cardiologist is trained to interpret an ECG derived from an exercise stress test. Transient arrhythmias may lead to an incorrect diagnosis of CHD. Monitoring bipolar leads may mislead due to postural ECG changes. A negative test result using one lead ECG monitoring does not necessarily exclude CHD, nor does the appearance of an occasional complex with depressed ST segment necessarily imply CHD.

Further, physical educators or physical therapists cannot be substituted for exercise physiologists since their training does not prepare them to develop exercise prescriptions, interpret oxygen consumption and energy cost measurements, operate the necessary laboratory instrumentation, or provide *exercise exchanges* for more flexible programming. Also, *lay leaders* or untrained instructors cannot generally substitute for the physical educator at the training station. The individuals at the training stations must have the professional background (not common in health clubs) and ethics necessary to accept medical recommendations, understand them, and adhere to such standards while providing motivation and leadership in their programs for promoting fitness.

Programmatically, in the New York community at least, exercise stress testing and exercise training programs serve the referring physician only in providing information about the exercise capacity of patients and not as part of a total overall medical approach to the patient. Physicians in this area prefer to provide the medical evaluation and laboratory studies required by their patients and they consider the exercise evaluation as contributory to their patient management plan.

Economic Considerations

Persons considering setting up such programs should seek consultation with individuals trained in business practices. The magnitude of the operation makes the usual private office methods too costly, whereas hospital administrators, in our experience, have little training in arranging what is essentially an outpatient operation, partially off premises and yet not a clinic.

Finally, some conflict may arise concerning expansion of the stress testing and training operation to include other remunerative activities. Sidelines such as developing a line of gymnasium clothing or selling exercise equipment may be attempted by non-medical people and should be discouraged.

Summary

At Montefiore Hospital, we have demonstrated that it is programmatically and economically feasible to operate an exercise stress test facility with at least three satellite training stations. Principles, policies, procedures, workload, and income data have been reviewed. The results of a questionnaire survey by participants in the program are presented and recommendations for the development of similar programs have been formulated.

TABLE I

How to use the target heart rate to guide your exercise program

1. *What is the "target heart rate"?*
   The target heart rate is that heart rate (in number of beats/min) which will provide sufficient challenge to your cardiovascular system to result in physical fitness, while remaining below the "too strenuous" level. Maintaining the target heart rate for 10-20 minutes supposedly provides an adequate "stimulus phase" in your exercise program. The preceding exercise or "warmup period" gives your circulatory system a chance to work up to the target gradually. The "cooldown period" after the stimulus phase at target heart rate permits the circulation to gradually slow down so that all parts of the body, including the heart, can accommodate to a lesser supply of blood (and oxygen) and thereby avoid a sudden deficiency in any one location.

2. *How to count the heart rate*
   Except under certain special circumstances (such as if an individual has irregular heart action or extra heart beats) the heart beats each minute are equal in number to the pulse beats each minute. Therefore, heart rate may be counted at any convenient pulse point—over the heart, over the carotid artery in the neck, at the wrist on the thumb side, inside the elbow towards the body, or even in the groin. It is important that the counting point be easy to feel, and the prospective exerciser should experiment until he finds a location on his anatomy at which the beat is readily accessible and easy to count. Sometimes a location with a weak beat at rest sports a bounding, easily countable beat on exercise so that selecting the counting point should be based on both a resting and exercising survey.
   Heart rate should be counted for 10 seconds only, and then multiplied by 6 to give the heart rate/min or minute heart rate. Taking one's own heart rate during exercise is

difficult; for practical purposes, therefore, we may assume that the rate counted during the first 10 seconds *immediately following* exercise is equivalent to the exercising rate, thus skirting the difficulty. However, this does *not* hold true for the entire first minute after exercise since the rate drops back towards the resting rate very quickly. In fact, one of the evidences of having attained physical fitness is the rapidity of this decline in rate *after* exercise; the more rapid the decline, the more fit the individual.

3. *When to count the heart rate*

To use heart rate as an effective guide in regulating your program you should analyze your exercise routine by developing a "heart rate profile" for yourself. That is, every 3-5 minutes of a new activity, you should stop for 10 seconds and count your heart rate. If these are written down or preferably drawn on a chart you will be able to determine at a glance how your exercise stacks up against your target rate.

Heart rate need not be counted every time one exercises, lest more time be devoted to counting than to exercising. Once you have established your "profile" it is reasonable to assume that if you are feeling well, your profile will be nearly the same today as yesterday. However, as you become more fit, your heart will have to beat less often and your profile will change. Therefore, examine your own profile again after 3-4 weeks of doing the same exercise program.

Similar principles apply if you are just beginning to exercise. Select a set of exercises or a sport which appeals to you and try it gradually. Monitor your heart rate at 3-5 minute intervals, then draw your profile. Certain activities get you up to high heart rates more quickly than others—for example, jogging or running raise the heart rate more swiftly than fast walking. Running upstairs or uphill does it even faster.

4. *How to use your target heart rate*

Once you have determined your heart rate profile for the type of activity you prefer to do, check it against the following guidelines:

a. The exercise period should last at least 30 minutes and need not be more than 60 minutes.

b. The first 10-20 minutes should result in heart rates which are somewhere in-between your resting heart rate and your target, but should not be in the target zone. During this "warmup period" the heart rate should be climbing gradually from resting to target.

c. The next 10-20 minutes should maintain the heart rate at the target level plus or minus about 5 heartbeats.

d. The last 10-20 minutes should permit the heart rate to gradually come down within 10 beats of the resting level—either above or below.

The exercise should be adjusted so that it results in the pattern described, either by eliminating the very strenuous exercises from the warmup and cooldown periods and doing them during the stimulus phase, or by doing the same activity at a slower or faster cadence.

5. *What kind of exercise is best?*

Exercise can be used to promote strength, skill or endurance. The desired goal dictates the type of exercise to be done. For example, weight lifting promotes strength predominantly rather than endurance. Running, cycling or swimming promote endurance. Endurance-building exercises are the most desirable for inducing cardiovascular fitness. Maintaining the heart rate in the desired target zone stimulates cardiovascular fitness by increasing endurance. Therefore, exercises which contract muscles and produce rhythmic, repetitive movements (isotonic exercises) are best since they promote endurance. Spurts of short-lived high-level exercise won't have the same desirable effect.

6. *How often should I exercise?*

Achieving physical fitness requires at least 30-minute exercise periods (of the right kind of exercise) at least 3 times weekly. Apparently there is only a small gain if exercise is done 5 or 6 times a week. However, there is a considerable loss of gains previously made if one does not exercise for more than 2 days. Alternate days of exercise seem to be the preferred pattern.

27

THE LAW AND CARDIAC REHABILITATION

A. LEGAL ASPECTS OF INFORMED CONSENT, STRESS TESTING, AND EXERCISE PROGRAMS

Gerald H. Siegel

The subject matter of exercise and heart disease is difficult to approach from a strictly legal perspective. In order to define a physician's responsibilities, minima of conduct should be established. This in turn requires that the legal advisor enter into the sphere of activity of a medical practitioner.

Thus, one is put in the seemingly anomalous position of advising a physician on the steps to take in the treatment of his patient. It is not my intention to encroach in any way on his prerogatives. However, acceptable norms of conduct or the so-called *standards of care* need to be discussed. To do so requires a detailed account of certain medical steps to be taken, or procedures to be followed. It is not the intention to imply that this is the only way; rather, it is hoped that a certain legally acceptable minimum can be established.

The law is not as universal as medicine. The standard of care varies from State to State, as, for example, does the time limit within which a legal action must be commenced. No attempt will be made to cover every contingency in every jurisdiction. Rather, a broad overview is sought. Similarly, no effort is made to set forth detailed rules of law and the reasons for them. Instead, broad generalizations are used in order not to become bogged down in an otherwise burdensome mass of citations and statutes.

Informed Consent[1]

Informed consent is but one consideration in the legal aspects of exercise stress testing and exercise programs. An exercise stress test should not be performed, nor an exercise program prescribed, without first obtaining the patient's informed consent *in writing*. Informed consent is a legal doctrine concerned with the patient's decision whether or not to undergo a procedure. Exercise stress testing is a diagnostic aid. Exercise programs are a form of medical treatment, either in the nature of preventive or rehabilitative medicine.

---

[1] Representative consent forms are on pages 392-394.

Not everyone should engage in an exercise program. Certain recognized conditions mitigate against it. Stress testing is designed to assist in detection of such conditions, and to set the limits of the program.

As a general statement, one should not prescribe an exercise program without first obtaining the results of an exercise stress test. A brief hypothetical case will serve to illustrate the reason:

> Assume that an individual had a condition detectable by stress testing which would contraindicate an exercise program. Assume further that this individual has such a program prescribed for him without first having stress testing.

> Assume further that as a result of the exercise program, acute pathology is precipitated by the exercise.

> Assume an action is brought as a result of this accident on the theory that stress testing is a recognized diagnostic aid and should have been performed.

The defense of such an action would be most difficult and the physician prescribing the exercise program might well have a sizeable verdict returned against him.

In general, when dealing with *elective* procedures a physician has two basic responsibilities:

1. That the patient be made aware of the foreseeable risks of the procedure and that with such knowledge he consents to them.

2. That the procedure be carefully performed and all steps to minimize the risks to the patient be taken.

Informed consent is the term given to the first. Failure to do the second is known as malpractice. Informed consent must be just that. The patient must voluntarily consent to the procedure after having been made aware of the risks known to the physician at the time he administers the procedure.

This imposes a further duty on the physician to make himself aware of dangers attendant in the test or treatment. A physician is held to the standard of care of the reasonably well-trained practitioner in similar circumstances. A physician who was not aware of a risk that he should be informed of may be responsible for that failure. That does not appear to be a real problem in stress testing or an exercise program where one is dealing with a reasonably accepted procedure in a well-defined area.

It should be noted that a physician may be held responsible in the event of an untoward event, where the test is carefully performed or the exercise carefully supervised, if consent is not first obtained. In such a case the action is based in part on an assertion that the patient would not have undergone the procedure had he been aware of the risks. A nonspecific or blank consent form is of little use because it does not inform. Two elements are necessary—knowledge and permission: knowledge of the risks and permission to perform the procedure, hence *informed consent*.

A properly prepared written informed consent when signed by the patient is evidence that he has been made aware of the risks. Some physicians have resisted the use of written informed consent. The resistance appears to be based, in part, on the feeling that he will frighten the patient needlessly.

In this regard, a study performed at the Cleveland Clinic [1] might be noted, the conclusion of which seems to indicate that the more detailed the disclosure, the more likely the patient is to sign it. This seems to be true, partly, because the patient feels that he is being taken into confidence by the physician. Experience indicates that there is little likelihood of an action where the doctor has established good personal relationship with the patient. Taking the patient into the doctor's confidence is the first step towards the development of such a relationship.

Experience shows further that the patient who refuses to undergo the test after having been made aware of the risks is often the one most likely to have an unfavorable result, and the most likely to commence an action.

Exercise stress testing is a diagnostic aid, the use of which is elective. Informed consent is important in this instance, because clearly, the test is not immediately necessary to the preservation of life. Informed consent could be dispensed within an emergency situation such as cardiac arrest during routine surgery.

Performance of Stress Testing

Stress testing should be carefully performed. That sounds like a fairly obvious statement, but what does "carefully performed" mean? In general, it should be performed only by personnel trained in the administration of the test and in dealing with those problems which may arise. Further, the patient should be taught those signs and symptoms which would indicate to him that he should terminate the test. The patient should be carefully monitored during the performance of the test. Emergency resuscitation equipment and personnel trained for its use should be available. A doctor should be in attendance or near enough to render emergency treatment. At the first sign of any nonacceptable irregularity the test should be terminated. The patient should not be permitted to shower for a substantial period of time following the test. A cool-down period should be encouraged. Tne test should not be administered before the patient has had a pretest physical examination.

Exercise Programs

Most of the foregoing applies to an exercise program. In general, informed consent is as important in an exercise program as in stress testing and largely for the same reason. The further removed from immediate lifesaving procedures, the more necessary the informed consent.

An exercise program should not be undertaken without a doctor's prescription. It should be preceded by a complete physical examination, again, to determine if there is any condition which would mitigate against participation in an exercise program and to set its limits. It is suggested that stress testing is an excellent safety device for use with an exercise program. If only one case is detected in stress testing where exercise would be contraindicated, its use is almost mandated.

The patient for whom an exercise program is prescribed should be carefully instructed by the doctor on the signs and symptoms which would alert him to discontinue the exercise, similar to that in stress testing. The program should be carefully designed to provide the patient with a gradual increase in exercise. It is important that the personnel supervising the exercise be trained to recognize danger signs in the person performing the exercise.

Likewise, it is most important that the supervisors of the exercise be trained in certain minimum resuscitation techniques. The least that a physical educator or other health professionals would be legally expected to know are:

1. Knowledge of mouth-to-mouth resuscitation and the ability to establish an airway.

2. The ability to render closed chest massage.

3. A planned program of action in order to have medical assistance obtained in the most expeditious manner.

The failure of the instructor to be trained could give rise to a cause for action against the instructor and the institution where the exercise is performed. Where certain risks are recognized, all reasonable steps must be taken to minimize them; failure to do so may be actionable at law.

Experience has indicated that some physicians are adverse to following some of the steps set forth. Mention was made in passing of the hesitancy of some physicians to obtain informed consent. It has not been the intention here to imply coercion, but rather to present my opinion of a way to save a doctor needless grief. To borrow a well-known medical phrase, "prevention is the best cure." The intention here is a form of preventive law, steps that can protect both the practitioner and patient. It is, of course, up to the individual physician which, if any, of these steps he chooses to follow. Just as a doctor cannot compel a patient to follow or take a prescription, so a lawyer cannot compel a client to follow his advice.

SUMMARY

The importance of informed consent cannot be overemphasized; it provides excellent protection for both the patient and the physician, and is in keeping with the most recent trends in the law of negligence and malpractice. The patient's signature on an informed consent form does not, of course, relieve the physician or physical educator from responsibility for acts of negligence or malpractice.

Emphasis should also be placed on pretest screening of patients who are to undergo exercise stress testing, on the necessity for careful administration of the test, and on monitoring the patient's vital signs during the test. Again, this is in keeping with recent trends, and failure to do so may be actionable at law.

With reference to the performance of exercise programs, emphasis should be placed on training the patient to recognize danger signs, on training the supervisor in emergency resuscitation procedures, and early detection of physical signs which indicate that the participant should stop.

In stress testing and exercise programs, the recognized minimum standards of conduct must be observed, and, as always, prevention is the best cure. By obtaining a patient's informed consent, carefully performing a test, having resuscitation equipment and trained personnel available, it is believed that one is reasonably safe legally from lawsuit based on an untoward event occurring in exercise stress testing or exercise programs.

REFERENCES

1. Alfidi, R.J. Informed consent—a study of patient reaction. *J.A.M.A.* 216(8):1325, 1971.

PROPOSED FORM FOR INFORMED CONSENT
For Exercise Testing
of the Apparently Healthy Subject

In order to determine an appropriate plan of medical management, I hereby consent to voluntarily engage in an exercise test to determine the state of my heart and circulation. The information thus obtained will help my physician in advising me as to the activities in which I may engage.

Before I undergo the test, I will have an interview with a physician. I will also be examined by a physician to determine if I have any condition which would indicate that I should not engage in this test.

The test which I will undergo will be performeu on a _____ (describe) with the amount of effort increasing gradually. This increase in effort will continue until symptoms such as fatigue, shortness of breath, or chest discomfort may appear, which would indicate to me to stop.

During the performance of the test, a physician or his trained observer will keep under surveillance my pulse, blood pressure and electrocardiogram. Oxygen intake may also be measured and _____ tests performed.

There exists the possibility of certain changes occurring during the tests. They include abnormal blood pressure, fainting, disorders of heart beat, too rapid, too slow or ineffective, and very rare instances of heart attack. Every effort will be made to minimize them by the preliminary examination and by observations during testing. Emergency equipment and trained personnel are available to deal with unusual situations which may arise.

The information which is obtained will be treated as privileged and confidential and will not be released or revealed to any person without my expressed written consent. The information obtained, however, may be used for a statistical or scientific purpose with my right of privacy retained.

I have read the foregoing and I understand it and any questions which may have occurred to me have been answered to my satisfaction.

SIGNED _____

Patient

_____

Witness

_____

Date

_____

Physician Supervising the Test

PROPOSED FORM FOR INFORMED CONSENT
For Exercise Testing of People with Heart Disease

In order to determine an appropriate plan of treatment to assist in my recovery from my recent heart attack, I hereby consent to voluntarily engage in an exercise test to determine the state of my heart and circulation. The information thus obtained will help to aid my physician in advising me as to the activities in which I may engage.

Before I undergo the test, I will have an interview with a physician. I will also be examined by a physician to determine if I have any condition which would indicate that I should not engage in this test.

The test which I will undergo will be performed on a _____ (describe) with the amount of effort increasing gradually. This increase in effort will continue until symptoms such as fatigue, shortness of breath, or chest discomfort may appear, which would indicate to me to stop.

During the performance of the test, a physician or his trained observer will keep under surveillance my pulse, blood pressure and electrocardiogram. Oxygen intake may also be measured and _____ tests performed.

There exists the possibility of certain changes occurring during the tests. They include abnormal blood pressure, fainting, disorders of heart beat, too rapid, too slow or ineffective, and very rare instances of heart attack. Every effort will be made to minimize them by the preliminary examination and by observations during testing. Emergency equipment and trained personnel are available to deal with unusual situations which may arise.

The information which is obtained will be treated as privileged and confidential and will not be released or revealed to any person without my expressed written consent. The information obtained, however, may be used for a statistical or scientific purpose with my right of privacy retained.

I have read the foregoing and I understand it and any questions which may have occurred to me have been answered to my satisfaction.

SIGNED   _____

                                 Patient

                                _____

                                 Witness

_____   _____

Date   Physician Supervising the Test

ADDENDUM TO PROPOSED INFORMED CONSENT
To Be Completed when Patient is Under Twenty-One

I am the (parent)/(legal guardian) of _____ the patient who is to
                                            Name
engage in the above described exercise test. I have read and understand the foregoing consent form, and I agree to the performance of the test.

SIGNED   _____
                              Parent/Legal Guardian

INFORMED CONSENT FOR EXERCISE AS TREATMENT

I desire to engage voluntarily in an exercise treatment program in order to improve my cardiovascular function. This program has been recommended to me by my physician, Doctor _____.

Before I enter such a program I will have a clinical evaluation including a medical history and/or physical examination which includes but is not limited to measurement of heart rate and blood pressure, EKG at rest and with effort. The purpose of this evaluation is to detect any condition which would indicate that I should not engage in an exercise program.

The program will follow an exercise prescription prepared by Doctor _____ and will be carefully followed by the supervisor of the treatment program. The amount of exercise will be regulated on the basis of my tolerance.

Before starting the program I will be instructed as to the signs and symptoms that will alert me to modify my activities. I will also be observed by the supervisor of the exercises who will also be alert to changes which would suggest that I modify my exercise.

The activities are designed to place a graduated increased workload on the circulation and thereby to improve its function. The reaction of the cardiovascular system to such activities cannot be predicted with complete accuracy. There is the risk of certain changes occurring during or following the exercise. These changes include abnormalities of blood pressure, increased, irregular or ineffective heart rate, and in rare instances "heart attacks" or "cardiac arrests."

Every effort will be made to avoid such events by the preliminary medical examination and by observation during the exercise. Emergency equipment and trained personnel are available to deal with and minimize the dangers of untoward events should they occur.

I have read the foregoing and I understand it. Any questions which have arisen or occurred to me have been answered to my satisfaction.

SIGNED   _____
                     Patient

_____
Witness

_____
Date

_____
Physician Supervising the Test

B. THE ROLE OF THE PHYSICIAN IN
EXERCISE TESTING AND EXERCISE TRAINING

Nanette K. Wenger, M.D.

The role of the physician in the legal aspects of exercise testing and exercise training in cardiac rehabilitation is, in my opinion, primarily educational. It includes formulation and implementation of a curriculum for himself and for other physicians; for his patients who participate in the rehabilitation programs; and for the health care personnel responsible for the patient's restoration to normal living.

Are physicians in need of a curriculum regarding exercise as a diagnostic and therapeutic modality? The results of a recent survey [1] indicate that only 12 to 14 percent of physicians (general practitioners, internists, and cardiologists) use formal exercise testing to evaluate cardiovascular function. The majority of physicians do not perceive exercise testing as more helpful than clinical judgment in patient evaluation. Other factors cited for not using the procedure are lack of familiarity with exercise tests and/or lack of available equipment or facilities for exercise testing. Approximately one-third of the physicians express concern for patient safety during exercise testing. This overconcern seems unwarranted in view of a recent analysis of the morbidity and mortality associated with approximately 170,000 exercise tests [2]. There were 2.4 episodes of myocardial infarction (MI) and one death within the week after exercise testing for each 10,000 exercise tests performed.

Exercise Testing

Considerable information is available about exercise testing. Contraindications to this procedure are known and include active or recent MI, new or progressive angina pectoris, many cardiac arrhythmias, high degree atrioventricular block, a fixed rate cardiac pacemaker, uncompensated congestive heart failure, significant obstructive valvular disease, uncontrolled diabetes mellitus or hypertension, and certain orthopedic and neuromuscular diseases.

It is generally accepted that exercise testing procedures can be performed with safety [2] when these guidelines are employed: The patient is given an appropriate examination by the physician just prior to exercise testing. Evaluation includes specific interrogation regarding recent chest pain or discomfort, palpitations or arrhythmia, and undue fatigue or other new symptoms. The physical examination is directed toward recording baseline cardiovascular data with attention to the presence or absence of arrhythmia, hypertension, heart failure, and thrombophlebitis. A resting ECG, obtained that day, is reviewed; this record serves as the baseline for comparison during the exercise test. Written, informed consent is obtained. Safety features, in addition to supervision by a physician and other appropriately trained personnel, include monitoring the ECG for heart rate response, ST segment changes, and for the appearance of arrhythmias. Other safety features include determination of the blood pressure response and observation of the patient for evidence of discomfort or dyspnea, an ataxic gait, or change in mentation. The instant availability of a DC defibrillator, emergency cardiac resuscitation equipment, and drugs is mandatory. Personnel must be familiar with ECG diagnosis of arrhythmias; with the administration of cardiopulmonary resuscitation; with the use of a DC defibrillator; and with other emergency care procedures. The physician is responsible for the training of the health care personnel in these procedures [3, 4].

Data obtained from standardized exercise test procedures are reproducible, both on repeated testing of the patient and from one laboratory to another. The adjusted age-predicted maximum heart rates can serve as guidelines for exercise testing levels. A heart rate which approximates 80 to 85 percent of this predicted maximal rate is apparently a safe level to which to test patients after MI. Most patients without specific contraindications to exercise can attain this heart rate level with safety from 8 to 12 weeks after sustaining an uncomplicated MI. The data obtained from exercise testing can be correlated with the established energy requirements of most jobs, and thus furnish an objective basis for recommendations regarding the safe return of the patient to work [4].

A number of facets of exercise testing require further evaluation. The relative merits of different testing methods and protocols are not established. Newer parameters of monitoring require evaluation to determine if they provide increased information of value in the care of the patient. These parameters include noninvasive evaluation of left ventricular function with systolic time intervals; ventricular volume studies determined by echocardiography or other external techniques; and high-frequency ECG monitoring. The value of measuring metabolic adaptation during exercise testing must be evaluated. The ability to detect malingering requires further study. Although it is known that an abnormal exercise ECG in an otherwise healthy individual has the highest predictive value of any of the established risk factors for the subsequent occurrence of a coronary event [5, 6], correlation of exercise test results must also be made with the subsequent functional performance of the patient, with recurrence of MI, with the occurrence of sudden cardiac death, and with total survival statistics.

Exercise Training and Cardiac Function

Exercise training programs can enhance cardiac function in normal individuals and in patients after uncomplicated MIs. Improvement in cardiac function after training, as measured by the cardiovascular response to the same workload, is characterized by lesser increase in heart rate, lesser increase in systolic blood pressure, decreased or absent angina pectoris, decreased ST segment changes on the ECG, and lesser increase in the calculated tension-time index for the same amount of external work. This response to physical training has been reproduced in many countries and in many populations [7, 8]. However, similar to any other therapeutic modality, the physician who prescribes exercise should know the indications and contraindications to its use, its expected advantages and possible disadvantages, and the guidelines for recommending the amount of exercise [9].

The contraindications to exercise testing mentioned earlier also apply to exercise training programs. The energy costs per kilogram of body weight for different physical activities are comparable for apparently normal individuals and for patients with clinical evidence of coronary heart disease, even those who have sustained MIs. This information can serve as a guide for introducing progressively more difficult and demanding physical activities in exercise training programs [9].

The intensity, duration, and frequency of exercise training required to induce a training effect in patients after MI and to maintain this training effect for at least several months, have been documented by several groups of investigators [9, 10, 11]. Whether similar benefit can be obtained with less prolonged or less intensive exercise training programs is not established. The *training effect* is primarily a peripheral circulatory effect, rather than one on the coronary collateral circulation.

There is little evidence that exercise training programs increase the inter-coronary collateral circulation. The physically trained individual is usually a more efficient organism, able to perform the same amount of external work at lesser cardiovascular cost [7]. The psychologic benefit of exercise training programs, as with in-hospital physical activity programs, is manifest by a reduction in anxiety and depression scores on standard psychologic tests and by an improved level of self-confidence and self-esteem [12, 13]. Whether this improvement, both psychologic and physical, is related to the exercise training programs per se, or whether it is attributable to other factors such as change in diet, discontinuation of smoking, loss of body weight, associated intervention regarding other risk factors, or change in intensity of stress, remains to be determined.

Exercise training programs must be critically evaluated to determine if there are significant differences between patients in formal exercise training programs and patients undergoing the "normal" process of recovery. It is controversial whether formal exercise training programs provide greater improvement and increased cardiac reserve [14, 15]. The intensity, duration, and frequency of exercise needed to maintain a *training effect* on a long-term basis must be investigated, as must the factors influencing adherence to an exercise program. The need for continued physician supervision and/or ECG monitoring during long-term exercise training programs, particularly those outside the hospital, must be determined.

The risks involved in exercise training programs must be assessed, even when preceded by exercise testing conducted under proper supervision, according to an exercise prescription, and with the availability of emergency equipment and appropriately trained personnel. The efficacy of exercise training programs in preventing recurrent MIs and sudden cardiac death, and its effect on total CHD mortality, return to work, and the eventual psychologic status of the patient are not well-established. The morbidity, such as orthopedic problems, non-life-threatening arrhythmias, development of left ventricular dysfunction or ventricular aneurysm, involved in exercise training programs must be assessed. The effect of exercise training programs on serum lipid levels and coagulation factors requires further study.

Educational Aspects

Exercise testing and training constitute a discipline characterized by rapidly changing and expanding information. Continuing educational programs must be available for physicians to periodically update their knowledge of this sphere of patient management.

In regard to patient education, the informed consent statement [16], legal implications of which have been defined by attorneys, may also be considered an educational document. The physician who transmits to his patient the information required for a true *informed consent* must be knowledgeable about exercise testing programs. The patient is made aware of the possible complications of the procedures and of the organization and programming that have been implemented to insure his safety. The training and quality of supervisory personnel, the availability of emergency equipment, and the standardization of procedures are explained to the patient.

Education of the Patient

The patient is taught the *patient end points* for exercise testing and training—the signs and symptoms which will signal the patient to terminate the exercise testing or training procedure. During exercise testing, the *patient end points* include unusual dyspnea or chest pain, lightheadedness or dizziness, and undue fatigue [17]. Patients are taught to follow their exercise prescription during exercise training programs. This requires that the concept of exercise prescription, determined by the results of prior exercise testing, for a program of gradually progressive physical activity be explained to the patient. He is reminded at periodic intervals that exercise training programs are noncompetitive and that he should not exercise when unduly fatigued or subjected to increased or excessive stress. Patients are specifically instructed to report the occurrence of chest pain, dyspnea, palpitations, dizziness, or other symptoms that might signal a temporary contraindication to exercise training programs, or a need for reduction in the intensity of physical activity. Hot showers should be avoided immediately after exercising [9]. Isometric exercises, which may increase blood pressure and impose an undue workload on the left ventricle [18], should also be avoided.

The character and quality of the supervision, the organization, and the safety features of the exercise testing and the exercise training programs are explained to the patient. The central concept of the emergency care system (equipment, procedures, and training) is the ability to reverse an episode of ventricular fibrillation or cardiac arrest immediately and to prevent its evolution to MI.

Education of the Health Care Team

The physician's responsibility also extends to educational programming for other members of the health care team. A repeatedly mentioned problem concerns the availability of a sufficient number of adequately trained individuals to perform the exercise testing required to identify coronary-prone individuals, to evaluate functional capacity of patients with angina pectoris or with healed MI, and to enable initial and serial exercise prescription for patients in exercise training programs designed to enhance function. A variety of non-physicians can fill this role if properly trained. These include physical educators, exercise physiologists, nurses (particularly those with Coronary Care Unit (CCU) training), and specialized technologists and technicians.

It is interesting to speculate that "rest and recreation" rotations for CCU nurses may include assignment to an exercise testing or exercise training facility, where their expertise in the ECG diagnosis of arrhythmias and emergency therapy of cardiac arrhythmias can be best utilized. Indeed, the CCU nurse training programs comprise a model for the training and retraining necessary for health care professionals involved in exercise testing and training. The advent of the CCU demanded availability of individuals with expertise in the identification and reversion of life-threatening arrhythmias. Equally specialized approaches were required for the problems of heart failure and shock. The need generated new and innovative training programs, particularly for nurses, but also for a variety of medical specialty assistants and physicians' assistants. The guiding concept of these programs was that the training be commensurate with the type of work and the degree of responsibility to be assumed. A goal-oriented training program, directed specifically toward the function an individual is required to perform, may be the answer to the persu̇nnel shortage in exercise testing and exercise training programs.

The recommended curriculum for the various members of the health care team varies with their prior training, with the degree of supervision available in their work, and with the degree of responsibility expected of them. An adequate curriculum includes information about:

- clinical characteristics of CHD and MI
- an explanation of coronary risk factors and the rationale for intervention
- varied aspects of cardiovascular physiology
- operation of equipment
- methods, measurements, and calculations used in exercise. testing and exercise training
- concept and elements of exercise prescription
- design of exercise training programs
- psychologic factors in CHD and MI
- emergency care training including diagnostic ECG, emergency procedures, cardiopulmonary resuscitation, cardiac defibrillation, and use of anti-arrhythmic and other cardiovascular drug therapy.

Emphasis is directed to training commensurate with the degree of responsibility to be assumed, practical and written testing to assess comprehension and application of the material presented, and periodic retraining for both presentation of new material and review of previously taught information. The importance of continuing education for both the physician and other health care personnel cannot be overemphasized.

The physician's pattern of delivery of health care should not reflect the attitude of "looking back over his shoulder, worrying that an attorney is gaining on him." Rather, the physician's approach to legal aspects related to exercise testing and exercise training programs should reflect his concern that the optimal procedures, performed by adequately trained personnel, have been designed and implemented to insure benefit for, and safety of, his cardiac patient. The information and guidelines described here are designed to help achieve this goal.

REFERENCES

1. Wenger, N.K., Hellerstein, H.K., Blackburn, H., and Castranova, S.J. Uncomplicated myocardial infarction. Current physician practice in patient management. *J.A.M.A.* 224:511, 1973.

2. Rochmis, P., and Blackburn, H. Exercise tests. A survey of procedures, safety, and litigation experience in approximately 170,000 tests. *J.A.M.A.* 217:1061-1066, 1971.

3. [Committee on Exercise] *Exercise Testing and Training of Apparently Healthy Individuals: A Handbook for Physicians*, 40 pp. New York, Amer. Heart Assoc., 1972.

4. Blomquist, C.G. Use of exercise testing for diagnostic and functional evaluation of patients with arteriosclerotic heart disease. *Circulation* 44:1120-1136, 1971.

5. Doyle, J.T., and Kinch, S.H. The prognosis of an abnormal electrocardiographic stress test. *Circulation* 41:545-553, 1970.

6. Blackburn, H.W., Taylor, H.L., and Keys, A. Prognostic significance of the post-exercise electrocardiogram: risk factors held constant. *Am. J. Cardiol.* 25:85, 1970.

7. Detry, J.-M.R., Rousseau, M., Vandenbroucke, G., Kusumi, F., Brasseur, L.A., and Bruce, R.A. Increased arteriovenous oxygen difference after physical training in coronary heart disease. *Circulation* 44:109-118, 1971.

8. Detry, J.-M., and Bruce, R.A. Effects of physical training on exertional S-T-segment depression in coronary heart disease. *Circulation* 44:390-396, 1971.

9. Fox, S.M., III, Naughton, J., and Gorman, P.A. Physical activity and cardiovascular health, I. Potential for prevention of coronary heart disease and possible mechanisms, II. The exercise prescription: Intensity and duration, III. The exercise prescription: Frequency and type of activity. *Mod. Concepts Cardiovasc. Dis.*, 41:17-30, 1972.

10. Redwood, D.R., Rosing, D.R., and Epstein, J.E. Circulatory and symptomatic effects of physical training in patients with coronary artery disease and angina pectoris. *N. Engl. J. Med.* 286:959-965, 1972.

11. Zohman, L.R., and Tobis, J.S. *Cardiac Rehabilitation*, 248 pp. New York, Grune and Stratton, 1970.

12. Wishnie, H.A., Hackett, T.P., and Cassem, N.H. Psychological hazards of convalescence following myocardial infarction. *J.A.M.A.* 215:1292-1296, 1971.

13. Hackett, T.P., and Cassem, N.H. The psychological adaptation of myocardial infarction patient to convalescence. *In*, Naughton, J., and Hellerstein, H., Eds. *Exercise Testing and Exercise Training in Coronary Heart Disease*. New York, Academic, 1973.

14. Kavanagh, T., Shephard, R.J., Pandit, V., and Doney, H. Exercise and hypnotherapy in the rehabilitation of the coronary patient. *Arch. Phys. Med. Rehabil.* 51:578-587, 1970.

15. Kellerman, J.J., Modan, B., Levy, M., Feldman, S., and Kariv, I. Return to work after myocardial infarction. Comparative study of rehabilitated and nonrehabilitated patients. *Geriatrics* 23:151-156, 1968.

16. *Exercise Testing Informed Consent Form*. New York, Amer. Heart Assoc., 1972.

17. Wenger, N.K., Gilbert, C.A., and Siegel, W. Symposium: The use of physical activity in the rehabilitation of patients after myocardial infarction. *South. Med. J.* 63:891-897, 1970.

18. Nutter, D.O., Schlant, R.C., and Hurst, J.W. Isometric exercise and the cardiovascular system. *Mod. Concepts Cardiovasc. Dis.* 41:11-15, 1972.

C. THE PHYSICAL EDUCATOR

1. PREPARATION OF EXERCISE PROGRAM DIRECTORS
FOR CARDIAC REHABILITATION PROGRAMS

William L. Haskell, Ph.D.

The successful long-term management of exercise programs for cardiac patients or others with symptoms of cardiovascular disease (angina pectoris, ischemic ECG changes, peripheral vascular disorders) requires a well-trained, highly motivated individual. An exercise program director must be more than an exercise demonstrator and leader to provide safe and effective reconditioning for cardiovascular disease patients. The exercise program director should be able to administer or, at least, effectvely assist in the exercise stress testing of patients; to design an appropriate exercise program for each patient based on his needs and capacities; to be aware of certain psychological problems associated with cardiovascular disabilities; to motivate program participants to modify other risk factors such as diet, body weight, and cigarette smoking, in addition to organizing and conducting a program of increased physical activity.

Short-Term Training Programs

Short-term or special training programs to prepare individuals to direct cardiac reconditioning programs should include classroom, laboratory, and practical experience. All participants should be evaluated separately on their performance in each three areas. Such a program probably would vary from 6 weeks to 9 months, depending on the participants' backgrounds and intensity of the instruction.

Areas that should be covered in the classroom sessions include:

Cardiovascular and respiratory physiology. Basic cardiovascular and respiratory function with emphasis on hemodynamics and electro-cardiographic measurements.
Cardiovascular pathology. The nature of major cardiovascular diseases and their appropriate management.

Exercise physiology. Particular emphasis on acute and chronic responses of the cardiovascular, respiratory, and metabolic systems to physical exertion.

Ergonomics. Analysis of factors influencing the energy requirement of various activities, and techniques for measurement of energy expenditure.

Kinesiology. Principles of human movement, proper action of selected muscle groups and joints.

Psychology. Review principles of motivation, behavior modification, psychological disorders associated with cardiovascular disease.

Physical activity program management. Design of individualized exercise programs, group exercise organizations, activity selection, facility and equipment selection.

Principles of measurement and evaluation. Methods of physical performance evaluation, test data collection and analysis, data interpretation.

Prevention and care of exercise-related injuries. Prevention and treatment of orthopedic problems, cardiopulmonary resuscitation.

The laboratory sessions should include (1) conducting various types of exercise stress tests, (2) analyzing exercise test data to determine an individual's capacity for exercise, (3) electrocardiographic waveform recognition, (4) exercise program leadership, and (5) cardiopulmonary resuscitation. Reasonably extensive laboratory experience is useful in developing a competent and confident exercise program leader. As much as 50 percent of the time in a training program might be spent in the practical application of knowledge.

The final phase of a training program for an exercise leader should be his participation as a student-leader in an ongoing adult exercise program with cardiac patients as participants. Under such circumstances of close supervision, the new leader can apply his knowledge and leadership abilities without fear that he might make potentially dangerous mistakes.

Exercise Program Director Certification

In order to provide a number of trained exercise program directors for cardiac rehabilitation groups, a certification procedure is advisable similar to the physical therapist certification system. Individuals who receive the special training to result in certification could have one of several educational backgrounds: physical education, physical therapy, recreation, or nursing. The specific courses and practical experience necessary in this type of special training program would depend upon the participant's previous education and job experience. For certification, however, each individual would be. required to demonstrate certain knowledge and proficiencies during a written and practical certification examination.

Certification might result in a single classification or in a graduated or multi-level system. An individual could then be designated as (1) *exercise leader*, (2) *exercise instructor*, or (3) *exercise program director*. For the classification, *exercise program director*, an individual might be responsible for exercise programs as well as training and certifying *exercise leaders* and *exercise instructors* on a local level.

A certification system of exercise leaders in the United States probably should be instituted by an organization such as the American College of Sports Medicine (ACSM) with cooperation or representation from the American Heart Association; American College of Cardiology; American Association for Health, Physical Education and Recreation; and similar professional organizations. The ACSM or delegated organization would establish minimum criteria for certification of exercise program leaders and define the type and number of educational institutions to be designated as training centers for this type of certification program. Ideally, training institutions selected to develop certification programs would have a physical education department with strong orientation in exercise physiology, a medical school or interested cardiologists in the community, and an ongoing adult fitness program. These requirements have already been met by the University of California, Davis; San Diego State University; University of Wisconsin, Madison; Wake Forest University; and Ball State University.

Continuing Education Programs

The establishment of selected centers for training exercise leaders should include a system of updating and retraining the individuals. Periodic workshops and seminars are needed to keep exercise program leaders aware of recent developments in this rapidly changing profession. Programs of this type have been made available during the past several years but a more systematic approach is needed. If certification becomes part of the training of exercise leaders, yearly participation in a certain number of these meetings (or acceptable educational substitutes) would be required to retain certification, which is similar to the continuing education point system of the American College of General Practice.

2. THE PHYSICAL EDUCATOR'S ROLE IN EXERCISE PROGRAMS

Karl G. Stoedefalke, Ph.D.

The information in this section, from the perspective of a physical educator, is meant to assist the medical doctor in understanding the physical educator's role in exercise programs of prevention, intervention, and rehabilitation. TABLE I identifies the relationships among the patient-physician-physical educator team.

TABLE I

The Physical Educator's Perspective
Physical activity as a therapeutic modality for man at risk

STAGE I   NEED AND ACCESSION

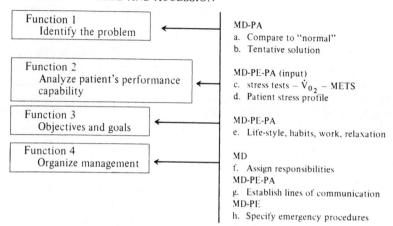

Function 1
Identify the problem

MD-PA
a. Compare to "normal"
b. Tentative solution

Function 2
Analyze patient's performance
capability

MD-PE-PA (input)
c. stress tests – $\dot{V}_{O_2}$ – METS
d. Patient stress profile

Function 3
Objectives and goals

MD-PE-PA
e. Life-style, habits, work, relaxation

Function 4
Organize management

MD
f. Assign responsibilities
MD-PE-PA
g. Establish lines of communication
MD-PE
h. Specify emergency procedures

STAGE II   PROGRAM PRESCRIPTION

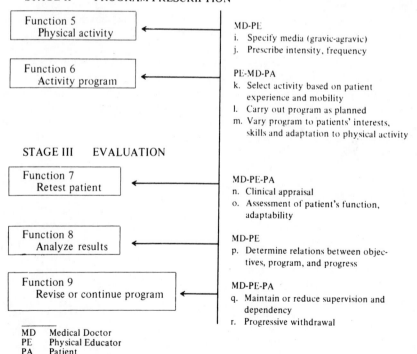

Function 5
Physical activity

MD-PE
i. Specify media (gravic-agravic)
j. Prescribe intensity, frequency

Function 6
Activity program

PE-MD-PA
k. Select activity based on patient
   experience and mobility
l. Carry out program as planned
m. Vary program to patients' interests,
   skills and adaptation to physical activity

STAGE III   EVALUATION

Function 7
Retest patient

MD-PE-PA
n. Clinical appraisal
o. Assessment of patient's function,
   adaptability

Function 8
Analyze results

MD-PE
p. Determine relations between objectives, program, and progress

Function 9
Revise or continue program

MD-PE-PA
q. Maintain or reduce supervision and
   dependency
r. Progressive withdrawal

MD   Medical Doctor
PE   Physical Educator
PA   Patient

Stage I – Need and Accession

Function 1, identifying the problem. The patient, during his medical examination, is diagnosed by the physician as a candidate for an exercise program. The patient may exhibit a variety of medical problems including elevated arterial blood pressure, hypercholesterolemia, excessive adipose tissue, or any condition which would lend itself to a prescription of physical activity. When the problem has been identified, the physician may recommend a series of solutions to alleviate or ameliorate the problem. If one of the recommended treatments is a supervised program of physical activity, the patient is referred to a laboratory unit to undergo assessment of his performance capability.

Function 2. The physician may personally conduct the exercise stress test or may supervise a qualified physical educator in administrating the graded exercise test. The physical educator may also be competent in obtaining the 12-lead electrocardiogram and other recommended tests for the patient's work capacity profile, which could include strength determination or flexibility testing. Upon completion of the test and evaluation of the records, the patient's stress profile is established. There is a cooperative sharing and input by the attending physician and physical educator.

Function 3. The physician is responsible for reporting the results of the test to the patient. He will also make recommendations on altering, or perhaps changing, life-style or habits, ingestion of food, occupational work capacity, or relaxation. The physical educator may interview the patient to determine his previous participation in physical activity and his leisure-time activity interests. A decision is made by the patient to enter a program of organized physical activity based on the recommendations of the physician and physical educator.

Function 4, organized movement. The physician has the ultimate responsibility for the care of his patient; he may delegate certain authority, but the command responsibility is vested in him. He establishes lines of communication with the physical educator and patient, and informs the physical educator on the need-to-know basis of possible patient problems which could be incurred in an activity program.

Stage II – Program Prescription

Function 5, physical activity. The physical activity prescription is a result of baseline determinations made during the graded exercise testing session. As the patient is accessed into the program, determinations on media, land or water, and the intensity, frequency, and the duration of the activity are decided.

Function 6, activity program. At this point, the physical educator plays an important role. Through his experience and knowledge, he selects activities based on the patient's previous physical activity and ability to sustain human movement. The physical educator supervises the patient's exercise program as planned, maintains open lines of communication with the physician, and varies the program to the participant's changing interests, skills, and adaptation to physical activity.

Stage III — Evaluation

Function 7, retest patient. At intervals from 3 to 6 months, the patient is retested to determine his functional adaptability to the exercise program. This entails a stress test or other determinations which the physician deems necessary.

Function 8, analyze results. Results of the stress test are evaluated to determine relationships among the objectives of the program, success of the program for the patient, and progress the patient has made in the restoration of his performance capability.

Function 9, revise or continue program. Revision of the program or increasing the intensity of the work is recommended through the cooperative efforts of the physician, physical educator, and patient. Recommendations may include a reduction in supervision or increased supervision while participating in an exercise program. The rehabilitative aspect is complete when the physician and physical educator can progressively withdraw their supervision and support.

The input and responsibility of accessing a high-risk man into an exercise program has been discussed. An attempt has been made to show continuity and flow from a physician's recommendation, the patient's acceptance, and the physical educator's direction. Rehabilitation rests with a mutual acceptance of expertise by the physician for the physical educator and the acknowledgement that the physician has the command responsibility for management of the patient's exercise prescription. Implicit in this discussion is the importance of the patient, his feelings, his adaptation to exercise, and his eventual ability to participate in physical activity safely and with enjoyment.

D. THE ALLIED HEALTH PROFESSIONAL

William L. Haskell, Ph.D.

If supervised exercise programs are to be included as part of comprehensive cardiac rehabilitation programs on a nationwide basis, a great many allied health professionals will be required to assist, and conduct, exercise stress testing and exercise training sessions. Legally, there is a need to define the services allied health professionals can provide, the type of physician direction and supervision they require, and their responsibility to minimize the occurrence of an untoward cardiovascular event during exercise testing or conditioning.

Legal Considerations

Conducting exercise tests, prescribing specific exercises or physical activities, and leading a supervised exercise program as a part of a cardiac rehabilitation program are considered the practice of medical care under the generally accepted legal definition of medical practice:

> Diagnosis, treatment, or correction or attempting or holding oneself out as being able to diagnose, treat or correct, prescribe for, palliate or prevent human diseases, injuries, ailments or infirmities, be they physical or mental, by any means, methods, devices or instrumentalities [1].

This definition obviously is quite broad and apparently includes those activities of a cardiac rehabilitation program that are either diagnostic or therapeutic. Thus, from a purely legal standpoint, conducting activities within this scope requires a licensed physician, or a direct agent of a physician who is defined as qualified to perform specific services as directed by the physician. Allied health professionals who are adequately trained in cardiac rehabilitation techniques can legally conduct selected aspects of the program when directed and supervised by a responsible physician.

The use of allied health personnel for conducting various aspects of a cardiac rehabilitation program has numerous precedents in other forms of medical practice. It was pointed out in the Bethesda Conference Report on the Early Care for the Acute Coronary Suspect, regarding the use of nonphysicians [2]:

This is not a new problem on the national or local level, and physicians in their offices and hospitals have coped with this in an obvious manner. They have delegated some part of their functions and prerogatives to individuals they deem qualified to carry them out, in accordance with their instruction, direction and supervision. Since this practice satisfied the concept of 'agent' and since they continue as responsible in law and fact for their agent's actions, this is a major solution to the problem of physician shortage.

However, within this agency procedure, the non-physician is carrying out an order by the physician according to the physician's advice and instruction, and is not making independent judgements such as prescribing, diagnosing, or evaluating. Further, there exists ample opportunity for instruction, guidance and supervision by the physician or a medical colleague.

When a physician is physically present at a rehabilitation program (testing or training), appropriate activities can be undertaken by a trained assistant. When a physician is not present, however, additional legal authority is required for him to delegate the performance of any medical activity to someone other than another physician. The legality of the delegation of this authority by a physician depends upon: (1) the statutory definition of the practice of medicine; (2) the mandatory nature of the legislation requiring licensure for the practice of medicine; and (3) the level of physician supervision and control over existing personnel [1].

Delegation of Selected Medical Services

From a practical or operational point of view, the delegation of selected medical services to allied health personnel is governed by prevailing custom and practice. In the United States at present, the prevailing practice regarding administration of exercise stress tests and supervised exercise programs by allied health personnel under physician supervision for cardiac patients has not been well-established. In many cases, exercise programs for individuals with cardiovascular disease have evolved from YMCA adult fitness programs, without those responsible taking into consideration the added risk and responsibility associated with exercise by symptomatic individuals. Many such exercise programs operate without physician supervision [3]. That many programs operate in this manner should not be considered the prevailing practice or endorsement for such an approach.

Recommendations made by several *expert groups*, representing different major medical associations, provide more desirable guidelines for the role of the allied health professional in exercise testing and training of cardiac patients. There is general agreement among these groups that when individuals with symptoms of cardiovascular disease exercise, a physician should either participate in the testing or be immediately available. Some specific recommendations regarding exercise testing from several groups are:

A physician should be present whenever possible during the testing of patients with known or potential cardiovascular disease [4].

A physician must be present during exercise tolerance testing of patients known to have ischemic heart disease [4].

However, if a simple exercise test is used involving stepping or pedalling a bicycle ergometer, with determination only of ECG wave-form, blood pressure and pulse rate, then one experienced person can cope with the whole procedure; but a physician should be at hand if the person in charge of the testing is not medically qualified [5].

A qualified physician should always be present [during exercise testing] and in direct visual and verbal communication with patients who have a cardiac or other diagnosis suggesting increased hazards above those usually found in their age group in good health [6].

Recommendations regarding the need or desirability of direct physician supervision during exercise training are not as consistent as those for the exercise testing of cardiac patients. Some impetus has been given to the concept that, if during the training of cardiac patients, exercise is performed at work intensities below the level attained during performance of the exercise stress test, a physician need not be present. On the other hand, experience so far in various exercise programs for cardiac patients indicates that untoward cardiovascular events do occur even when the physical activity is well-controlled. When promptly and appropriately treated, there is full recovery without clinical evolution of myocardial infarction, it has been reported. A most desirable situation appears to be one where a physician is either on-site or within several minutes of the exercise facility.

As plans for operating a cardiac rehabilitation program are developed and a decision is made to delegate certain tasks to allied health professionals, it is important to remember that, as a result of court decisions, a professional custom is not an adequate defense for contravention of medical licensure statutes. Prevailing custom and practice, if contrary to explicit law, do not provide legal sanctuary [1]. Only five states (Arizona, Colorado, Kansas, Oklahoma, and California) provide a general exemption allowing the delegation of medical functions to non-physicians. The general trend of most State medical boards is to exclude delegation of exemption in medical practice.

Use of Medical Equipment

A second legal question relates to the use of various types of medical equipment or drugs by allied health personnel when a physician is not present for supervision. The availability to non-physicians of defibrillators, other emergency equipment, and drugs to treat a cardiac event which might arise during exercise testing or training is of particular concern. In regard to this situation, Cooper and Willig have stated [1]:

All instruments and apparatus intended for medical use are subject to the 'device' provisions of the Federal Food, Drug and Cosmetic Act and must therefore be compliant with the applicable provisions of that act. The definition of the term 'device' in the act is quite broad and includes such diverse articles as heating pads, phonograph records and electrical defibrillators. An individual who is not a physician and uses such a device on a patient is subject to criminal prosecution. Most devices that would be used by non-physician personnel in coronary emergencies are prescription devices; whenever they are used without the prior prescriptive direction of a physician, they are technically used in violation of federal law. However, there has apparently been no instance in which an individual has been charged with such a violation. Further, federal law defers to the state's right to determine who in that state may prescribe or administer prescription drugs and devices. Therefore, a state can qualify by its own laws any practitioner to prescribe or administer prescription drugs and devices, and conceivably could do so for paramedical assistants as well.

The consensus of individuals working in cardiac rehabilitation and cardiopulmonary resuscitation is that if a reasonable expectation exists that an emergency requiring electrical defibrillation or drug administration might occur during an organized program of medical care, a physician should be immediately available to provide such care.

Professional Liability Insurance

Professional liability insurance covering allied health professionals working in cardiac rehabilitation programs usually is provided by the organization (hospital, clinic, YMCA, university) employing them. Individuals employed in YMCAs, YMHAs, and similar organizations with new cardiac rehabilitation programs should investigate the nature and extent of their insurance coverage. The medical-legal implications of a known heart disease patient dying while performing in an exercise program designed to improve his health compared with the sudden death of an apparently healthy participant in an unsupervised or supervised activity in which no medical clearance or examination is required may be substantially different.

Avoiding Medical-Legal Encounters

Since any large-scale implementation of cardiac reconditioning programs will require the participation of numerous allied health professionals, appropriate action must be taken to minimize the frequency of untoward cardiovascular events and to manage appropriately those events that do occur in association with exercise testing and training. It is important to accept the possibility at the outset, that even under the best circumstances, when large numbers of symptomatic individuals begin to participate in supervised exercise programs, potentially fatal cardiac emergencies may not be uncommon. Thus, procedures for the effective management of a sudden cardiac dysfunction are extremely important elements in exercise program implementation.

Certain actions should be taken to insure as safe an environment as possible for the exercising cardiac patient.

1. All exercise leaders or allied health professionals conducting or assisting with exercise stress testing must be properly trained. Details of suggested educational requirements and experience are provided in other chapters of this volume.

2. Appropriate attention to numerous details of cardiac reconditioning programs is necessary to substantially reduce the risk of negligent action on the part of the exercise leader.

3. Develop an effective two-way working relationship with the physician supervisor of the program. Know what he expects you to do and not to do.

4. Establish open communications with physicians in the community who refer patients to the rehabilitation program. Apprise them of any changes in the health status of their patients and request that they do the same for you at regular intervals. Invite the referring physicians to visit the exercise program or testing sessions so that they have a better understanding of what their patients are doing.

5. Insist that all patients sign an informed consent for participation in the exercise program, as well as for exercise testing, and that this signature is witnessed by a relative or close friend of the patient.

6. Define criteria for patients' entrance into the exercise program. Also, contraindications for participation in any specific exercise session should be established, which all patients should fully understand and the reasoning for them.

7. Encourage patients to avoid psychological and environmental stresses in conjunction with their exercise program. This includes highly competitive situations (against his own accomplishments, as well as others') and the use of sauna baths, steam baths, or extremely hot or cold showers.

8. Acquire proper emergency equipment, and maintain it in excellent working order. Make sure all members of the exercise testing and training team know how to use the equipment effectively. Develop proficiency in treating emergencies through periodic unannounced drills. It is useful to teach all exercise program participants basic cardiopulmonary resuscitation.

Thus, the allied health professional's best protection against legal action resulting from his involvement in the exercise phase of cardiac rehabilitation programs is close supervision by a knowledgeable physician; to be well trained in the areas of exercise testing, prescription, and program leadership; and to develop an effective program of emergency treatment to care for any untoward events.

REFERENCES

1. Cooper, J.K., and Willig, S.H. Nonphysicians for coronary care delivery: Are they legal? *Am. J. Cardiol.* 28:363, 1971.

2. Bethesda Conference Report: Early care for the acute coronary suspect. *Am. J. Cardiol.* 23:603, 1969.

3. *Directory: Exercise Programs for Cardiacs.* New York, Am. Heart Assoc., 1970.

4. Proceedings: National Conference on Exercise in Prevention Evaluation and Treatment of Heart Disease. *J. S.C. Med. Assoc.* 65(Suppl. 1):73, 85, 1969.

5. Andersen, K.L., et al. *Fundamentals of Exercise Testing*, p. 43. Geneva, World Health Organization, 1971.

6. Fox, S.M., III. *Exercise Test Methodology.* Draft document. International Society of Cardiology, Council on Cardiac Rehabilitation, May, 1971. Unpublished report.

28

VARIOUS TYPES OF EXERCISE PROGRAMS

A Discussion

PANELISTS: *K.K. Datey*, M.D.; *Henri Denoline*, M.D.; *Samuel Fox*, III, M.D.; *Patrick A. Gorman*, M.D.; *Herman K. Hellerstein*, M.D.; *Jan Kellerman*, M.D.; *Mohamed Alumgir Khan*, M.D.; *Nasirud Din Azam Khan*, M.D.; *Cedomil Plavsic*, M.D.; *Karl Stoedefalke*, Ph.D.

Editors' Note: Although discussions were not to be part of this volume, this discussion was considered of more than routine interest and accordingly has been included.

DR. PLAVSIC: I would like to speak about a very simple and practical method of exercise—walking. Walking is a type of physical activity in which patients are trained by changing the speed and the route. This exercise is performed outdoors; paths are marked with different degrees of steepness. By selecting a path we can determine the degree of effort a person should tolerate or reach. During the walking exercise session, periodic repose is interspersed, but rest periods are not strictly determined.

Short walking periods are alternated with rest periods instead of continuous loading. However, longer continuous walking exercises are not completely abandoned. According to the results and experience gained, walking exercises are justified, with regard to both favorable influence on cardiovascular function and as a type of training suited to many people.

DR. STOEDEFALKE: My current interest is in coeducational rehabilitative programs. I think exercise programs have tended to include predominantly men, and the women have been slighted. Our programs consist of games and activities performed with partners, at a low-to-moderate degree of intensity. They are performed outdoors whenever possible, the participants being sufficiently acclimatized to sustain this activity even during the snow season. The activity is continuous, 30 to 40 minutes, three times weekly, and includes a wide variety of movements involving all types of sport. It is medically supervised. Although it is not always performed within the proximity of help, we do maintain radio contact with physicians and the assistants have been trained to administer emergency care.

DR. DATEY: Most people exercise to keep fit, to avoid illness, and perhaps to delay death. In the usual avocations of life, most people, barring those whose work involves strenuous exercise or exertion, do not exceed about 6 to 9 METS and this may be excessive. The exercises of the submaximal tests are oriented mainly toward the muscles of the extremities. We attempt to orient exercises toward the different organs of the body which should be kept fit. The exercises are very easily and comprehensively achieved by a series of yogic exercises.

In addition to the effect on the body, yogic exercies include certain mental exercises as well. Various speakers, including Dr. Khan, have pointed out the importance of the mind in relation to the body. Dr. Hackett noted yesterday that on the third day after myocardial infarction, depression is an important factor and is not easily controlled.

The results of our work [1] indicate that some yogic exercises such as Shavasan, nispandebawh, and even transcendental meditation reduce the patient's reaction to stress. Therefore, we have performed a comparative study of yoga with other forms of physical exercise as it is performed in the western world to determine the effects on these patients.

To evaluate them, we do not use the MET system. One of the speakers pointed out that he considered himself very fit, but when it came to sawing he found that an older man was more fit, because he was not trained for that. So when these people are not trained for this sort of exercise, the evaluation is directed toward the determination of the morbidity and mortality of the two groups of patients.

DR. KELLERMAN: Our program in Israel began 10 years ago. When it was initiated, we had mostly welfare people who had not worked for 5 to 9 years. The original objective was to determine whether a physical conditioning program, not only by means of exercise and calisthenics, but also through gardening and farming, could help rehabilitate people capable of working, but who were misguided by their physicians. Some were suffering, of course, from angina pectoris as well as from other functional disorders of the cardiac system.

In the beginning, we had a cardiac garden. Cardiac patients worked there for 4 months, then were discharged with a work "prescription." We learned very soon that the prescriptions were not filled. People had neither motivation nor discipline to go on with their exercise. Finally 4½ years ago, we changed the program to a group effort which simulates many of the programs currently underway in the United States. The patients meet three times weekly for exercise.

DR. HELLERSTEIN: I think it would be wrong to gain the impression that in the exercise intervention programs there is sole preoccupation with physical fitness. Plato, in emphasizing the importance of gymnastics, said that the more gentle arts and muses should not be forgotten. My associates and I have heeded this advice in the design of exercise programs for patients in institutional facilities and out in the community—often at great distances. The evaluation is individualized and personalized; it includes psychological, vocational, social apsects; an account of sleep and family problems; as well as physiologic assessment.

Coronary arteriography is also done because much time was wasted in approximately 18 percent of the coronary patients who have extensive multivessel disease and extremely low levels of performance. Such subjects do not respond to physical reconditioning.

In summary, our program in Cleveland, Ohio, has dealt basically with the physiologic and psychologic, vocational and personal aspects. While I would not discourage you from developing a specialized institution with exercise facilities in your community, ultimately we will come back to the fact that exercise prescription can be developed in most instances by a well-informed physician and a well-informed physical health educator who work in collaboration.

DR. KHAN: I would like to pose questions as a rough guide for prescription effort. Would it be appropriate to inform our patients that they should take an exercise which will make them a little breathless, but yet they should be able to communicate verbally with their partners?

What about conditioning for sexual activity? How much time should elapse between the acute attack and the permission to engage in such activity?

DR. PLAVSIC: In my opinion, regarding the sexual life, if a patient is rehabilitated, his way of life should be normal and there is no limited prescription for sexual life.

DR. KELLERMAN: I would not advise a patient to exercise to the point of breathlessness. There are many testing procedures suitable for large populations. As Dr. Hellerstein has reported, we should deal with exercise as though it were a "drug." We should know the indications, the contraindications, and the dosage. You cannot estimate this from symptoms alone.

DR. HELLERSTEIN: In a study made by Dr. Ernest Friedman and me [2], middle-aged men had an average peak heart rate response of 117 beats per minute during sexual activity. Their physiologic responses, therefore, approximated 70 percent of their age-predicted maximal heart rate, which was maintained for only 30 seconds. Many patients can withstand 30 seconds of high level effort (maximal or even supramaximal) because the oxygen intake does not increase within such brief periods and an oxygen deficit is incurred. Furthermore, they showed no more ST changes during sexual activity than in ordinary life activity. This was documented while they wore a tape recorder.

The subjects who had more sexual activity prior to their infarct from age 25 years on returned sooner to sexual activity than those who reported lesser activity.

In answering Dr. Khan's question, an enormous decline in sexual activity occurs from age 25 to age 50. The mean number of orgasms per week decreases from 4.4-4.2 (Kinsey report and our report) to about 2.5 times in men who are ostensibly well at least 1 year prior to the infarct or to the onset of other manifestation of coronary disease.

Certainly, "sexercise stress" should never be considered to be so great that the physician routinely prevents his patient from returning to conjugal sexual activity. However, extraconjugal sexual activity may be harmful according to Ueno in Japan. He reported that in nonviolent sudden deaths, cardiac death related to sexual activity occurred once in 500 deaths and usually occurred in a geisha house. We have studied several subjects during extramarital sexual activity, and found their responses to be comparable to those of the other study subjects.

Briefly, if you, the physician, have doubts about whether your patient should return to sexual activity, monitor the patient with a tape recorder, and do what I call the "sexercise" tolerance test. If you are going to forbid sex, forbid other activities such as brisk walking down the street, climbing a flight of stairs, or getting into an argument, as well, because the stresses of sexual activity in middle-aged people are certainly not as great as are many other aspects of living.

With reference to the question of breathlessness, yes, on a mass-scale symptoms can be used as a crude monitor. However, in our modern era some type of stress test is preferable. I would urge you to go beyond the symptomatic approach. Dr. Bruce and Dr. Levenson have reported that clinical judgments can be in error in 10 or 20 percent of the people in estimating exercise capacity on clinical grounds alone. Therefore, objective testing is really required as an adjunct to patient evaluation.

DR. FOX: Dr. Datey, we have seen some very stimulating cave carvings across the bay from Bombay during the visit some of us made some years ago. Can you tell us what the appropriate therapy is in your culture to prepare people to return after infarct to marital relations?

DR. DATEY: Those people who are excessively sexual will return to sexual activity. For those who develop symptoms, it might be best to advise them to let the healthy partner share the major portion of the work. This is the prescription which is followed by a number of people, at least in the initial stages.

DR. KHAN: Would you advise them to return to marital relations within 2 or 3 weeks of the infarct?

DR. DATEY: It is not a matter of advice. The patient will inquire about that when he has developed confidence in you. Therefore, he is indicating the desire to reassure himself that he is still vital. So from that point of view many are ready to resume sexual activity after about 3 weeks.

DR. KAHN: Our experience is different, sir, because people are afraid. They consider it strenuous exercise. The patients I deal with ask again and again, and they usually delay returning to normal sexual activity for a longer time than I have suggested.

DR. DATEY: May I point out that the amount of exercise will depend upon which partner is the major participant. If the healthy partner is doing the major share, the amount of exercise is minimized.

On the second point, about the stress testing, we use spot walking as a guide. On spot walking the blood pressure can be measured and the ECG monitored for irregularity.

DR. HELLERSTEIN: Dr. Datey has stressed an important point: there are intercultural differences. For example, in Yugoslavia, the coronary patients have higher cholesterols than those of the noncoronary patients, but the values of the former are much lower than in American normals. We need comparative data. It may well be that Pakistanis have a different energy requirement for the performance of sexual activity than do the Indians.

I recall that north of New Delhi there are monuments that indicate a great expertise of certain Indians of the past. Maybe we can learn more about this problem from them.

DR. FOX: In regard to the question about breathlessness, Dr. Paul Dudley White said many years ago that exercise should be pursued to the level that produces shortness of breath, a perspiration, an increase in the heart rate, an undefined and pleasant sense of fatigue not lasting in severity or time to any great extent. This is probably still a worthwhile guideline.

DR. GORMAN: What is the place of yoga in the rehabilitation of the post-myocardial infarction patient and in coronary individuals in western society?

DR. DATEY: We have not used it in the preventive program because it is not easy to collect the data. We have initiated certain exercises on the second day, provided the postcoronary patient is uncomplicated. They first learn shavasan. The technique was published in *Angiology* [1]. This helps them develop mental relaxation, with the result that the reaction to a given stress is reduced. Active movements of the legs are begun the next day. On the third or fourth day, the patient sits up in a chair and begins to take short walks around the bed.

This is, of course, a project where patients are telemetered to determine their adaptations to gradually increased levels of physical activity. If the heart size is normal and if they do not show any evidence of cardiac failure within about 10 to 15 days, they are permitted to walk about. That is probably one of the earliest types of mobility that we can give to these patients.

The number of patients who respond successfully within 15 days is only about 19 to 20 percent. Others have a number of problems which delay their rehabilitation. Different yogic exercises are used for various organs.

DR. HELLERSTEIN: Years ago I was very much impressed with how anxious the coronary patients were, and when I met their physicians I understood the reason. Anxious doctors have anxious patients. There is a subtle transfer of attitude from doctor to patient. We are not seeing as much depression in acute myocardial infarction as we did 10 years ago. In large part, this is due to the greater confidence of the physicians. Excessive restrictions can be eliminated. We do not have to tell an able-bodied coronary patient who was working the day before how to move his arm or his leg. Such coddling is nonsensical. There is no reason to go to passive movements in most cases. There is no reason to over-restrict. As a result of our changed attitude, the depression that was seen earlier is disappearing or decreasing because we are more secure and less anxious.

There is a biochemical basis for setting an atmosphere to relieve anxiety and depression whether by shavasan, or by understanding and therapeutic words. Lennart Levi of Stockholm has reported that people exposed to pastoral scenes and tranquil music such as Brahms showed a decrease in catecholamine excretion. When they saw violent movies of war and atrocities of primitive tribes, the catecholamines rose. However, when he showed the test subjects a hilarious French movie, their catecholamines rose equally high.

The point is that one can change the responsiveness of people to their environment, and in several ways reduce the biochemical determinants of myocardial oxygen needs.

DR. DENOLIN: If sexual activity is one of the important aspects of rehabilitation, I think we also have to discuss some results. I would like to have information from the panel about the results of the different programs in terms of physical conditioning, return to work, morbidity, and mortality. We lack information on these very important aspects of the different types of programs. Perhaps the question is a little too broad for a few moments, but it is very important.

DR. PLAVSIC: In a group of 1,350 patients, we had only 20 deaths during the rehabilitation period. Usually they were due to heart failure or other sudden death and usually occurred in the night. There was no death during actual exercise performance.

DR. DATEY: So far, our observations indicate that the patients are able to sleep without any medication. They are happier and more contented. That is the sort of impression I can give you.

DR. KELLERMAN: I can give you the results in 230 patients who recovered from a single myocardial infarction. They were divided into three groups. Group I, consisting of 92 patients, was not formally rehabilitated. The mortality in a followup of 8.9 years revealed that 21.7 percent sustained cardiac deaths. Group II (85 patients), trained for 4 months. Their mortality after 8.9 years was 22.3 percent. Group III (53 patients) conditioned for 54 consecutive months. Their followup extended over a period of 7.2 years, and their mortality rate was 5.7 percent.

As to the physical capabilities of these three groups, Groups I and II experienced a decrement in performance, while Group III improved and reached 130 percent of our normal of healthy individuals.

DR. HELLERSTEIN: Our data indicated that the mortality rate in a group of 254 coronary patients at the end of 3 years was 2.11 per 100 person years. When the group was subdivided into those patients who had both a transmural myocardial infarct and angina pectoris, the mortality rate was 2.9 per 100 person years. In contrast, populations which were drawn from the same community and from the same social class to form a comparable but not a true control group had a mortality rate of 4.3 per 100 person years. The latter data are comparable to the Coronary Drug Project data. The more severe cases had a mortality rate of around 6 per 100 per year. There is a need for a well-controlled randomized prospective study to quantitate the effects of physical conditioning on morbidity and mortality in ASHD.

REFERENCES

1. Datey, K.K., Deshmukh, S.N., Dalvi, C.P., and Vinekav, S.L. Shavasan—a yogic exercise in the management of hypertension. *Angiology* 20:325-333, 1969.

2. Hellerstein, H.K., and Friedman, E.H. Sexual activity and the postcoronary patient. *Arch. Intern. Med.* 125:987-999, 1970.

29

AIRLIE POSTGRADUATE COURSE

A. THE CORONARY RISK FACTORS AND EXERCISE TOLERANCE OF PARTICIPANTS

J. E. Merriman, M.D., F.R.C.P.(C), and *M. E. Donegan*

Introduction

The Airlie Postgraduate Course on Exercise Testing and Training was planned to provide maximum educational benefit for those attending. The participants, from different disciplines including cardiology, physiology, rehabilitation medicine, and physical education, were interested in exercise testing and training, especially in patients with coronary artery disease.

Each participant was given an opportunity to have his personal coronary risk factors assessed and to have an exercise tolerance test performed, either on the bicycle or on the treadmill. This chapter assesses the coronary risk factors of the Airlie participants.

Methods

Each participant completed a specially designed form which documented his history in regard to family, weight, and smoking. Other significant aspects of the medical history were also noted. The height and weight were recorded without shoes. The skinfold thickness was measured at the triceps, subscapular, and suprailiac sites using Harpenden calipers and International Biological Programme methodology [1]. Durnin's modified formula was used to estimate the percentage body fat [2].

Ventilation volumes were recorded using the Vertek VR-5000 spirometer. Each patient's total vital capacity (TVC) and forced expiratory volume in 1-second (FEV-1) were expressed as a percentage of predicted normal.

A resting 12-lead electrocardiogram was obtained before an exercise test. Each participant had been asked to bring to the course the results of a recent fasting blood lipid analysis.

421

Exercise tests were conducted using either the treadmill or a bicycle ergometer. The treadmill tests were performed under the direction of the course teachers (Drs. Bruce, Naughton, and Buskirk) and bicycle tests were done using Dr. Hellerstein's methodology. Cuff blood pressures were measured at rest and during exercise. Maximum oxygen intake was estimated and expressed as milliliters per kilogram per minute (ml/kg/min).

Results

TABLE I shows the test results of 123 males and 13 females in the study. The majority of these participants had all determinations done although only 89 males and seven females had skinfold measurements for percentage body fat determination.

TABLE I

Test results of participants in the study

	MALES n = 123		FEMALES n = 13	
	Mean	S.D.	Mean	S.D.
Age (in years)	43.6	12.0	38.3	8.5
Height (in inches)	69.0	2.7	64.8	2.8
Weight (in pounds)	171.5	20.6	133.9	24.2
Percentage body fat	21.6	4.5	27.6	4.0
Blood pressure–systolic	133.3	15.9	122.8	14.5
Blood pressure–diastolic	84.3	11.3	83.2	9.8
TVC (in liters)	4.39	0.81	3.27	0.53
FEV-1 (in liters)	3.49	0.78	2.72	0.42
TVC as a percentage of predicted normal	90.6	12.4	99.4	13.1
FEV-1 as a percentage of TVC	79.9	12.8	83.5	6.8

TABLE II shows comparative figures for some of the important coronary risk factors from three studies. In the Airlie study of 123 males, on only 25 were blood lipids determined. The data from Canadian physicians were compiled from studies made in coronary screening clinics in Saskatoon and at different medical association meetings. These two studies are compared with the recently published U.S. Drug Study on patients with myocardial infarction [3].

Abnormal diagnoses. From the medical questionnaire, the diagnoses noted were:

Hypertension–6; Coronary artery disease–5; Diabetes–2; Mitral insufficiency–1; Auricular fibrillation–1; Asthma–1; Others–1.

Thus, of 136 participants, 17 diagnoses were other than *normal*, an incidence of 12.5 percent.

Anthropometry. Percentage body fat. On the basis of Saskatchewan data, we used the calculated percentage body fat to classify subjects into different weight groupings as outlined in TABLE III.

TABLE II

Coronary risk factors in a male population

	Airlie Study n = 123	Canadian Physicians n = 563	U.S. Drug Study n = 8338
Age	43.6 ± 12.0	47.6 ± 11.5	52.4 ± 7.1
Height	69.0 ± 2.7	68.8 ± 2.9	68.2 ± 2.4
Weight	171.5 ± 20.6	172.4 ± 22.2	172.2 ± 25.0
Percentage fat	21.6 ± 4.5	19.5 ± 3.7	
Percentage smoking	35.6	34.6	86.5
Blood pressure–S	133.3 ± 15.9	125.0 ± 17.1	129.9 ± 18.8
Blood pressure–D	84.3 ± 11.3	81.8 ± 9.9	81.9 ± 10.9
Serum cholesterol	206.0 ± 35.6	231.5 ± 38.5	250.8 ± 48.0
Serum triglycerides	100.2 ± 51.4	160.4 ± 111.3	188.0 ± 147.0 [1]

[1] Quoted mean 6.10 ± 4.79 mEq/L.

TABLE III

Percentage body fat of participants

	Percentage body fat	No.	% of total
Normal	10-15%	9	9.4
Tendency to overweight	15-20%	24	25.0
Overweight	20-25%	43	44.8
Obese	>25%	20	20.8
		96	100.0

Note: For normal females the percentage body fat is 20-25% of total body weight. An obese female has a percentage of body fat greater than 35%.

Thus, using this criterion, more than 65 percent of the participants at the Airlie Postgraduate Course would be classified as overweight or obese. Only 9.4 percent of the participants had a normal percentage body fat. In a study of 299 normal Saskatoon males, 41 percent were of normal weight.

Calculation of ideal weight. Body weight can be subdivided into two main compartments: (1) fat; and (2) the non-fat compartment which has been called lean body mass. Using the three skinfold measurements and Durnin's formula, the percentage body fat can be computed and the lean body mass can be derived. Assuming the upper limit of normal percentage body fat for males is 15 percent, an ideal weight can be calculated for an individual patient.

Weight history. The medical history asked the patient's weight at different times—aged 20, 5 years ago, 1 year ago, and his all-time maximum. TABLE IV shows these values together with the calculated ideal weight. For this group, the maximum weight occurred 8.5 ± 9.1 years previously.

TABLE IV

Weight history (values in pounds)

	Males	Females
At age 20	158.4 ± 22.3	128.5 ± 23.0
Maximum weight ever	181.8 ± 23.8	145.2 ± 32.1
5 years ago	170.4 ± 22.5	133.7 ± 33.4
1 year ago	169.7 ± 19.5	136.2 ± 33.4
Weight now	171.5 ± 20.6	133.9 ± 24.2
Ideal weight	156.4 ± 17.7	126.1 ± 14.7

It will be noted that the average maximum weight was 25.4 lbs above the present ideal weight for males and 19.1 lbs for females. The close similarity between the ideal weight as determined now and the weight at age 20 is noted. These results are in agreement with other observations from our laboratory.

Smoking history. A smoking history was obtained from 136 participants. (TABLE II shows that 35.6 percent of the 123 males were smokers.) Fifty percent had never smoked, 14.7 percent had quit smoking, and 33.8 percent were now smoking. The smoking history was not recorded in 1.5 percent. In the coronary drug project it is noted that 86.5 percent of the patients were smokers prior to their entry into the project.

Blood pressure. Blood pressures were determined in the sitting position using a sphygmomanometer cuff. The blood pressures were read to the nearest 5 mms of mercury. A value of 140/90 was considered the upper limit of normal. A systolic value of 145 or greater, and/or a diastolic value of 95 or greater was considered as abnormal. Using these criteria, there were 21 individuals with elevated resting blood pressure readings.

Blood lipids. Very few individuals submitted the results of their blood lipids. However, of the 25 that did, there were four instances where the serum cholesterol was resported in excess of 250 mg percent and three values where the serum triglycerides were greater than 150 mg percent.

Resting electrocardiogram. A 12-lead resting electrocardiogram was obtained from 108 of the participants. Seventy-nine tracings were within normal limits; 12 were probably within normal limits; in eight instances the tracing was considered as a borderline curve; and in nine instances it was definitely an abnormal curve. Thus 84.3 percent of the electrocardiograms were normal and 15.7 percent were abnormal.

Physical activity. In the history form, three questions were asked which were graded as: rarely or never, sometimes, or frequently. The three questions were: Do you walk in good weather? Do you work around the house? Do you take part in any high-intensity physical activity? TABLE V shows the results from the physical activity questionnaire. The range of scores is from 1 to 7.

The mean score was 4.10 ± 1.50 suggesting that the population was fairly representative and that the physical activity of these individuals ranged from very unfit to very fit.

TABLE V

Assessment of physical activity from history

		(Sedentary)				(Active)		
Score		1	2	3	4	5	6	7
Male		5	16	15	38	26	13	10
Female		1	2	0	1	4	4	1
TOTAL		6	18	15	39	30	17	11

Exercise tolerance study. The mean maximum oxygen intake ($\dot{V}_{O_2}$ max) for 40 individuals from a bicycle test was 32.68 ± 10.42 ml/kg/min. The mean values for 21 treadmill studies was 32.20 ± 8.12 ml/kg/min. The $\dot{V}_{O_2}$ max was expressed as a percentage of normal for the age. TABLE VI summarizes our results.

TABLE VI

Maximum oxygen intake as a percentage of predicted normal

% of Normal	50-59	60-69	70-79	80-89	90-99	100-109	110-119	120-129	130-139
Bicycle	3	6	6	5	5	9	2	3	1
Treadmill	2	1	1	4	1	5	5	1	1
TOTAL	5	7	7	9	6	14	7	4	2
% of Total		31.2			24.6		34.4		9.9

Exercise electrocardiogram. The exercise ECGs were graded as:
1. No change.
2. Not abnormal—indicating some ST segment changes not considered to be ischemic
3. Abnormal

There was one abnormal ischemic exercise electrocardiogram, 20 which were not abnormal, and 19 which showed no change.

Exercise blood pressure. The criteria for abnormal exercise blood pressure response were: systolic blood pressure should not be greater than 120 plus 1/10 of the workload in kilogram meters per minute (kg/m/min). If an individual was able to perform a 600 kg/m/min workload, he could have a normal exercise systolic blood pressure of 180 during that exercise. An abnormal diastolic exercise blood pressure of 100 or more was considered abnormal.

Using these criteria, 16 of the 40 participants (40 percent) had an abnormal blood pressure response to bicycle exercise. Twelve individuals had abnormal systolic and diastolic responses, three had only an abnormal systolic response, and one had only an abnormal diastolic response.

Summary

The coronary risk factors of 136 Airlie Postgraduate Course participants were assessed. Of these participants, 65.6 percent were overweight or obese; 15.4 percent had systemic hypertension (145/95 or greater), and 33.8 percent were cigarette smokers. There were 12.5 percent of the participants whose diagnoses were other than normal, and 15.7 percent exhibited an abnormality in the resting electrocardiogram. Thirty-one percent of the subjects tested had maximum oxygen intake values less than 80 percent of predicted normal for age, and 40 percent of the subjects tested, using a bicycle ergometer, had an abnormal blood pressure response to exercise.

This study indicates that a significant number of abnormalities will be detected during medical screening for coronary risk factors in an apparently healthy population.

REFERENCES

1. Weiner, J.S., and Lourie, J.A., Eds. *Human Biology: A Guide to Field Methods.* (International Biological Programme Handbook 9) Philadelphia, Davis Co., 1969.

2. Durnin, J.V.G.A., and Rahaman, M.M. The assessment of the amount of fat in the human body from measurements of skinfold thickness. *Br. J. Nutr.* 21:681-689, 1967.

3. The Coronary Drug Project: Design, methods and baseline results. *Circulation* 47(3): Suppl. No. 1, March, 1973.

B. CARDIOPULMONARY RESUSCITATION TRAINING COURSE:

Format, General Comments, Test Results

Nanette K. Wenger, M.D.

Cardiopulmonary resuscitation (CPR) is an emergency first aid measure designed to maintain life in a patient who has sustained a respiratory and cardiac arrest until definitive therapy can be instituted. The ABC steps include: (A) opening and maintaining of a patent Airway; (B) restoration of Breathing by means of artificial ventilation; and (C) restoration of Circulation by external cardiac compression.

All health care personnel involved in exercise testing and in exercise training programs must be competent in the recognition of cardiorespiratory arrest and in the performance of artificial ventilation and closed chest compression. Therefore, the decision was made to offer a CPR training course, leading to certification, to all Airlie House conference participants. Eighty-nine of the 146 conference participants attended the CPR sessions.

The format of the CPR course, which followed the American Heart Association recommendations, included: lecture, slide, and film presentations; demonstration of procedures; and actual practice by the participants on training manikins under the supervision of certified instructors. These certified instructors included the CPR Project Director of the Virginia Heart Association and several nonphysician volunteers, all members of local fire departments, and most involved in community emergency care services. The CPR practice sessions enabled the course participants to demonstrate that they were capable of identifying a cardiopulmonary arrest and performing artificial ventilation and external cardiac compression in proper sequence, both when a single individual and when two rescuers were available.

Fifty-nine Airlie Conference attendees volunteered to take a CPR pretest to assess baseline information. The CPR course content was completed in an intensive 2-hour session, with additional manikin practice time and/or question-answer sessions available if desired. A postcourse written examination and an actual performance test were criteria for certification. All 89 CPR course participants were certified, and appropriate training course diplomas awarded. The results of the postcourse examination were compared with pretest data.

Several senior physicians from abroad questioned the propriety of a practice session, working in shirtsleeves, kneeling on the floor. The role of the layman-fireman as an instructor of physicians also appeared disquieting to many. However, once assured that this was accepted and routine procedure in the United States, and after the U.S. Professor(s) of Medicine had knelt on the floor to assist in training practice, physician cooperation and involvement was genuine and enthusiastic. Indeed, some of the senior physicians from abroad commented that they had never actually performed CPR on a patient, but had taught and then delegated this procedure to their junior associates and trainees; others expressed new appreciation of the competence of nonphysicians (both the instructors and other course participants) in cardiopulmonary resuscitation. For a few physicians it was an initial opportunity to practice using the defibrillator (which was available for demonstration during the CPR course), as this equipment, while on order, was not yet available in their medical communities. Interestingly, an additional number of attendees, who had not originally planned to participate in CPR training, did so when they learned a diploma was to be given as evidence of certification. Both during and after the course, considerable interest was engendered by the teaching aids used—slides, films, pamphlets, practice manikins—and questions raised as to their cost and availability.

The mean group pretest score was 74.8 percent and the mean group posttest score was 95.17 percent, an increase in the mean score of 21.9 percent (Fig. 1). The matched (paired) pre- and posttest scores were available for 46 individuals and showed an increase in the mean score of 20.8 percent. The professional classification of these 46 individuals was as follows: cardiologist—6, internist—4, physiologist—4, physical educators—10, graduate students—2, other (nurses, physicians in rehabilitation medicine, etc.)—4, and not stated—16. One of the physical educators had a perfect score on the pretest. The four physiologists and the 10 physical educators had the highest final scores. As a group, the cardiol-

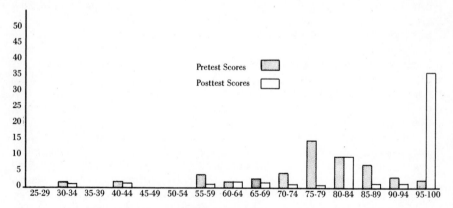

Fig. 1. Distribution of pre- and posttest scores for cardiopulmonary resuscitation examination (Coronary Exercise Conference).

ogists improved least, because they started from a slightly higher level (TABLE I). The major significant error evident on the written (as well as on the practical) examination was in the sequence of performance of cardiopulmonary resuscitation—failure to indicate that the initial step was opening of the airway by raising the neck and tilting the head backward.

TABLE I

Comparison of pre- and posttest data

	Number	Pre- Posttest Average Increase	Pretest Average	Posttest Average
Cardiologist	6	+2.15	12.15	14.3
Internist	4	+3.25	10.75	14.0
Physiologist	4	+2.75	11.75	14.5
Physical Educator	10	+3.5	11.0	14.5
Graduate Student	2	+1.5	12.5	14.0
Other	4	+3.5	11.5	15.0
Not Stated	16	+3.2	11.0	14.2

It is recommended that a course in cardiopulmonary resuscitation, leading to certification or recertification, be incorporated in educational programs dealing with the use of exercise testing and exercise training for patients with heart disease.

30

SELECTED CASE HISTORIES

University of Saskatchewan—University Hospital

CASE HISTORY: B.N.—U.H.#211382

A 53-year-old college instructor, born in Denmark, was in good health until the spring of 1970, when he experienced exertional dyspnea and a burning sensation in his throat with radiation to both arms. It was always immediately relieved by rest, and was not related to meals, cold, or emotional upset. Occasionally it was experienced during sexual intercourse.

On further questioning, the patient added the information that for the past 4 years he had some exertional dyspnea and had complained of mild fleeting chest pain—not related to exertion.

Physical examination was within normal limits.

Special Studies:

1. Coronary Risk Factors (Fig. 1)
2. EKG—Rest (Fig. 2)
3. EKG—Exercise and Recovery (Fig. 3)
4. Coronary Arteriograms (Fig. 4)

History:

December 1970. Diagnosis of angina confirmed. Abnormal coronary risk factors treated. Patient's diet was changed to reduce the saturated fat intake. Exertional dyspnea and angina still bothersome.

April 1971. Cholesterol—275; triglycerides—145. An exercise prescription was written for a noon-hour training program in the hospital gymnasium. This prescription consisted of calisthenics, volleyball, and walking. The patient was closely supervised and EKG monitored during the first month on the program. In view of the improved performance when nitroglycerin was used prophylactically, this principle was incorporated in his training program.

June 1971. Clinically—greatly improved. The patient noted dyspnea and angina *only* on very strenuous exertion.

Coronary Angiograms:

Left — complete occlusion of the proximal portion of anterior descending and circumflex. Note the greatly enlarged branch of the obtuse margin.

Right — a long and fairly stenotic segment of the proximal portion. Note the intraluminal filling defects proximally. Note the multiple collateral vessels.

June 1971–Cardiac Conference. The surgeons and half of the cardiologists present favored surgical treatment. Clinically the patient was greatly improved and he declined surgery.

March 1972. The patient has continued on the exercise program 3 times/week. He is still not bothered by dyspnea or angina. He will be restudied in the next few months.

TABLE I

Summary of patient's history

Date	Weight	MAXIMUM Work–kgm/min	H.R.	$\dot{V}O_2$ max ml/kg
Dec./70	193	500	112	18.8
April/71	188	500	103	15.4
June/71	176	600	120	22.9

EXERCISE AND CORONARY ARTERY DISEASE
RESEARCH PROJECT

University of Saskatchewan   University Hospital

CORONARY RISK FACTORS

		Date:	December 18, 1970
Name:	B.N.	**Age:**	52
Diagnosis:	Ischemic Heart Disease	**Hosp. #:**	211382
	Angina — Mild		
	Exertional Dyspnea — Moderate		

I.   **Family History:** Parents are both alive and well at 79 and 73

    Body Build: Medium-Tall   **Height:**   71 inches

    Blood Group: A_1, Rh Positive

II.   **Diet:**   Formerly ate a great deal of eggs, cheese, and meat

    Weight: % Body Fat 21.6   **Present Weight:**   193

                                          Ideal Weight: 170

    Smoking: Does not smoke

    Fitness: **Maximum Workload**   500

                                                Percentage of

        Maximum Oxygen Intake—ml/kg 18.8   **Normal:**   59.0

III.   **Blood Pressure:**   **Rest**   100/70

                            On <u>500</u> Exercise   160/90

    Lipids: **Uric Acid**   6.6

               Cholesterol   330

               Triglycerides   176

    Tension: Mild   **Resting Heart Rate:**   50

IV.   **Heart Size:**   Normal

    Electrocardiogram:

        Rest -   Axis +30. Suggestive of old lateral wall MI. Definitely abnormal
                curve.
        Exercise- See tracing

    Other Factors: Coronary arteriogram — June 3/71

*Abnormal values are starred   Nov., 1971

Fig. 1.   Coronary Risk Factors.

B.N. - # 211382 - 53 YEARS - MALE

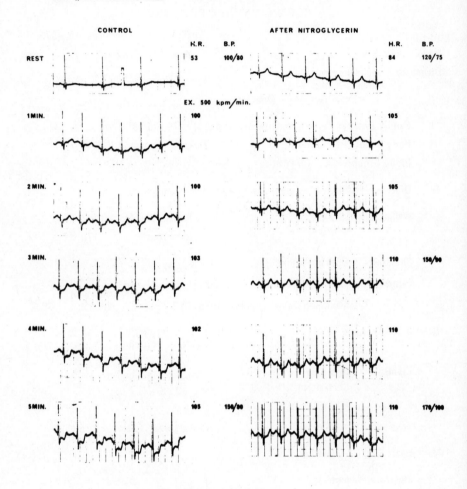

Fig. 2.   EKG at rest.

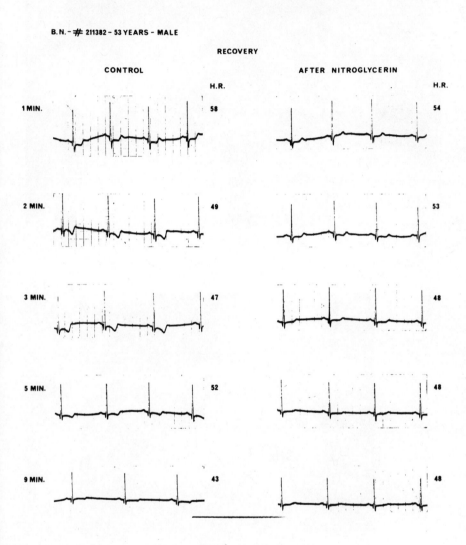

B.N.-# 211382 - 53 YEARS - MALE

RECOVERY

CONTROL   AFTER NITROGLYCERIN

H.R.   H.R.

1 MIN.   58   54

2 MIN.   49   53

3 MIN.   47   48

5 MIN.   52   48

9 MIN.   43   48

Fig. 3. EKG—exercise and recovery.

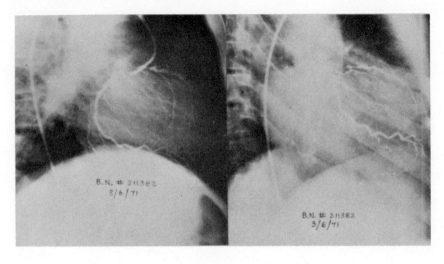

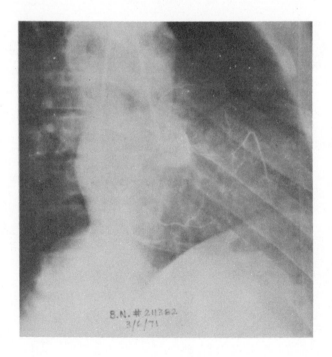

Fig. 4. Coronary arteriograms.

University of Saskatchewan–University Hospital

CASE HISTORY: A.D.–U.H.#210991

A 52-year-old carpenter first noted the onset of typical exertional angina in *March 1970.*

In June 1970 he developed sudden chest pain while watching T.V. This pain was more severe than his anginal pains, lasting for a half-hour, and was associated with pallor and sweating. He did not consult his physician. The next day he noted that his angina occurred with much less intense activity. He then remained relatively free of pain until . . .

September 1970 when he collapsed while pouring cement and later complained of chest pain. He continued working but again noted his angina with very limited activity. He was hospitalized but continued to have episodes of chest pain at rest, as well as on exercise. He has not been able to return to work. His angina is induced by exercise, sexual intercourse, and emotional upset. It is usually relieved by rest and responds very well to nitroglycerin.

Medications: Danilone, Stellazine, Inderal, and nitroglycerin.

Physical examination was within normal limits.

Special Studies:

1. Coronary Risk Factors (Fig. 1)
2. EKG–Rest (Fig. 2)
3. EKG–Exercise and Recovery (Fig. 3)
4. Coronary Arteriograms (Fig. 4)

History

December 8, 1970. Evaluated. Booked for coronary studies. Patient strongly advised to stop smoking.

January 14, 1971. Repeat exercise test showed a definite improvement in exercise tolerance. No chest pain but on the 500 exercise patient was very dyspneic and sweaty. (The only known change in therapy was that he had stopped smoking 5 weeks before.)

Coronary Arteriogram:

Left — There is diffuse atherosclerotic change in the left coronary system with a severe, localized zone of stenosis in the proximal portion of the anterior descending branch. This vessel proceeds distally in a non-, or minimally tapering fashion, indicating that this vessel serves a major role as an anastomotic channel to the base of the heart. Late in the study, portions of the posterior descending branch at the crux are visualized and apparently are fed in part by this vessel. The circumflex shows atherosclerotic change and a multitude of small collateral vessels which proceed distally, eventually terminating in the posterior descending artery of the right coronary artery.

Right — The right coronary artery is totally occluded some 5.5 to 6 cm from its orifice. All the branches off the right coronary proximal to this stenosis are enlarged and some collateral circulation is present distally, but the posterior descending branch is never visualized from this side.

At the Cardiac Conference it was suggested that surgery might help him. He had shown frequent ventricular premature systoles and a hypotensive response on exertion and he had severe three-vessel coronary artery disease.

May 18, 1971. Repeat exercise tolerance test showed marked limitation. A double aortocoronary bypass was performed to the right coronary artery distal to the crux and to the left anterior descending in its proximal third.

Postoperatively the patient noted marked subjective improvement and he had not experienced any anginal pain.

September 9, 1971. As noted, his exercise tolerance showed no objective change until the 6-month postoperative study (November 16/71). At that time his $\dot{V}_{O_2}$ max had shown a definite improvement. However, the hypotensive response to exercise associated with marked dyspnea persisted.

January 27, 1972. Repeat angio studies showed that the right saphenous bypass graft was patent. However, the left graft could not be visualized.

Hemodynamic Data–January 27, 1972:

Pressures		RV	LA	LV	Ao	
		$\dfrac{26}{7}$	8	$\dfrac{100}{9}$	$\dfrac{114}{73}$	· 85
Volumes	Systolic	29 CM^3/M^2				
	Diastolic	73 CM^3/M^2				

Ejection Fraction   60%

Cardiac Index $1.7 \ L/min/M^2$

TABLE I

Exercise tolerance data

Date	Weight	Maximum Workload	Maximum H.R.	$\dot{V}O_2 \ max$ ml/kg	Comment
Dec. 8/70	173	200	122	14.4	Frequent VPS, Angina Smoking 8 cigs/day
Jan. 13/71	177	500	155	21.4	Angina: Not smoking
May 14/71	182	300	112	14.6	Angina − ℞ NG No AP
May 18/71	Surgery				
May 27/71	174	200	118	14.2	
July 6/71	172	300	132	15.6	Angina − ℞ NG No AP
Sept. 9/71	172	300	138	15.4	Angina; Hypotension ℞ − NG No AP
Nov. 16/71	172	600	162	19.1	BBB & Hypotension, yet no angina
Jan. 26/72	177	600	160	20.4	Slight chest pain

EXERCISE AND CORONARY ARTERY DISEASE
RESEARCH PROJECT

University of Saskatchewan   University Hospital

CORONARY RISK FACTORS

Date: December 8, 1970

Name: A.D.   **Age:**   51

Diagnosis: Ischemic Heart Disease   **Hosp. #:**   210991

I. **Family History:**   Nil

   Body Build: Small-Medium   **Height:**   68.5 inches

   Blood Group: O, Rh Negative

II. **Diet:** Lots of butter, cheese, & pork; 18 eggs/week   **Present Weight:** 173

   Weight: % Body Fat 16.9   **Ideal Weight:**   171

   Smoking: 10 cigarettes/day

   Fitness: **Maximum Workload** 200- 5 minutes   **Percentage of**
            Maximum Oxygen Intake - ml/kg   14.4   **Normal**   44.5

III. **Blood Pressure**   **Rest**   125/95
                          On 200 Exercise   155/100

		Dec. /70	Jan./71
Lipids:	**Uric Acid**	5.9	8.5
	Cholesterol	285	265
	Triglycerides	270	280

   Tension: Moderate   **Resting Heart Rate:**   62

IV. **Heart Size:**   Normal

   Electrocardiogram: **Rest** - Nonspecific ST-T changes
                Exercise- See tracing

   Other Factors: Coronary Arteriogram — January/71

*Abnormal values are starred   Nov., 1971

Fig. 1. Coronary risk factors.

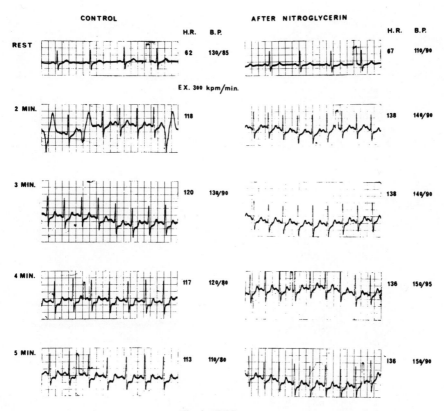

Fig. 2. EKGs at rest.

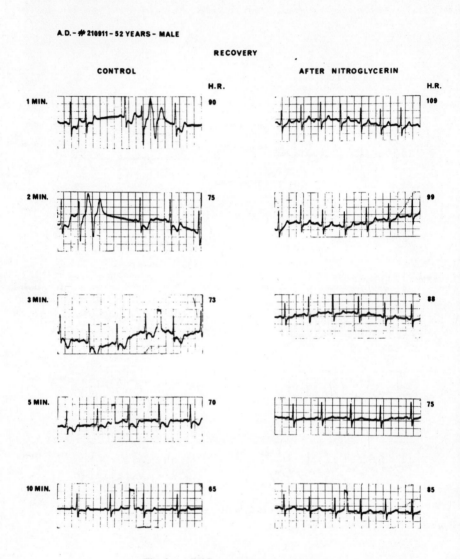

A.D. - # 210911 - 52 YEARS - MALE

RECOVERY

CONTROL   AFTER NITROGLYCERIN

                              H.R.   H.R.

1 MIN.   90   109

2 MIN.   75   99

3 MIN.   73   88

5 MIN.   70   75

10 MIN.   65   85

Fig. 3.   EKG—exercise and recovery.

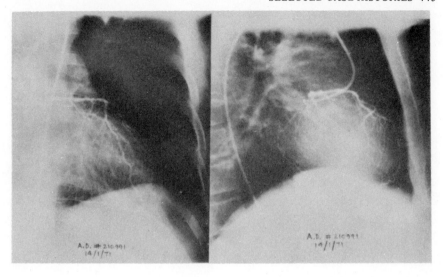

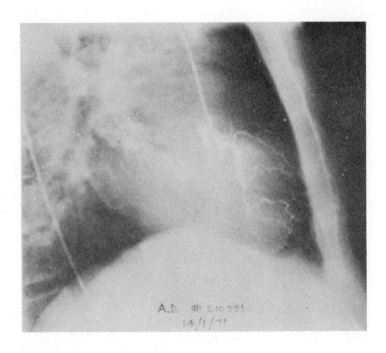

Fig. 4. Coronary arteriograms.

PARTICIPANTS

Bojan Accetto, M.D.
Richarjeva 24, Yugoslavia

Amjad Ali, M.D.
Chicago, Illinois

Michael Angelo
Washington, D.C.

William J. Armstrong, M.D.
Butler, Pennsylvania

Theodore W. Arnold, M.A.
Cleveland, Ohio

Zdzislaw Askanas, M.D.
Warsaw, Poland

Mohamed Attia, M.D.
Cairo, Egypt

C. William Bell, B.A., M.S.
Pittsburgh, Pennsylvania

Abdesattar Ben Hamida, M.D.
Tunis, Tunisia

Herbert E. Bessinger, M.D.
Chicago, Illinois

Steven N. Blair, B.A., M.S., P.E.D.
Columbia, South Carolina

W. Vincent Blockley, B.A.
Malibu, California

Alston W. Blount, Jr., M.D.
Richmond, Virginia

Arthur Bobruff, M.D.
Washington, D.C.

Richard L. Bohannon, M.D.
Dallas, Texas

Bernardo Boskis, M.D.
Buenos Aires, Argentina

Judythe Boswell, R.N.
Washington, D.C.

Alan D. Bram, B.A., M.A.
Cleveland, Ohio

Demetrios K. Calogirou, M.D.
Athens, Greece

Emil J. Carazo, B.S.
Ridgewood, New Jersey

William H. Carter, M.D.
Charleston, West Virginia

James C. Carver, Jr., M.D.
Bloomfield, New Jersey

Ned H. Cassem, M.D.
Boston, Massachusetts

Gaston Choquette, M.D.
Montreal, Canada

James F. Conner, M.D.
St. Petersburg, Florida

Manuel N. Cooper, M.D.
Seattle, Washington

Theodore Cooper, M.D.
Bethesda, Maryland

Thomas F. Coyle, M.D.
Bridgeport, Connecticut

Don E. Craig
  Woodbridge, Virginia

David E. Cundiff, Ph.D.
  Bowling Green, Kentucky

William C. Day, M.A.
  Cambridge, Massachusetts

Robert F. DeBusk, M.D.
  San Francisco, California

Michael M. Dehn, B.A., M.S.
  Seattle, Washington

Daniel J. Diana, M.D.
  Washington, D.C.

Hadi Dizadji, M.D.
  Chicago, Illinois

Bozidar S. Djordjevic, M.D.
  Belgrade, Yugoslavia

Mary Therese Doherty, R.N., M.S.
  Chicago, Illinois

Joseph Dorchak, M.D.
  Spartanburg, South Carolina

Leonard Dudka
  Greensboro, North Carolina

Michael Donegan
  Saskatoon, Saskatchewan, Canada

Lloyd Elliott, Ph.D.
  Washington, D.C.

Norma Ellman
  New York, New York

Blair D. Erb, M.D.
  Jackson, Tennessee

George H. Feil, M.D.
  Cleveland, Ohio

Joseph Fenton, Ed.D.
  Washington, D.C.

Ronald James Ferguson, Ph.D.
  Montreal, Quebec, Canada

Stanley H. Fisher, Ed.D.
  Storrs, Connecticut

Jesse W. Fowler
  Washington, D.C.

Glenn M. Friedman, M.D.
  Scottsdale, Arizona

Newton J. Friedman, M.D.
  Ventura, California

Rufus S. Gardner, Jr., M.D.
  Fishersville, Virginia

James F. Garrett, Ph.D.
  Washington, D.C.

L. H. Getchell, Ph.D.
  Muncie, Indiana

John W. Gruber, M.D.
  Reading, Pennsylvania

Walter D. Gundel, M.D.
  Burlington, Vermont

John A. Hagan, M.A.
  New York, New York

Michael Halberstam, M.D.
  Washington, D.C.

Bent B. Hansen, B.P.T.
  Winnipeg, Manitoba, Canada

Antoine Harovas, M.D.
  New York, New York

Walter H. Hasbrouck, M.D., F.A.C.C.
  Montclair, New Jersey

Javid A. Hashmi, M.D.
  Karachi 35, Pakistan

Philip K. Hensel, M.D.
  Harrisburg, Pennsylvania

Gerald Herbison, M.D.
  Philadelphia, Pennsylvania

T. G. Hiebert, M.D., Ph.D.
  Hines, Illinois

Marvin Hines
  Richmond, Virginia

James Hodgson
  University Park, Pennsylvania

Frank W. Jackson, M.D.
  Harrisburg, Pennsylvania

Amer I. Jafari, B.S., Ed.M.
  Buffalo, New York

Thomas J. Janicki, M.D.
  Institute, West Virginia

Michael Jelinek, M.D.
  Boston, Massachusetts

Maurice Jette, Ph.D.
Ottawa, Canada

Rudolf Jirka, L.L.D.
Anderson, Indiana

Sarah A. Johnson, M.D.
Chicago, Illinois

Robert H. Jones, M.D.
Rochester, New York

David B. Jordan, Ph.D.
New York, New York

V. S. Josipovic, M.D.
Belgrade, Yugoslavia

Gabrijel Kastelec, M.D.
Radenci, Yugoslavia

Jay T. Kearney
Boone, North Carolina

David Keegan, M.D., F.R.C.P.
Saskatoon, Saskatchewan, Canada

George Kelser, M.D.
Washington, D.C.

Mohamed Alumgir Khan, M.D.
Lahore, Pakistan

Nasirud Din Azam Khan, M.D., F.R.C.P.
Peshawar, Pakistan

George R. Kinnear, M.A.
College Park, Maryland

John F. Kirby, Jr., M.D.
Seattle, Washington

Irvin Klein, M.D.
New York, New York

Robert M. Kohn, M.D.
Buffalo, New York

Knut Konig, M.D.
Freiburg, West Germany

Frederic J. Kottke, M.D., Ph.D.
Minneapolis, Minnesota

Lawrence Krohn, M.D.
Detroit, Michigan

Scottie Kuse
Cleveland, Ohio

Kenneth S. Landauer, M.D.
Ridgewood, New Jersey

Fernand Landry, Ph.D.
Quebec, Canada

Jules H. Last, M.D., Ph.D.
Chicago, Illinois

Charles N. Leach, Jr., M.D.
New Britain, Connecticut

Hillard E. Leetma, M.D.
New York, New York

Irving M. Levitas, M.D., F.A.C.P.
Hackensack, New Jersey

Valdemar A. Lindquist, M.D.
Denver, Colorado

James W. Long, M.D.
Washington, D.C.

J. Loomis
University Park, Pennsylvania

Laura C. Lowe, MPH; M.S. Ed.
Greensboro, North Carolina

Ross MacKenzie, M.D., F.R.C.P.
Montreal, Quebec, Canada

Sy Mah, B.P.E., M. Ed.
Toledo, Ohio

K. M. Malik, M.D.
Chicago, Illinois

Vasil William Masica
Springfield, Illinois

William P. McCahill
Washington, D.C.

Martin McCavitt, Ed.D.
Washington, D.C.

Anna Delores McWilliams, B.S.
Washington, D.C.

Sander H. Mendelson, M.D.
Washington, D.C.

William Miller
Chicago, Illinois

Kenneth Morgan
Richmond, Virginia

Max Morton, R.P.T.
Fort Collins, Colorado

Frank Naso, M.D.
Philadelphia, Pennsylvania

Arlene Niccoli, R.N., B.S.
Denver, Colorado

W. Channing Nicholas, M.D.
University Park,, Pennsylvania

Donald E. Noble
Washington, D.C.

Simon Ohanessian, M.D.
Cleveland, Ohio

Donald G. Pansegrau, M.D.
Dallas, Texas

Frederick W. Parker, III
Washington, D.C.

Raymond E. Phillips, M.D.
Bronx, New York

Franklin Plotkin, M.D.
Cleveland, Ohio

Willard Pushkin, M.D.
Charleston, West Virginia

R. S. Rajagopalan, M.D.
Madras, India

Michael M. Rand
New York, New York

Jim Reedy, M.A.
Bridgewater, Virginia

Leon Reinstein, M.D.
Philadelphia, Pennsylvania

Suzanne Rodgers, Ph.D.
Rochester, New York

Martha Rotstein
Washington, D.C.

Sujoy Roy, M.D.
New Delhi 16, India

Vincenzo Rulli, M.D.
Rome, Italy

Nancy Saxon, R.N.
Pittsburgh, Pennsylvania

Joel P. Schrank, M.D.
Charlottesville, Virginia

Lewis P. Scott, M.D.
Washington, D.C.

Chandrakant V. Shah, M.D.
Bombay 8, India

Ramakant Shah, M.D.
Washington, D.C.

Alan J. Shalleck,
New York, New York

Marc L. Siditsky
Washington, D.C.

Wesley Sime, M.S.
Pittsburg, Pennsylvania

Mary Z. Skorapa, M.D.
Atlanta, Georgia

Paul M. Snapper, M.D.
Catskill, New York

Seth William Snover
Washington, D.C.

Thomas J. Solon, M.D.
Chestertown, Maryland

Bernard S. Staller, M.D.
Charlottesville, Virginia

David Sterling
Washington, D.C.

Merritt Stiles, M.D.
Spokane, Washington

Dusan Surzic, M.D.
Krusevac, Yugoslavia

Shauket Ali Syed, M.D.
Karachi 35, Pakistan

Tal T. Talibi, M.D.
Edmonston, Alberta, Canada

Irene Tamagna, M.D.
Washington, D.C.

Abdeslam Tazi, M.D.
Rabat, Morocco

Anne Teunis
Bethesda, Maryland

Pate D. Thomson, M.D.
Berkeley, California

Charles S. Tidball, M.D.
Washington, D.C.

Alan H. Tinmouth, M.D., F.R.C.P.
Montreal, Quebec, Canada

Charles Tipton, Ph.D.
Iowa City, Iowa

William J. Tomik, Ph.D.
Cortland, New York

Malcolm Van Kirk
Washington, D.C.

Richard C. Warner, M.Ed., A.B.
Bronx, New York

Herb Weber, Ph.D.
Stroudsburg, Pennsylvania

Martin H. Wendkos, M.D., F.A.C.P.
Philadelphia, Pennsylvania

Hal N. White
Wilmington, Delaware

Melvin H. Williams, Ph.D.
Norfolk, Virginia

Linda Woolsey
Washington, D.C.

Donald Youngblood
Washington, D.C.

Elihu York, M.D.
Portland, Maine

Michael Yuhasz, Ph.D.
London 72, Ontario, Canada

L. N. Ziecheck
Bethesda, Maryland

Arlene Zupp
Cleveland, Ohio

SUPPORTING STAFF

Theresa Breen
Washington, D.C.

Stephanie DeCoste
Washington, D.C.

Richard LeClair
Washington, D.C.

Josefina Magno, M.D.
Washington, D.C.

Carolyn Mills
Washington, D.C.

Barbara Moriarity
Washington, D.C.

Evelyn Parker
Washington, D.C.

Mary Portman
Washington, D.C.

Richard Reeves
Washington, D.C.

Mary Tonoda
Washington, D.C.

Sandra Wood
Washington, D.C.

GLOSSARY

A

adenosine diphosphate (ADP), component of nucleic acid, which is found in muscle tissue

adenosine monophosphate (AMP), component of nucleic acid, functions as a coenzyme in the breakdown of glycogen (animal carbohydrate) stored in the liver

adenosine triphosphate (ATP), coenzyme, valuable in transfer of phosphate bond energy

adenyl cyclase, enzyme

adenylate kinase (myokinase), enzyme, catalyzes breakdown of ADP

adipose tissue, fat storage in connective tissue; cells distended by fat droplets

ADP, *see* adenosine diphosphate

aerobic, living, active, or occurring only in presence of oyxgen

ambulation, walking, or ability to walk

amino acid, organic acid containing amino group NH_2; especially alpha-amino acids—chief components of proteins

AMP, *see* adenosine monophosphate

anaerobic, living or active in the absence of free oxygen

aneurysm, a sac formed by the walls of an artery or vein and filled with blood

angina, disease marked by spasmodic attacks of intense suffocative pain

angina pectoris, paroxysmal thoracic pain

angiography, an invasive technique for diagnosing atherosclerosis involving x-ray examination of the heart and great blood vessels to visualize the course of a fluid opaque to x-rays which has been injected into the blood stream

anticoagulant, a drug which delays clotting of the blood; when a blood vessel is plugged by a clot, the drug tends to prevent new clots from forming or existing clots from enlarging, but does not dissolve an existing clot

anoxia, hypoxia, especially of such severity as to result in a permanent damage

aortic stenosis, narrowing of aortic orifice of heart, or of aorta itself

arrhythmia, alteration in rhythm of heartbeat either in time or force

arteries, *see* artery

artery, (pl. arteries), tubular branching muscular and elastic-walled vessels that carry blood from heart through body

arteriovenous, both arterial and venous; pertaining to or affecting an artery and a vein

asthenia, lack or loss of strength or energy; weakness

atheroma, lipid deposits in the inner lining of the arteries, lesions characteristic of atherosclerosis; plural, atheromata

ATP, *see* adenosine triphosphate

ATPase, adenosinetriphosphatase, an enzyme which catalyzes splitting of adenosine triphosphate autonomic nervous system, part of the nervous system that innervates smooth and cardiac muscle and glandular tissue; governs actions more or less automatic

AVO_2, arteriovenous oxygen

azide, compound containing group N_3 combined with an element or radical

B

biochemical, *see* biochemistry

biochemistry, chemistry of living organisms and of vital processes

blood lipids, *see* lipids

blood pressure, pressure exerted by blood on walls of blood vessels

brachial artery, continuation of axillary (hollow beneath arm at shoulder) artery; distribution: shoulder, arm, forearm, and hand

bradycardia, abnormal slowness of heart beat, evidenced by slowing of pulse rate to 60 or less per minute

bruit, a sound or murmur heard in auscultation, especially an abnormal one

bundle branch block, heart block due to lesion in one of the bundle branches (atrioventricular bundles passing to ventricles)

C

calcium, element found in nearly all organized tissues in the form of calcium ions or bound in compounds (organic and inorganic)

cannulation, insertion of cannula (tube) into hollow organ or body cavity

capillary, any of the minute hairlike vessels of the blood-vascular system, connecting arterioles with venules, forming networks throughout the body

CAPRI, Cardio-Pulmonary Research Institute

cardiac, of or relating to the heart

cardiac arrest, cessation of cardiac function, with disappearance of arterial blood pressure

cardiac catheterization, passage of a small catheter into a vein in arm and through blood vessels into heart; for blood samples, determining intracardiac pressure, and detecting cardiac anomalies

cardiac index (CI), CO per square meter body surface area=$(CO/M^2$ B.S.A.) in liters per minute

cardiac muscle metabolism, metabolism of principal muscle of heart

cardiac output (CO), minute output of blood from the heart in liters per minute

cardiogenic shock, shock resulting from sudden diminution of cardiac output, as in myocardial infarction

cardiopulmonary, pertaining to heart and lungs

cardiovascular, pertaining to the heart and blood vessels

cardiovascular system, heart and blood vessels

catabolism, *see* catabolize

catabolize, or oxidize, subject to catabolism, destructive metabolism

catecholamines, compounds secreted by adrenal cortex, such as adrenaline

cerebral, relating to the brain or cerebrum; *see* cerebrum

cerebrum, the expanded anterior portion of the brain that, in higher mammals, overlies the rest of the brain

CHD, coronary heart disease

cholesterol, fat-soluble crystalline steroid alcohol, essential constituent of animal cells and body fluids, important in physiological processes cholinergic, stimulated, activated, or transmitted by choline (acetylcholine)

chronotropic, affecting time or rate, especially of the heartbeat

citric acid, tricarboxylic acid obtained especially from lemon and limes, or by fermentation of sugars

clavian, referring to the clavicle; *see* clavicle

clavicle (or clavicula), a bone, shaped like the letter *f*, that is part of the formation of either anterior half of the shoulder girdle. Also called collar bone

CoA, coenzyme A

conditioned reflex, a reflex that does not occur naturally but as a result of conditioning or association with a physiological function

congestive heart failure, prolonged impairment of ability of heart to maintain adequate flow of blood to the tissues

coronary, encircling in the manner of a crown: term applied to vessels, nerves, ligaments, etc.

coronary angiography, roentgenographic visualization of coronary arteries

CP, *see* creatine phosphate

CPK, *see* creatine phosphokinase

creatine phosphate (CP), phosphocreatine; phosphagen; acid compound occurring in muscle metabolism, being broken down into creatine and inorganic phosphorus

creatine phosphokinase (CPK), enzyme, catalyzes reaction of ATP and chromium

cristae, plural of crista, projection or projecting structure, or ridge, especially one surmounting a bone or its border. Also called *crest* or *ridge*

cyanide, a compound containing the cyanide ion bonded to an organic or inorganic group. The cyanide ion is obtained

sometimes from cyanogen. Cyanide ion forms poisonous complexes

cyclic AMP, adenosine monophosphate in which the phosphate group can migrate by means of a cyclic intermediate

cytochrome oxidase, an iron-porphyrin enzyme important in cell respiration; also called *respiratory enzyme*

cytochrome reductase, iron-containing enzyme catalyzing cellular reduction

D

defibrillator, apparatus to counteract fibrillation by application of electric impulses to the heart

diastolic [blood] pressure, lowest arterial blood pressure of a cardiac cycle (*see also* systolic)

digitalis, the dried leaves of *Digitalis purpurea* (foxglove): causes elevation of blood pressure, increase of systole, lengthening of diastole, and contraction of arterioles; used as heart tonic and diuretic

dinitrophenol, benzene derivative containing nitro and phenolic functional groups. It is a starting material in the syntheses of dyes and medicinals

diphosphopyridine nucleotide (DPNH), a coenzyme, transports hydrogen in metabolic reactions. DPNH is the reduced form of the enzyme

dopamine, drug to increaase cardiac output

dP/dt, rate expression, used in kinetics, shows rate of change of pressure with time

DPN (diphosphopyridine nucleotide), coenzyme which is a hydrogen acceptor in biological oxidations

DPNH, *see* diphosphopyridine nucleotide

dyspnea, difficult or labored breathing

E

ECG, *see* electrocardiogram

ECG recorder, *see* electrocardiograph

ejection fraction (EF), LV end diastolic volume - LV end systolic volume

$$\frac{}{\text{LV end diastolic volume}}$$
expressed as a percentage

ejection time index (ETI), SEP corrected for heart rate = SEP + .0016 HR in seconds

EKG, *see* electrocardiogram

electrocardiogram (EKG), also ECG; graphic tracing of electric current produced by contraction of heart muscle; obtained with electrocardiograph

electrocardiograph, instrument for recording changes of electrical potential occurring during heartbeat; used in diagnosing heart action

enzymes, any of numerous complex proteins produced by living cells which catalyze metabolic reactions at body temperature

epinephrine (adrenaline), adrenal hormone used especially as heart stimulant, vasoconstrictor, and muscle relaxant. It is the prototype of sympathomimetic substances

ergometer, apparatus measuring work performed by a group of muscles

F

fibrillation, exceedingly rapid contractions or twitching of muscular fibrils, but not of the muscle as a whole; commonly occurs in atricles or ventricles of the heart as well as in recently denervated skeletal muscle fibers

free fatty acids, saturated and unsaturated aliphatic monocarboxylic acids, naturally occurring, usually in fats, waxes, and oils

G

gallop rhythms, cardiac rhythm with an accentuated extra sound; usually heard only when the heart rate is rapid

gastrocnemius, largest and most superficial muscle of calf of leg

glucagon, a protein, is the hyperglycemic-glycogenolytic factor secreted by the α-cells of the pancreas

glucose, monosaccharide containing six carbons found abundantly in nature and easily absorbed in the gastrointestinal tract

glucose tolerance test, a laboratory test used in diagnosis of diabetes mellitus; sugar is given in the form of glucose; at periodic intervals, urine and blood are examined for amount of sugar present

α-glycerophosphate dehydrogenase, an enzyme, which functions with DPN and transports hydrogen from compounds

glycogen, a polysaccharide, the chief carbohydrate storage material in the animal is found in liver and muscles. It is the counterpart of starch

glycogenesis, formation of glycogen

glycogenolysis, splitting up of glycogen in the body tissues

glycolysis, enzymatic breakdown of glucose, glycogen, or other carbohydrate by way of phosphate derivatives

glycolytic, *see* glycolysis

H

hematocrit, laboratory procedure which determines relationship of cell volume to plasma volume

hemodynamics, study of the movements and forces concerned with blood circulation

hemoglobin, conjugated protein consisting of colorless basic proteins (globins) and ferroprotoporphyrin (heme). It is the oxygen-carrying complex of erythrocytes (red blood cells)

histotoxic anoxia, anoxia resulting from disturbance in cells that makes oxygen utilization impossible

homogenates, finely divided human (animal, plant) tissue

hormone, chemical substance secreted into body fluids by an endocrine gland; has specific effect on activity of organs

humor, fluid or semifluid substance, designating certain fluid materials in the body

humoral, see humor

hydrolysis, a chemical process of decomposition involving splitting of bond and addition of the elements of water

hyperlipidemia, abnormally high concentration of lipids in the blood

hypertension, abnormally high blood pressure, especially arterial; also, systemic condition accompanying high blood pressure

hypertrophy, morbid enlargement or overgrowth of an organ or part

hypoxia, low oxygen content or tension; deficiency of oxygen in inspired air

hypoxic, see hypoxia

I

I^{131}, Iodine 131, radioactive iodine of mass number 131; used as a tracer in chemical analysis and metabolic studies

infarct, an area of dead or necrotic tissue resulting from obstruction of circulation to the area

infarction, myocardial (see myocardial infarction)

inotropic, affecting force or energy of muscular contractions

intercoronary anastomoses, so-called collateral circulation which consists of small arterial channels which develop, circumventing coronary artery obstructive lesions, to enhance blood supply to hypoxic areas of the myocardium

intramyocardial tension, pressure times stress

ischemia, local and temporary deficiency of blood, chiefly due to contraction of a blood vessel

ischemic, see ischemia

isocitric dehydrogenase enzyme, catalyzes breakdown of isocitric acid in the presence of triphosphopyridine nucleotide (TPN) as coenzyme which accepts hydrogen

isometric, of equal dimensions; not isotonic (of equal tone, tension, or activity)

isotonia, condition of equal tone, tension, or activity; equality of osmotic pressure between two elements of a solution or between two solutions

isotonic, see isotonia

K

kcal, see kilocalorie

ketone bodies (a substrate), any organic compound containing the carbonyl group

kilocalorie (kcal), unit of energy contains 1000 calories. A calorie measures the heat needed to raise the temperature of one gram of water, $1\,^{\circ}C$.

Krebs (citric acid, or aerobic) cycle, tricarboxylic acid cycle; cyclic metabolic mechanism by which complete oxidation of the acetyl moiety of acetyl-coenzyme A is effected

L

lactate, a derivative (salt or ester) of lactic acid (found in milk) lactic acid, a hygroscopic organic acid present normally in tissue, also produced in carbohydrate decomposition usually by bacterial fermentation

lactic dehydrogenase (LDH), enzyme, obtained from heart muscle

LDH, *see* lactic dehydrogenase

left ventricular efficiency index (LVEI), $\dfrac{LVMWI}{TTI} \times 1000$

left ventricular mean systolic pressure (LVSPm), mean pressure during SEP

left ventricular minute work index (LVMWI), index of left ventricular mechanical work per minute = (LVSPm - LVED) $\times$ CI $\times \dfrac{1.36}{100}$ kg meters/min/M^2

left ventricular stroke work index (LVSWI), index of left ventricular mechanical work per stroke = (LVSPm - LVED) $\times$ SI $\times \dfrac{1.36}{100}$ kg meters/beat/M^2

left ventricular volume (LVV), volume of blood contained by left ventricle (usually at end diastole)

linoleate, a salt or ester of linoleic acid

lipids, any of various substances including fats, waxes, phosphatides, cerebrosides, and related and derived compounds, that with proteins and carbohydrates constitute principal structural components of living cells

M

malic dehydrogenase, an enzyme which catalyzes oxidation of malic acid to oxaloacetic acid

mean systolic ejection rate index (MSERI), index of mean rate of ejection from left ventricle during systole = $\dfrac{SI}{SEP}$ ml/sec/beat

metabolism, chemical changes in living cells providing energy for vital processes and activities; new material is assimilated to repair cells

metabolite, any substance produced by metabolism or by a metabolic process; *see also* metabolism

metabolize, *see* metabolism

metronome, instrument designed to mark exact time by a regularly repeated sound

mitochondria, granular or globular chondriosomes (structures occurring in cytoplasm of cells)

$M\dot{V}O_2$, minute cardiac oxygen consumption

myocardial, of primary cardiac insufficiency; *see* myocardium

myocardial infarction, coronary thrombosis; blocking of coronary artery of heart by thrombus

myocardial oxygen intake, oxygen absorption by muscular tissue of heart

myocardium, middle muscular layer of heart wall

myofibril, muscle fibril; especially one of the slender threads, rendered visible in a muscle fiber by maceration in certain acids

myoglobin, a red iron-containing protein pigment in muscle; contributes to color of muscle and acts as a store of oxygen. Also called myohemoglobin

myohemoglobin, *see* myoglobin

myosin, a globin which is the most abundant protein (68 percent) in muscle. With actin, is responsible for contraction and relaxation of muscle

N

neural, pertaining to a nerve or the nerves

nitroglycerin, a drug (one of the nitrates) which relaxes and widens the muscles in the blood vessels (vasodilation); often used to relieve attacks of angina pectoris and spasm of coronary arteries

non-isometric, not of equal dimensions; *see* isometric

norepinephrine, hormone secreted by the adrenal medulla. It increases systolic and diastolic blood pressure

O

oleate, a salt or ester of oleic acid

oscilloscope, instrument in which variations in a fluctuating electrical quantity appear temporarily as a visible waveform on the fluorescent screen of a cathode-ray tube

oxidation, oxidizing, to combine or cause to combine with oxygen; loss of one or more electrons from an element or a compound

oxidative, related to or characterized by oxidation; *see* oxidation

oxidative phosphorylation, oxidation of a tissue metabolite substrate with simultaneous formation of a high-energy phosphate

P

pacemaker, an emergency device for stimulating the heart

palmitate, a salt or ester of palmitic acid; *see* palmitic acid

palmitic acid, saturated, 16 carbon fatty acid found in most of the common fats and oils

paramedical personnel, people with limited training related to science or practice of medicine; assisting physicians. (Paramedical services include physical, occupational, and speech therapy, and activity of medical social workers.)

pathologic, altered or caused by disease

phosphate, any inorganic salt of phosphoric acid or esters obtained by reaction with organic alcohols

phosphofructokinase, enzyme, catalyzes the phosphorylation of fructose phosphate

phosphorylase, specific enzymes which catalyze reversibly the cleavage of polysaccharides (glycogen, starch) to glucose-1-phosphate

phosphorylation, conversion of an organic compound into an organic phosphate

Pi, inorganic phosphate

placebo, a preparation containing a substance that can neither help nor harm; in testing new drugs, the experimental group is given the drug and a control group is given a placebo that looks and tastes the same

procainamide, analgesic compound used in treatment of cardiac arrhythmia

propranolol, a drug, an adrenergic blocking agent

psoas muscles, muscles of the loin—flexes the trunk

pulmonary, relating to the lungs; carried on by the lungs

pyruvate, salt or ester of pyruvic acid, *see* pyruvic acid

pyruvic acid, a liquid ketoacid; important imtermediate in metabolism and fermentation

Q

quadriceps, the great extensor muscle of the thigh divided into four parts

R

respiratory enzyme, *see* cytochrome oxidase

S

sartorius muscle, crosses front of thigh obliquely, assists in rotating leg; longest muscle in man

serum, clear yellow watery portion of animal fluid remaining after clotting serum cholesterol, *see* serum *and* cholesterol

serum enzymes, enzymes such as creatine phosphokinase and S.G.O.T. which are released into the circulation from myocardial muscle when cell death takes place

serum glutamate-oxaloacetate transaminase (SGOT), an enzyme which catalyzes the intermolecular transfer of an amino group from glutamic acid to oxaloacetic acid. The level of the enzyme in blood indicates whether myocardial infarction took place

serum glutamate-pyruvate transaminase (SGPT), an enzyme which catalyzes intermolecular amino group transfer

SGOT, *see* serum glutamate-oxaloacetate transaminase

SGPT, *see* serum glutamate-pyruvate transaminase

sodium amytal, a barbituric acid derivative of intermediate length of action as a hypnotic (sleep-producer)

sphygmomanometer, instrument for measuring blood pressure, especially arterial blood pressure

splanchnic [region], pertaining to the viscera

stethoscope, instrument to detect and study body sounds

stroke index (SI), SV/M^2 B.S.A. in milliliters

stroke volume (SV), amount of blood ejected with each beat in milliliters per beat

substrates, substance(s) upon which ferment or enzyme acts or on which a reaction takes place

succinate, salt or ester of succinic acid

succinic acid, a crystalline saturated dicarboxylic acid; found widely in nature, active in biological energy-yielding reactions

succinic dehydrogenase, iron-containing enzyme, catalyzes removal of hydrogen from succinic acid

synergism, cooperative action of discrete agencies such that the total effect is greater than the sum of the effects taken independently

synergistically, *see* synergism

systolic ejection period (SEP), time during which blood is ejected during systole

systolic [blood] pressure, highest arterial blood pressure of a cardiac cycle (*see also* diastolic)

T

tachycardia, excessive rapidity of heart action; term is usually applied to pulse rate above 100 per minute

telemeter, electrical apparatus for measuring a quantity (pressure, radiation intensity, speed, or temperature), transmitting results especially by radio

telemetry, *see* telemeter

tension time index (TTI), an important determinant and approximate equivalent of myocardial oxygen consumption = (LVSPm $\times$ HR $\times$ SEP)

thromboembolism, embolism, or blocking, of a blood vessel with a thrombus which has broken loose from its site of formation

triglycerides, a triester of glycerol with one, two, or three acid molecules

V

vagal, pertaining to the vagus nerve; *see also* vagus nerve

vagus nerve, the 10th cranial nerve

vascular, pertaining to, or full of, vessels

vaso-, prefix denoting a vessel, or duct (e.g., vasodilation, vasoconstriction)

ventricle, chamber of heart which receives blood from a corresponding atrium and from which blood is forced into the arteries

ventricular aneurysm, aneurysmal dilation of a ventricle of the heart; *see* aneurysm *and* ventricle

ventricular contractions, shortening or tensing of one of the lower chambers of the heart (ventricle)

ventricular fibrillation, fibrillary twitching of the ventricular muscle

W

waveform, curve representing condition of wave-propagating medium at a given instant

workload 150 (WL150), work performance or work tolerance as an index of fitness, measured as the power (kg meters per min) at which a subject's heart rate (HR) reaches or would be expected to reach 150 beats per minute

INDEX